Textbook of Complete Dentures

SIXTH EDITION

Textbook of Complete Dentures

Arthur O. Rahn
Professor Emeritus
Department of Oral Rehabilitation
Medical College of Georgia
School of Dentistry
Augusta, Georgia

John R. Ivanhoe
Professor Emeritus
Department of Oral Rehabilitation
Medical College of Georgia
School of Dentistry
Augusta, Georgia

Kevin D. Plummer
Associate Professor
Section Director of Removable Prosthodontics
Department of Oral Rehabilitation
Medical College of Georgia
School of Dentistry
Augusta, Georgia

2009
PEOPLE'S MEDICAL PUBLISHING HOUSE
RALEIGH, NORTH CAROLINA

People's Medical Publishing House-USA
5711 Six Forks Road, Suite 210
Raleigh, North Carolina 27609
Tel: 919-502-4220
Fax: 919-502-7673
E-mail: info@pmphusa.com

PMPH-USA

18 19 20 21 25/KING/9 8 7 6 5

ISBN-13   978-1-60795-025-7
ISBN-10   1-60795-025-1
eISBN-13   978-1-60795-099-8

Printed in the United States of America by King Printing.
Editor: Jason Malley; Copyeditor/Typesetter: Spearhead; Cover designer: Mary McKeon

Sales and Distribution

Canada
Login Canada
300 Saulteaux Cr.
Winnipeg, MB R3J 3T2
Phone: 1.800.665.1148
Fax: 1.800.665.0103
www.lb.ca

Foreign Rights
John Scott & Company
International Publisher's Agency
P.O. Box 878
Kimberton, PA 19442, USA
Tel: 610-827-1640
Fax: 610-827-1671
rights@johnscottco.us

*United Kingdom, Europe, Middle East,
Africa, Singapore, Thailand, Philippines,
Indonesia, Vietnam, Pacific Rim, Korea,
Australia,
New Zealand, Papua New Guinea, Fiji,
Tonga, Solomon Islands, Cook Islands,
Malaysia*
Eurospan Limited
3, Henrietta Street, Covent Garden,
London WC2E 8LU, UK
Tel: Within the UK: 0800 526830
Outside the UK: +44 (0)20 7845
0868
http://www.eurospanbookstore.com

Jaypee Brothers Medical Publishers
Pvt. Ltd.
4838, 24 Ansari Road, Darya Ganj
New Delhi- 110002, India
Phone: +91 11 23272143
Fax: +91 11 23276490
www.jaypeebrothers.com

People's Republic of China
People's Medical Publishing House
International Trade Department
No. 19, Pan Jia Yuan Nan Li
Chaoyang District
Beijing 100021, P.R. China
Tel: 8610-67653342
Fax: 8610-67691034
www.pmph.com/en

This book is dedicated with love

■ ■ ■ ■ ■

This textbook is dedicated to all students of the clinical practice of complete denture prosthodontics. The rehabilitation of completely edentulous patients requires skill, compassion and perseverance in order to arrive at a point that improves a patient's life both in social situations and in healthy dietary function. The "basics" are so truly important when other options might fail and the editors and authors have strived to put those "basics" at your finger tips in this book. We hope that this textbook will improve your ability to provide solid care for the complete denture patients in your practice.

This book was the work of many individuals and the original concept was built on Dr. Arthur Rahn's work over many years. His dedication to the dental profession and the education of dental students is renowned and was the inspiration to the new editors to undertake this project. His advice and friendship is greatly appreciated.

Sadly my co-editor, Dr. John Ivanhoe passed away shortly after the manuscript was finished and he will not get to see the textbook in production. During this project, John's enthusiastic spirit kept all of those involved excited and hopeful that this textbook would be a reference helpful to both dental students and practitioners providing those skills so important in complete denture prosthodontics. He is missed as a colleague and most importantly as a close friend. His sweet wife Alice supported John in all of his work and I'm sure John would give her credit for her inspiration to him during all their time together.

I would like to acknowledge my friends who are authors of the various chapters for their time and effort to support this project. We all know this type of work is a labor of love for dental education. Of course, as always, my wife Connie keeps me on track and provides the support and loving family life that sustains me in all I do.

And thanks to you—students of the dental profession

Kevin D. Plummer

■ ■ ■ ■ ■

Contents

C h a p t e r   3
Anatomy of the Edentulous Ridges   25

C h a p t e r   4
Diagnosis and Treatment Planning   45

C h a p t e r   5
Pre-prosthetic Surgical Considerations   65

Clinical and Technical Procedures

Preface

The editors have felt for many years that there was no simple textbook designed for the undergraduate dental student or family dentist that explains the fundamental treatment needs for completely edentulous patients. This textbook was not designed to contain all the information a graduate student or prosthodontist might desire, but provides the basic information for consistent and quality treatment of the typical denture patient seen in dentist's offices every day. It is arranged in typical chapters with information in text and figure format. The primary chapters relate to the second portion of the textbook, which is an Atlas of figures and legends to supplement the chapter information. The figures are all new and in color, which supplements the text nicely. The material is easy to read and clinically related to place the fundamental steps in denture fabrication in an easy-to-use reference. Our hope is that this textbook will help make the treatment of denture patients a rewarding aspect of your clinical practice.

Kevin Plummer

Contributors

Philip S. Baker, DDS
Associate Professor
Department of Oral Rehabilitation
Medical College of Georgia
School of Dentistry
Augusta, Georgia

Henry W. Ferguson, DMD
Associate Professor
Vice Chair, Director of Post Graduate
  Training
Department of Oral and Maxillofacial
  Surgery
Medical College of Georgia
School of Dentistry
Augusta, Georgia

John R. Ivanhoe, DDS (Deceased)
Professor Emeritus
Department of Oral Rehabilitation
Medical College of Georgia
School of Dentistry
Augusta, Georgia

Dennis W. Kiernan, DMD
Prosthodontist
Private Practice
Augusta, Georgia

Carol A. Lefebvre, DDS, MS
Professor; Associate Dean for Strategic
  Initiatives and Faculty Development
Department of Oral Rehabilitation
Medical College of Georgia
School of Dentistry
Augusta, Georgia

W. Jack Morris, DMD
Assistant Professor
Department of Oral Rehabilitation
Medical College of Georgia
School of Dentistry
Augusta, Georgia

Kevin D. Plummer, DDS
Associate Professor
Section Director of Removable Prosthodontics
Department of Oral Rehabilitation
Medical College of Georgia
School of Dentistry
Augusta, Georgia

Arthur O. Rahn, DDS
Professor Emeritus
Department of Oral Rehabilitation
Medical College of Georgia
School of Dentistry
Augusta, Georgia

Frederick A. Rueggeberg, DDS, MS
Professor
Section Director of Dental Materials
Department of Oral Rehabilitation
Medical College of Georgia
School of Dentistry
Augusta, Georgia

Mohamed Sharawy, DDS, PhD
Professor
Departments of Oral Biology and Oral
  Maxillofacial Surgery
Medical College of Georgia
School of Dentistry
Augusta, Georgia

1

Introduction and Definitions

Dr. John Ivanhoe

Introduction

The effect of new, well-fitting esthetic, functional complete dentures on a patient's social life, sense of well-being, and quality of life is often dramatic. On post-insertion visits you may note new hairstyles, makeup, a new job, a change in dress and/or a personality change. Changes such as these justifiably make clinicians proud of their work and skills. Many of these patients are reasonably simple straight-forward denture patients who are easily managed. However, it must be remembered that every patient requiring opposing complete dentures is a "full-mouth rehabilitation" patient, and the treatment of some will be very difficult.

Understanding these patients and providing the services necessary to achieve excellent results requires well-trained, capable, and caring experts. Unfortunately there is a feeling among some that, with the advances in the dental education of patients and dental materials and techniques, complete denture patients will become rare in the immediate future, and therefore complete denture prosthodontics is a dying art. This lack of appreciation has resulted in a decreased emphasis in this specialty area within the curriculum of dental schools to the point that some schools question the need for complete dentures in their curriculum.

Contrary to those opinions, data indicates that the number of patients requiring complete dentures will continue to increase over at least the next fifteen years and then stabilize for the foreseeable future. The number of patients in need of one or two complete dentures will increase from 33.6 million in 1991 to 37.9 million by 2020. Unfortunately these facts have been lost on some state legislatures and senior dental educators resulting in a decreased quality of health care in some areas allowing laboratory technicians with no diagnostic skills or clinical experience to legally fabricate complete dentures.

The diagnosis and fabrication of complete dentures is often a very difficult area of dentistry because of the uniqueness of the average denture patient's physical and mental condition. The dentist must attempt to restore, most often an elderly patient with physical, mental and/or financial difficulties, to an acceptable level of esthetics and function. This may be difficult because completely edentulous patients have lost all of the natural teeth that would have provided valuable guidance on vertical and horizontal relationships, tooth size and color, and tooth position. They have lost the esthetics and function of natural teeth anchored securely in strong bone. They may have lost large amounts of ridge structure, which might have provided stability to their dentures. Many of these patients have lost muscular structure, which makes chewing food difficult. Most have lost tissue elasticity resulting in poor muscular support of the lower face.

Mental stresses may also be devastating. Elderly patients are not as mobile as they once were; many can't drive themselves and are totally dependant on others for their needs. They are often on multiple medications, which may be creating a severe financial burden. Additionally these drugs often result in xerostomia, which often makes wearing dentures very difficult. Some patients are seeking mates and they feel that dentures make them less of a person. Many are embarrassed over the possibility that their spouses will see them without their dentures. Many are depressed over loss of a spouse or close long-time friend. Others are depressed due to the loss of "feeling good and young." Some are concerned because they recognize that they have developed a significant loss of short-term memory. These mental stresses contribute to how cooperative these patients may be during the denture fabrication process.

Functionally these patients may also be quite compromised. Proprioception and a stable occlusion have been lost with the removal of the last natural teeth. Food may be unappetizing because of the lost taste buds and changes in salivary flow, perhaps resulting in weight loss. Often these patients are debilitated and their tissues are abused from wearing poorly fitting dentures or not wearing dentures at all.

How did these patients reach this condition? The familial history of some will indicate neglect because dentistry wasn't important or perhaps the family simply couldn't afford dentistry. Some are the result of a history of lack of concern for their own oral hygiene or the importance of preventive dentistry. Some may simply be facing the effects of advanced age and a combination of conditions leading to edentulism.

It becomes very important to differentiate between what can and can't be done for patients with these physical, mental, and personal problems. Obviously a dental professional cannot reverse the age-related changes, however dentists are able to diminish the effects of these changes in many patients. Patients cannot be restored to the esthetics and functional level of a dentate patient; however compromised function and esthetics can be adequately addressed in most patients. Unrealistic expectations cannot be achieved and clinicians are on dangerous ground if they do not objectively recognize capabilities and ensure that the patient understands limitations. Even the most skillful and caring of clinicians is doomed to failure if patients cannot be educated and made to understand the degree to which their oral conditions have been compromised. It has been said that some patients with unrealistic expectations must be made to understand that complete dentures are not a replacement for the missing natural dentition; they are a replacement for having no dentition at all.

In reaching a prognosis a clinician often focuses in on the condition of the oral cavity and loses sight of the physical, mental, and financial difficulties of the patient. Because of compromised denture stability, the use of a denture adhesive is often recommended—forgetting that the patient may not be able to afford the denture adhesive and also how difficult it is for a physically challenged patient to apply and remove from both the dentures and the ridges. To increase the stability clinicians may recommend that the patient attempt to chew food on both sides of the arch simultaneously forgetting the difficulty in achieving such a feat for even the physically capable patient with their natural dentition. Satisfactory denture function is a combination of both the fabrication of excellent prostheses and managing the emotional and physical conditions of the patient.

Yes, completely edentulous patients may be very difficult to manage, however, once the initial hesitancy of treating these patients is overcome and clinical skills developed, this is an extremely rewarding area of dentistry from both a financial and professional standpoint. Because many dentists never developed the skills and appreciation of treating edentulous patients, those who do will become an important referral base for their colleagues and other patients alike.

Definitions

The editors have intentionally not been consistent in using the Glossary of Prosthodontic Terms for all terminology in this textbook. While the terminology, as defined in the Glossary, is excellent for usage by specialists, it does not reflect many of the common and accepted terms as practiced and understood by the average dentist or clinician. Therefore terms such as balanced occlusion, crossbite, and occlusal prematurities continue to be used in place of balanced articulation, reverse articulation, and deflective occlusal contacts.

Articulator—A mechanical instrument that represents the temporo-mandibular joints and jaws, to which maxillary and mandibular casts may be attached to simulate some or all mandibular movements.

Balanced occlusion—The bilateral, simultaneous, anterior, and posterior occlusal contact of teeth in the eccentric position and the bilateral simultaneous occlusal contact of posterior teeth *only* in centric occlusion.

Centric occlusion—The occlusion of the opposing teeth when the mandible is in centric relation.

Centric relation—The maxillomandibular relationship in which the condyles articulate with the thinnest avascular portion of their respective disks with the complex in the anterior-superior position against the shapes of the articular eminencies. This position is independent of tooth contact. This position is clinically discernible when the mandible is directed superior and anteriorly. It is restricted to a purely rotary movement about the transverse horizontal axis. The clinician must be able to manipulate the patient's mandible to this position, as it is: 1) the starting reference point for complete denture fabrication, 2) repeatable and can be verified, and 3) is a functional position for denture occlusion. The definition provided above is accurate but sometimes very difficult to determine clinically. Remember, centric relation is located by detecting the only retruded position of the mandible to the maxilla in which a clinician can obtain a purely vertical hinge movement of the mandible in relation to the maxilla.

Christensen's phenomena—Eponym for the space that occurs between opposing occlusal surfaces that occurs during mandibular protrusion.

Closest speaking space—The clearance between the anterior teeth when the patient makes sibilant sounds. It is generally 1–2 mm.

Combination syndrome—The characteristic features that occur when an edentulous maxilla is opposed by natural mandibular anterior teeth, including loss of bone from the anterior portion of the maxillary ridge, overgrowth of the tuberosities, papillary hyperplasia of the hard palate's mucosa, extrusion of the lower anterior teeth, and loss of alveolar bone and ridge height beneath the mandibular removable dental bases; also called anterior hyperfunction syndrome. Initially described by Kelly.

Compensating curve—The anteroposterior curving and the mediolateral curving within the alignment of the occluding surfaces and incisal edges of artificial teeth that is used to develop balanced occlusion.

Crossbite—The relationship of the opposing posterior teeth when the buccal surfaces of the mandibular teeth are more buccally positioned than those of the maxillary teeth. The maxillary buccal cusps are often occluded with the central grooves of the mandibular teeth. (Reverse articulation)

Hinge axis—An imaginary line between the two condyles around which the mandible rotates when the patient is in centric relation. It is seen in the sagittal plane. (Transverse horizontal axis)

Immediate denture—Any removable dental prosthesis fabricated for placement immediately following the removal of a natural tooth or multiple teeth.

Incisal guidance—1. The influence of the contacting surfaces of the mandibular and maxillary anterior teeth on mandibular movements. 2. The influences of the contacting surfaces of the guide pin and guide table on articulator movements.

Interim complete denture—An immediate denture that is fabricated to serve only during the healing phase following extractions. It will be replaced by a more definitive denture following healing. It is generally less costly than a conventional denture, and the master cast is often fabricated from an irreversible hydrocolloid impression.

Interocclusal clearance—The arrangement in which the opposing occlusal surfaces may pass one another without any contact.

Interocclusal distance—The distance between the occluding surfaces of the maxillary and mandibular teeth when the mandible is in a specific position.

Monoplane occlusion—An occlusal arrangement wherein the posterior teeth have masticatory surfaces that lack any cusp height.

Nonworking side—That side of the mandible that moves toward the medial line in a lateral excursion.

Occlusal vertical dimension—The distance measured between two points when the occluding members are in contact. (Vertical dimension of occlusion)

Overdenture—Any removable dental prosthesis that covers and rests on one or more remaining natural teeth, the roots of natural teeth, and/or dental implants; a dental prosthesis that covers and is partially supported by natural teeth, natural tooth roots, and/or dental implants.

Overextended—Being excessively long or deep. The term usually applies to an impression tray or impression, which may eventually lead to the final denture being overextended.

Physiologic resting position—1) The mandibular position assumed when the head is in an upright position and the involved muscles, particularly the elevator and depressor groups, are in equilibrium in tonic contraction, and the condyles are in a neutral, unstrained position, 2) the position assumed by the mandible when the attached muscles are in a state of tonic equilibrium. The position is usually noted when the head is held upright, 3) the postural position of the mandible when an individual is resting comfortably in an upright position and the associated muscles are in a state of minimal contractual activity.

Protrusion—The position of the mandible anterior to centric relation.

Rebase—The laboratory process of replacing the entire denture base material on an existing prosthesis.

Relining—The procedure used to resurface the tissue side of a removable dental prosthesis with new base material, thus producing an accurate adaptation to the denture foundation area.

Resting vertical dimension—The distance between two points (one of which is on the middle of the face or nose and the other of which is on the lower face or chin) measured when the mandible is in the physiologic resting position. (Vertical dimension of rest)

Retention—The quality of a denture that resists movement of the denture away from the tissue.

Stability—The quality of a denture that resists movement of the denture in a horizontal direction.

Support—The quality of a denture that resists movement of a denture toward the tissues.

Underextended—Being excessively short or shallow. This term usually applies to an impression tray or impression. Being underextended may result in a denture with lack of stability or retention.

Working side—The side toward which the mandibles moves in a lateral excursion.

References

Douglass, C.W., Shih, A., Ostry, L.: Will there be a need for complete dentures in the United States in 2020? J Prosthet Dent. 2002;87:5-8.

The Nomenclature Committee, The Academy of Prosthodontics. The Glossary of Prosthodontic Terms. J Prosthet Dent. 2005;94:1-92.

The Glossary of Prosthodontic Terms. J Prosthet Dent. 2005 July;94(1):23.

CHAPTER

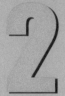

Dental Materials for Complete Dentures

Dr. Fred Rueggeberg

The fabrication of dentures involves a wide range of materials and products. The varieties of processing methods for the denture base and the range of materials from which denture teeth are made provide the clinician with many decision-making steps. Knowledge of the underlying materials used for denture base construction, the principles of their use, and the selection of ancillary products available help the clinician provide the most effective, appropriate treatment for each patient.

Denture Base Materials

When the natural teeth are extracted, the underlying, supporting bone that previously supported the tooth eventually disappears, leaving only a dense, "basement" type (alveolar) bone covered with oral mucosa. The elevated contour of this tissue that remains is termed the "edentulous" or "residual" ridge. Previous to tooth extraction, the contours of the face were largely determined by the presence of alveolar bone and teeth beneath them. Loss of these tissue results in the typical "sunken" appearance of edentulous patients. In addition, when teeth and boney structures are in good health, their positions greatly aid in the ability of the patient to speak naturally, as well as to chew and appreciate textures and temperatures of food.

In considering replacing the missing natural teeth, not only do artificial teeth need to be provided, but they must also be positioned to provide for correct articulation and an esthetic facial contour. The bulk, form, and contour of missing hard, boney structures also need to be replaced to help hold the artificial teeth in these positions.

The purpose of the "denture base" then is to cover the existing residual ridge, provide facial contour, and hold the artificial denture teeth in the correct position. In addition, the denture base must provide an intimate contact with the underlying mucosa without interfering with movements of the cheeks and tongue. The thin layer of saliva that exists between the tissue-bearing side of the denture base and the oral mucosa helps form a hermetic seal, aiding in holding the denture to tissues through capillary action. Because the denture base replaces mucosa-covered bone and will be visible to others, this part of the prosthesis should also have life-like features, both in color and in contour.

Denture bases are fabricated of either polymeric materials or metal. The most popular material for denture base construction is a polymer. Polymers are very easily shaped and formed, and do not weigh as much as (are less dense than) the metallic materials. In most denture base materials, the same basic chemistry is involved. The liquid monomer (methyl methacrylate) is added with ground, powdered, pre-polymerized material. The resulting polymer consists of strands of newly polymerized material (polymethyl methacrylate) surrounding (but not chemically bonded to) the pre-polymerized material originally added. The result is a very tangled mass of polymer chains that provides strength. Various types of monomers (resins) are used in different products to control physical properties. Some products include a rubber-like molecule that provides elasticity to the denture and decreases the potential for fracture, should it be dropped against a hard surface: high-impact denture base materials.

Resin-Based Dentures (Heat- and Auto-Polymerized Materials)

Denture base materials are "processed" (polymerized) in a variety of ways. The most common method has been used for more than 60 years and includes a heat-polymerized resin. In this method, the dentist initially constructs a denture using wax as a base material to temporarily hold the artificial teeth. This assembly is made outside of the patient's mouth, on stone casts that replicate the patient's oral mucosa (master casts). Using interocclusal records, these casts are positioned on an articulator. The artificial teeth are positioned in wax on the casts to have the angulation desired in the final denture. The wax is also sculpted to simulate the form and natural contours of the gingiva and mucosa that were present prior to tooth extraction. Once the teeth are in their desired location and the wax denture base has been sculpted, the cast and denture are invested in a large, brass flask (flasking), and the wax denture base is removed by using boiling water. The base resin polymer and monomer are mixed to a dough-like consistency, and packed into the void left when the wax was removed. The flask halves are closed and pressed together, which forces the unpolymerized dough to flow into all the empty spaces within the stone mold. Pressing also helps to extrude and eliminate excess, unpolymerized dough. The brass flask is placed into water and heated to a specific temperature at a specific rate. The warmth of the water eventually reaches the unpolymerized dough where it activates a setting mechanism of the polymer (heat-polymerized resin).

The dough-like material could have been specially formulated so that the polymerization process would not require any heat to react, but instead, the components, when added and mixed, undergo a polymerization reaction at room temperature inside of the flask (autopolymerizing resin). After the material inside the flask has maximally polymerized, the flask sections are separated, and the "processed" (cured, polymerized) denture is separated from the master cast, trimmed, polished, and stored in water. Because of resin shrinkage during polymerization (approximately 0.3 to 0.5%), dimensions of the denture are slightly smaller than prior to polymerization. Fortunately, the denture will absorb water from its storage fluid, and expand slightly (0.1 to 0.2%), making its final dimensions almost exactly the same as those of the mouth. For this reason, dentures must be kept wet when removed from the mouth for soaking, cleaning, or storage.

A polymer denture base can also be made from different types of materials. In the "fluid-pour" technique, instead of mixing components into a dough-like consistency, the same basic materials are mixed to provide a much less viscous (more water-like) product. This material is also formulated to undergo an autopolymerization setting reaction. The denture is "flasked" in a similar manner, heated, and the wax is removed as mentioned previously (for the heat-polymerized and autopolymerized methods). Rather than pressing the dough into the mold, the unpolymerized, fluid-like uncured resin is poured through a specially created hole in the flasking material, and the void is filled until the fluid flows out another hole. The flask is then allowed to sit at room temperature where the autopolymerizing reaction takes place. After the denture base material has polymerized, the denture is recovered as described above, and finished.

Another type of denture base is also mixed into a dough and flasked like those dentures mention above. Instead of being inserted into the conventional brass flask, however, the assembly is contained in a special flask material that does not interfere with microwave penetration. Polymerization of the resin denture base inside the special flask is caused by exposure to microwave radiation. A conventional, consumer microwave oven can be used. This process is easy, requires no special equipment for processing, and has been found to result in accurate, durable, clinically acceptable denture bases.

The final type of polymeric denture base material comes in thin sheets of unpolymerized material. The product is placed directly onto the master cast, molded, and teeth are placed. The assembly is then placed into a large unit where it is exposed to very intense light, causing the denture base to polymerize (a light-polymerized denture base).

Metal-Based Dentures

A different type of denture base material is metal. Usually, only the side of the denture that will be next to the oral mucosa (the tissue-bearing side) will be metal, and a polymer material will be added to stimulate gingiva and hold the denture teeth in place. The metal base is fabricated in a process that involves replacement of the wax form of the desired metal base with one that is made of metal using the lost wax technique. This technique is similar to that described previously for replacing wax with a material that is polymerized, but instead uses a special high-heat process that involves depositing molten metal into the void. Advantages of the metallic base are that it provides a much more accurate fit to the underlying mucosa, and it also transfers heat from foods and fluids to the palatal area (there is usually no polymer coating on this area). This added sensation provides a great enhancement of the pleasure gained from eating for many edentulous patients. An additional advantage of a metal-based denture is its added weight. For the mandibular denture, this weight helps to keep the denture in place. However, for metal-based maxillary dentures, the added weight may compromise the retention of the prosthesis.

Denture Teeth

Tooth Retention

The function of an artificial tooth in a denture is to provide esthetics, function, and articulation that were present in the natural state. The teeth are retained to the denture base by either a mechanical undercut (with no chemical bonding), or by means of micromechanical retention.

In mechanical bonding, the denture base flows into an internal void in the surface of the tooth. This void has small vent holes into which the unpolymerized denture base material flows during packing, polymerizes, and becomes mechanically locked in place. Also, some denture teeth use pins with heads that will be covered by the unpolymerized denture base, and will be mechanically retained in place after polymerization.

There is no method to chemically bond any type of denture tooth to the denture base. However, treatments of the underside of plastic teeth do allow a shallow infusion of denture base material into this surface, where it polymerizes around the existing polymer network of the denture tooth, and is this held in place micromechanically (mechanical retention, but on a very small, microscopic scale).

Porcelain Teeth

Denture teeth are made of either porcelain or plastic (a polymer). Within each type of material, there is a very wide range of shapes, colors, and compositions. Porcelain teeth were the first to be developed. These teeth are made of ceramic material and are quite hard and wear resistant. Disadvantages of porcelain denture teeth include their hardness, which can be a factor in excessive wear of any natural teeth to which they may articulate. Porcelain teeth also tend to transmit impact forces from biting to the underlying mucosa, which helps to increase in the rate of bone resorption occurring in the under-lying residual ridge. Because these teeth are fabricated of ceramic material, they are subject to fracture with minimal trauma. Again, because of the ceramic material, oppos-ing porcelain teeth that touch during speech often make a distinctive and disturbing clicking sound. Being ceramic, these teeth are difficult to contour to fit ridges and to adjust when inserting. The hardness of the material can also be an advantage because patients with porcelain denture teeth are less likely to demonstrate a loss of occlusal verti-cal dimension caused by wear of the denture teeth. However, one note of caution is in order: The hardness of the porcelain teeth may direct forces to the underlying bone and cause a loss of occlusal vertical dimension because of bone loss. Many clinicians would prefer that patients exhibit a loss of denture tooth material as opposed to loss of bone.

Polymer (Plastic) Teeth

The other type of denture teeth are made from polymers (called "plastic teeth"). These teeth are much softer than are their porcelain counterparts, and therefore do not impart as high an impact force to alveolar bone. Because of their comparative softness, plastic teeth are thought to lessen the stresses to the residual ridge resulting in less ridge resorp-tion. Being softer, plastic teeth are also less wear resistant than their porcelain equivalents and therefore, when placed to occlude against natural dentition, plastic teeth will not cause the natural teeth to wear; instead the plastic tooth will bear most of the wearing process. Plastic teeth are easily contoured to fit the underlying ridges and are easy to adjust at insertion. They are less likely to fracture than porcelain teeth, but their occlusal surfaces do wear more rapidly.

Plastic teeth can be classified into a variety of types, based on their composition and method of polymerization: conventional plastic teeth and IPN (Interpenetrating Polymer Network). Conventional plastic teeth are homogeneous in their composition and contain a polymer network that is basically only one type of resin. IPN teeth, however, are composed of a unique combination of materials and offer enhanced physi-cal properties (increased hardness and wear resistance) over their conventional analogs. In IPN teeth, two different polymers do not chemically bond to one another, but instead form totally independent polymer networks, where they become mechanically tangled. The combination of the different properties of these polymers as well as their mechani-cal entanglement help to enhance their properties compared with conventional teeth.

Plastic teeth are retained to the polymerizing denture base using a micromechani-cal interlocking of the new denture polymer enmeshing the polymer network of the denture tooth in contact with the curing base.

Denture Liners

Over time, the residual bone remaining after tooth extraction continues to slowly resorb resulting in a space between the tissue-bearing side of the denture and the residual ridge. Because of this space, the support, retention, and stability of the denture are all compro-mised. Excess movement of the denture base against the underlying mucosa (loose-fitting dentures) occurs, and the force delivered to the residual ridge is directed to only small areas instead of being spread uniformly. Because of the high stresses and lateral movements imposed on the delicate oral mucosa, the patient experiences "sore spots," which are localized areas of irritation that can cause extreme discomfort. Often, these discomforts are great enough to cause the patient not to wear the denture, except perhaps for social purposes.

To alleviate this ill-fitting condition, the clinician has two choices: making an entirely new denture, or adding only a small amount of new polymer that will take the place of the voids and return intimate contact and stability of the denture base to a large area of the underlying mucosa. The decision ultimately rests upon the amount of ridge loss and resulting space. If the space is large and occlusal vertical dimension has been lost, then making a new denture would seem appropriate. However, if the space is relatively small, a thin layer of new plastic can be added to the existing denture base. This later treatment is called a "reline" and can be performed either directly on the existing denture at chairside, or the denture can be sent to a laboratory where new material will be added using more sophisticated polymerizing techniques.

Chairside Reline Materials

If performed chairside, the clinician again has a decision to make: whether to add either a hard or a soft material to the existing denture. Both of these products consist of a powder and liquid that, when mixed, is very similar in content to that used when making the autopolymerizing denture base material. The difference is that the hard material sets to a relatively inflexible consistency, and the softer type polymerizes to more flexible mass. This flexibility helps to decrease biting forces on the underlying tissues by creating a soft cushion, while lessening tissue irritation and increasing overall patient comfort.

In this reline process, the tissue-bearing side of the denture base is roughened to provide a fresh, clean surface for the new material, and the product components are mixed and spread over the freshened denture surface. The denture is placed into the patient's mouth and held in position until the polymerization process has been completed. Extreme care must be taken because the heat released during the polymerization reaction occurring immediately against the oral mucosa is high enough to cause pain and scalding. Thus, it is not uncommon to remove and replace the denture several times during its process of intraoral polymerizing. When polymerized, the excess material flowing out of the denture is removed, and the junction of the old denture to the new is polished. Even though the basic components and chemistry of many of these types of lining agents are the same as those of the processed denture base, the extent of polymerization of the reline is not as thorough as that of the processed denture base. Thus, the reline materials have inferior properties: weaker and more prone to absorb fluids, and to discolor over time.

Recently, a new type of delivery system has been developed for extruding, mixing, and placing reline materials directly onto the old denture base chairside. In this system, the components to be dispensed are present in a single cartridge that is placed into a delivery gun. When the trigger is pressed, a plunger moves and forces both materials to be released, where they are directed into a nozzle that contains a special auguring device that thoroughly mixes them prior to extrusion from the tip end. The mixed material is placed directly onto the denture base, which is then inserted into the mouth and allowed to polymerize as stated previously. Both hard and soft reline materials are available using this type of delivery system.

Laboratory Reline Materials

Denture reline materials that are sent to the laboratory for processing polymerize to a higher degree than those that are used chairside. For the lab-processed relines, the old denture surface is roughened as before, an impression material is placed directly on the denture base, and the denture is inserted into the patient's mouth. Thus, the old base is used much as an impression tray would be. The denture/impression is then sent to the laboratory, where technicians encase the old denture in stone, much like in the conventional denture-making process previously described. The new denture base material is added and polymerized directly against the old base under heat and pressure. The resulting polymer from this laboratory processing is much stronger, bonded more tenaciously, and is more resistant to fluid absorption and color change than are the ones polymerized directly in the patient's mouth: the chairside products.

Laboratory methods are also used to process a "permanent," soft, silicone-based reline material. For this process, a piece of flexible liner is placed directly against the tissue-bearing side of the master cast, painted with an adhesive, and the case is then treated like a conventional heat- or autopolymerized, flasked denture. The resulting liner has the advantage of staying flexible for considerably longer periods than those made totally of a modified methacrylate-based polymer. However, a silicone surface is fairly porous and, over time, tends to accumulate bacteria and fungi; it must be treated to reduce this potential. Instead of using silicone, a modified resin-based, soft polymer can be placed on the tissue-bearing areas of the master cast in a similar manner as silicone. The conventional denture polymer is placed directly over this soft material, and the two are polymerized together. In this manner, there is a chemical bond formed between the two materials. This bond is more durable than the adhesive bond upon which the silicone material relies.

Denture Tissue Conditioners

It is not uncommon for a patient to present with a denture that has been in service for a very long time. As a result of this long-term use, the tissues of the residual ridge are often very irritated and inflamed. If impressions were made for a new denture at this time, the resulting master casts would only duplicate inflamed and irritated mucosa. A method must be used that allows these tissues to heal, while also permitting the patient to continue to wear and use their existing dentures. This is the function of a "tissue conditioner," which may be thought of as a temporary denture liner that provides a cushioning effect. The sponginess of this material absorbs loads to the underlying residual ridge, and allows those tissues to heal during function.

If tissue conditioner is allowed to remain on the patient's denture for too long, it may become hardened, resulting in recreation of the irritated state of the residual ridge seen prior to treatment. This loss of resiliency is the result of dissolution (leaching) of a component (plasticizer) that helps to keep the material flexible. Thus, it is typical that tissue conditioners must be frequently replaced during the course of a new denture fabrication.

These materials do not undergo any type of polymerization when "curing." The process by which they change from a fluid mass to a very viscous, flexible, and sponge-like solid is based on gelation of the components.

Denture Repair

Denture repair usually involves either replacement of a lost tooth or rejoining pieces of a fractured denture base (or both). In each situation, the pieces are joined using an autopolymerizing resin.

When joining broken sections, one must keep in mind that the success of the repair results on formation of both marcomechanical and micromechanical retentive mechanisms. Macromechanical aspects involve the purposeful fabrication of mechanical interlocks or undercuts, so that when the repair material is polymerized, it cannot be physically separated from the joined sections. Micromechanical retention involves application of a liquid, usually the liquid monomer of the repair material, on the outer surface of the pieces to be joined. The liquid is spread on the broken sections to cause only the outer layers of polymerized denture polymer to absorb the fluid and then physically swell. When the fluid repair resin comes into contact with this swollen surface, the polymerization process will also involve the fluid monomer that had been absorbed into only the very outer portions of the broken surface. Once again, additional strength is given to the repair at this site because of the formation of a new polymer network being formed around that of the old denture base: an interpenetrating polymer network.

If the repair resin is allowed to polymerize under high pressure and heat, the physical properties of the resulting joint will be greatly improved over one that is polymerized under ambient conditions. To create such conditions, the dental office laboratory will typically have a "curing" pot into which hot water and the unpolymerized repair resin are placed. Pressure is applied to the pot by using the existing in-house compressed air supply. This technique will produce a more dense, stronger polymer. The transverse strength of heat-polymerized repairs is approximately 80% of the unbroken material, whereas it is only 60% of the original strength for the chemically polymerized product.

Impression Materials

In order to fabricate a denture, exact replicas of the patient's edentulous jaws must be made. Basically, three different types of impression materials are used to capture the negative image of the patient's ridge. The selection of each type material is based on the degree of accuracy needed, as well as for the ability to mold the impression intraorally.

Alginate Hydrocolloid

Alginate hydrocolloid (an irreversible hydrocolloid) is usually packaged as pre-measured powder to which a specified volume of liquid (water) is added. Typically, room-temperature water is placed into a flexible, rubber mixing bowl, and the pre-packaged powder contents are sprinkled into the water. The components are actively mixed, using a wide-bladed spatula in a manner designed to eliminate incorporation of air bubbles. This mixed mass will have the consistency of very heavy dough, and is placed into a "stock" impression tray. These trays are generally available either in disposable plastic or reusable metal. Each tray will have some method of retaining the impression material, usually by the presence of small holes, through which the unset paste flows, hardens, and becomes locked. In addition, prior to placing the impression material, the tray may be sprayed with a special adhesive that further strengthens the bond between the impression tray and set alginate.

The tray is seated on the ridge, and held in a stable position, while the material sets. This process usually takes a few minutes, and can be accelerated by using warm water, or it can be lengthened by using cold water. In addition, the powder packet is available in regular and fast-set varieties. Once set, the impression and tray are removed by grasping the front handle lifting the vestibular tissue, to break the seal around the impression and exerting a rapid, snapping motion. The alginate may be difficult to remove because of excellent adaptation to the ridges. Fast removal of the impression is necessary because alginate is weak and may distort or tear if slowly pulled off the ridges during withdrawal.

The impression is examined to make sure that all desired areas were captured, rinsed to remove superficial debris and saliva, and is then sprayed with a solution of water-based disinfecting agent and placed into a sealed plastic bag as soon as possible. The impression should not be immersed in disinfectant because alginate can easily absorb water and swell, resulting in a distorted impression.

An alginate impression should be poured immediately. However, if the impression cannot be poured for several minutes, the set material should be wrapped in a wet paper towel, which provides a 100% humidity environment. The major component of alginate is water, and if not protected, fluid may evaporate prior to stone being poured into the impression. Even with good intentions, water may be lost from the impression and therefore, in all situations, an alginate impression should be poured within 10 minutes. Dental stone is poured into the impression and vibrated to remove air bubbles and allow the stone to cover all impression surfaces. The impression should be immediately separated from the set dental stone and not allowed to remain in contact with the stone. Alginate will absorb water from the set stone, resulting in a weak, powdery, soft superficial cast surface. If left for too long, dried alginate will become very hard, and may actually break the fine, delicate stone reproductions when the two items are separated.

Polyvinyl Siloxane (PVS) and Polyether (PE)

Most clinicians feel a more accurate impression and master cast are required when making complete dentures. These dentists will use the preliminary casts derived from alginate impressions to fabricate plastic custom or final impression trays. The tray is adjusted intraorally and the borders are correctly adapted to the ridges using some type of semi-solid impression material or a heavy-bodied polyvinyl siloxane or polyether. Once the borders of the trays are corrected, the tray is then removed and dried.

The tray is then painted with a specific adhesive material, which is allowed to dry for a specified period. This waiting time is necessary to allow the volatile components of the adhesive to evaporate and to allow the adhesive to slightly soften the surface of the impression tray. This softening allows the adhesive to diffuse into the outer portions of the tray, allowing for a more tenacious bond.

A synthetic, elastomeric impression material (either a polyvinyl siloxane known as PVS or a polyether-based product) is often used for making final impressions. These materials are known for their high degree of accuracy over the alginate products. PVS materials are available in a range of viscosities: light-bodied (a more fluid-like material), medium-bodied, heavy-bodied (much thicker consistency), or a putty (very dough-like and nonfluid). The viscosity to be used is based on the consistency of the tissues to be captured: the more unsupported and movable the tissue, the more fluid (the more light-bodied) the impression material desired so as to minimize distortion of the movable tissues. Polyether has an inherent heavy consistency, although there are modifiers that can be used to make it more fluid. It is not, however, available in the range of viscosities that the PVS products are.

Each material is packaged as two different pastes that, once mixed uniformly, start a setting reaction. The pastes can be mixed by hand using a spatula, or they can be extruded from a gunlike device that dispenses the two different pastes and thoroughly mixes them when they flow through a delivery tip. In either case, the mixed components are placed as a thin layer into the adhesive-coated custom tray, which is then placed in the patient's mouth. Once set, these types of materials are removed with a slow, teasing motion, rather than a snapping one because they are strong and stiff when set, and if removed quickly, they might scratch or tear delicate oral tissues.

For disinfection, the PVS material may be soaked in any type of disinfectant for any length of time, because it does not absorb water (is hydrophobic). Polyethers, however, do absorb water (are hydrophilic), so they must be spray disinfected, and placed in a plastic bag (similar to alginate disinfection technique).

These materials do not need to be poured immediately, and may be shipped to a laboratory for pouring if necessary. Once poured, neither material should be separated from the stone cast quickly, but instead a slow, steady force should be used. The PVS material is strong enough to withstand multiple pours of stone, but the polyether material is relatively weak, and would tend to tear under such repeated stress.

Dental Stones

The major component in all types of dental stones (calcium sulfate hemihydrate) is actually mined from the earth as the mineral gypsum. By treating the ground mineral in various manners (heating and application of pressure), different densities and hardness of stone powders are formed. When dental stone sets, there is a volumetric expansion, depending greatly on the type of stone used. Thus, the different types of stones arising from the various processing techniques vary in hardness, strength, surface detail reproducibility, and setting expansion.

To obtain maximal properties of these gypsum products, the proportioning of water and powder as well as the method of mixing are highly influential. Manufacturers provide detailed guidelines on the ratio of powder-to-water that should be present to provide optimal stone quality. To help develop the proper consistency, manufacturers provide dental stones in prepackaged, weighed, sealed bags, and also supply graduated cylinders for water measurement.

Reduction of air incorporation is a goal when mixing the powder and liquid components. For this purpose, special motor-driven mixing devices are available that also supply vacuum action during the mixing process: vacuum spatulation. The concept of filling the impression with stone is one that stresses displacement of trapped air and replacement with the stone slurry mixture. Thus, the impression may need to be tilted and the stone applied to the highest side, while the impression is placed in a vibrating table and the stone is allowed to flow downward using gravity. To help the stone wet (cover) the impression material surface and to reduce the possibility of bubbles forming at this interface, PVS materials are sometimes painted with a surfactant (a type of soap) prior to being poured.

Once the impression is filled, it needs to sit undisturbed while the chemistry of the setting reaction occurs. All types of dental stones release heat (are exothermic) during curing. Once the heat maximum occurs, and the stone temperature has declined to near room temperature (no longer warm to the touch), the impression and stone cast can be safely separated.

Types of Stones

Dental gypsum products range from a very soft, weak "impression plaster" (Type 1), to a very hard, strong, wear-resistant, and low expansion high-strength stone (Type IV). Most master casts for fabrication of indirect restorations (restorations not made directly in the patient's mouth, but instead, are made on stone reproduction casts) are made from one of the two hardest types of stone (Types III or IV). Type III stone (dental stone) is less strong that Type IV, and also expands slightly more. However, this type stone is used most often to fabricate master casts as well as articulating (working) casts because it has a relatively high strength, its surface reproduction is as good as that of the higher strength stones, and costs less than the higher strength products. Type II products (model plaster, mounting stone), have the highest setting expansion, and are weaker than Types III and IV materials. Model plaster is used mostly for stabilizing master casts in position to articulators.

Interocclusal Registration Materials

It is essential not only to obtain exact replications of the oral tissues captured in stone master casts, but also to have the opposing casts oriented in space precisely as they are in the patient's head. The dentist has a wide variety of mechanical devices (articulators) to which these casts can be attached that will not only correctly orient the casts, but will also allow the casts to very closely mimic the mandibular movements when in function. In this manner, the artificial teeth can be properly placed into a denture when in the wax-up stage, and they will very closely match the location as well as functional position when placed in the patient's mouth. However, for proper cast orientation, a facebow must be used to attach the maxillary cast to the articulator and some type interocclusal recording material must be used to relate the opposing casts to each other. This material is also used to orient the completed dentures at insertion. A variety of materials are used for this purpose.

Registration Materials

A variety of materials are used for the registration process. Generally the materials consist of either a moldable thermoplastic material or a polyvinyl siloxane. The thermoplastic materials are usually a fiber-reinforced, cloth-mesh encased, tough wax (Aluwax) or a mixture of resins and waxes (impression compound). These materials may be softened in warm water and harden readily when cooled in the mouth when a stream of air or cold water is directed at them. However, their ability to retain dimension is related to not being heated again nor flexed. Thus care needs to be taken in handling these registration materials once used. A light-bodied polyvinyl siloxane material (much like the PVS impression material previously mentioned) can also be used to capture the registration of the arches through their overlying appliances. Advantages of this material are that, once set, its dimensions are stable and not affected by temperature, and the material will not distort or break with flexure. A disadvantage is that the material is not rigid, and the casts may not be properly oriented because of this flexibility.

 ## Dental Waxes

Among other uses, dental waxes serve as replacement for missing bone and mucosa prior to denture fabrication, are used to join casts together, hold the denture teeth in position following the tooth arrangement, and for making specific type impressions. These materials are mixtures of natural and synthetic hydrocarbons specifically designed to soften at pre-desired temperatures. Once cooled and hard, they also have a variety of flexibilities and hardness.

The most typical type of wax used for denture base fabrication is termed "baseplate" wax. This type of wax is available in three different levels of hardness, each having a different flowability at specific temperatures (room temperature, body temperature, and an elevated temperature). Type 1 wax is used mostly in denture base construction, appears moderately soft at room temperature, and has a moderate flow when heated.

The other type of wax commonly used in denture base fabrication is "sticky wax" and is known for its ability to adhere to casts. Thus, master casts can be temporally held together using small pieces of tongue blade that have been attached to each cast using sticky wax. At room temperature, this material is hard and brittle, but it readily flows when heated.

Lastly, a special, low-melting impression wax can be used to help capture sections of oral mucosa in a nonfunctional state. In the warm, fluid state, this material can be painted over the impression tray to capture delicate, distortable tissues. When cooled, the material becomes hard and can be removed to provide a negative image of the tissues in their relaxed, unloaded state. These waxes are easily distorted, should be handled with great care, and the casts poured immediately.

As is the case for all types of waxes used in denture fabrication, care must be exercised not to expose the completed wax setup to temperature extremes, as wax has the highest level of thermal expansion or contraction of all materials used. If warmed, stresses that had been locked into the "frozen" solid wax may be released, causing the wax to flow and allowing distortion of any impression or denture tooth movement.

 ## Denture Cleansers

Proper denture cleaning is essential for maintaining denture base color and the general health of the patient's mouth. If the dentures and underlying mucosa are not maintained, tissue irritation, fungal infections, inflammatory papillary hyperplasia, and halitosis are possible. Often, patients clean only the visible, outside portion of the denture and neglect cleaning the tissue-bearing side, or also ignore cleaning the tissues upon which the denture rests. It is the clinician's responsibility to educate the patient in proper cleansing methods as well to recommend specific types of ancillary cleaning products. Patients should be warned to avoid use of high levels of heat to clean dentures because the dentures may warp irreversibly, resulting in a loss of correct fit.

Cleaning of the denture at office check-up visits should be used to reeducate the patient to the procedures and products recommended by the office. Efforts to reinforce compliance with proper cleaning of all surfaces of the denture, as well as the oral mucosa should be made.

Denture bases retain plaque and accumulate debris that should be periodically removed. Cleansing of the tissue-bearing side of the denture is often overlooked. Even with the unending list of denture cleansers that are commercially available, patients can obtain excellent results with the use of an ordinary soft-bristle tooth brush and a mild soap. This method of cleaning causes the least abrasion and discoloration of the denture base and provides a much cleaner surface. Another excellent method of cleaning dentures is through the use of an ultrasonic cleaner specifically made for denture cleaning and home use. The use of an ultrasonic cleaner in conjunction with any of the following materials will yield excellent results. Denture cleansers can be divided into two groups: abrasives and solutions.

Abrasive Cleansers

The abrasiveness of conventional toothpastes (especially the "whitening" formulations) is excessive for the relatively soft polymer of denture bases, and will easily scratch and cause excessive wear to the dentures. Thus, special formulations of paste-based cleansers are marketed specifically for cleaning these prostheses. Also, soft-bristled brushes are recommended, as they help to decrease the potential for the cleansing process to abrade the relatively soft denture polymer.

Solution Cleaners: Hypochlorites, Oxygenating Agents, Mild Acids

Hypochlorites Sodium hypochlorite is a well-known antibacterial agent, and in mild concentration, can be used to remove adherent protein from the denture surface as well as kill organisms present. However, caution must be used, as this fluid is also highly corrosive to the metal framework of removable partial dentures and therefore cannot be used on these restorations. In addition, the color characteristics of the denture base (basic tint as well as inclusion of colored fibers to simulate blood vessels) may be irreversibly oxidized, resulting in a loss of color and a general whitening.

Oxygenating Agents Solutions of oxygenating agents (such as peroxides, perborates, and percarbonates) are made by dissolving tablets or powders containing these compounds into water, in which the dentures are immersed for a period of time. The bubbling activity developed from the tablet dissolution also creates a small agitation that helps cleanse debris from the denture surface. However, the "cleaning power" of these agents is really only superficial, and a denture base can only be truly "cleaned" through the mechanical action of a paste and brush or an ultrasonic cleaner. These oxygenating agents should not be used if the denture base contains a soft liner, as the reaction of this type cleanser tends to irreversibly harden the liner.

Mild Acids The mechanism of "cleaning" of some products relies on creation of mildly acidic solutions: hydrochloric or phosphoric acids. These agents dissolve calculus deposits, however they may also attack metals used in partial denture frameworks and are therefore not recommended for routine use.

Denture Adhesives

If the tissue-bearing surface of the oral cavity is not in intimate contact with the denture base (through a thin layer of saliva), the denture becomes unstable and is easily dislodged. Increased space between the denture base and underlying tissues arises from resorption of underlying bone over time, or from improper denture construction. Relining the denture is often the best method of resolving this problem, however this is not always possible. To alleviate this misfit, a variety of products are made that fill these gaps as well as adhere to the denture and overlying mucosa. It should be mentioned, that in the majority of cases, these adhesive materials are not needed if careful attention is given to the details of the entire denture fabrication process. However, these products may be of use in emergency situations where immediate denture stabilization is desired.

Denture adhesives are often "self-prescribed" by the patient and are readily available in a variety of over-the-counter formulations. Basically, these products will be either a paste or a powder. There is no clear advantage to either type of product in their ability to help stabilize a lose-fitting denture. Adhesives are also useful for those patients with little-to-no remaining residual ridge to help supply resistance to lateral denture movement (stability), for edentulous patients with cleft palates, and for patients who wear post-cancer treatment intraoral prostheses.

Patients who use these types of supplementary products should be educated about the need for frequent removal of the products from both the denture base as well as the tissues upon which they rest. It is not uncommon that patients continue to place additional product to help "tighten their teeth," and the old material is never really eliminated. These products work best if used as a thin layer, and many times a patient will consider "more is better," and place too much, which results in a denture even more unstable than prior to the adhesive addition.

Two studies indicate that dentures adhesives may cause problems to a limited number of patients. First, sodium may leach from some of these materials and potentially be detrimental to those patients on sodium-free or reduced-sodium diets. Powder based adhesives allow more sodium to be released into the saliva because of the increased surface area of the powders: therefore a paste may be more appropriate for these patients. Second, some denture cleaners may allow a mild acid buildup in the saliva and could potentially etch (remove superficial enamel and dentin) the dentition in those patients with retained natural teeth.

Powder-Based Products

Powder-based denture adhesives contain vegetable gums or special types of polymers that become viscous and form a mucin-like gel when mixed with water. The resulting stickiness to both tissues and denture material helps to retain the dentures. The powdered material is sprinkled over the surface of a wet denture base and is then inserted into the mouth.

Paste-Based Products

Paste adhesives are based on a combination of natural tree-gums, a thick heavy organic gel, coloring, and flavoring agents. As opposed to the powdered products, these materials are water-resistant and attempt to displace surface water between the denture and the tissues and seal further water from seeping in. Paste is extruded directly onto the denture base and is spread until it forms a thin layer, after which the denture is inserted.

References

Beaumont, A. J., Tupta, L. M., Stuchell, R. N.: Content and solubility of sodium in denture adhesives. J Prosthet Dent. 1991; 65:536-40.

Craig, R. G., Powers, J. M., Wataha, J. C.: Plastics in Prosthetics. In: Craig, R. G., Powers, J. M., Wataha, J. C., editors. Dental Materials, Properties and Manipulation, 8th ed, St. Louis: Mosby; 2004, p. 270.

Garcia, L. T., Jones, J. D.: Soft Liners. In Agar, J. R., Taylor, T. D., eds. Removable Prosthodontics. Dental Clinics of North America. Philadelphia: W. B. Saunders Company; 2004; 48:709-20.

Grasso, J. E.: Denture Adhesives. In Agar, J. R., Taylor, T. D., eds: Removable Prosthodontics. Dental Clinics of North America. Philadelphia: W. B. Saunders Company; 2004; 48:721-33.

Koran, A., III.: Prosthetic Applications of Polymers. In Craig, R.G., Powers, M., editors: Restorative Dental Materials, 11th ed, St. Louis, MO: Mosby; 2002, p. 635.

Love, W. B., Biswas. S.: Denture adhesives -pH and buffering capacity. J Prosthet Dent 1991; 66: 356-60.

Rahn, A. O., Heartwell, C. M., Jr.: Complete Denture Impressions. In: Rahn, A. O., Heartwell, C. M. Jr, editors: Textbook of Complete Dentures, 5th ed, Philadelphia: Lea & Febiger. 1993; p. 228-31.

QUESTIONS

1. List three of the four methods of polymerizing denture base resin.

2. What is the approximate shrinkage of a denture base resin during polymerization (processing)?

3. Denture resin will absorb water from its storage fluid, and expand slightly (0.1 to 0.2%). Why is this important?

4. List four advantages of resin denture teeth over porcelain denture teeth.

5. What are some of the advantages of a laboratory denture reline as opposed to a chair-side reline?

6. Why should a tissue conditioner be replaced reasonably frequently?

7. How does the strength of a repaired denture compare to the original unbroken denture?

8. Why must an irreversible hydrocolloid (alginate) impression be poured within 10 minutes?

9. Why should the adhesive for an impression material be allowed to set for the manufacturers suggested time (often 10 minutes), when visually it appears fine after only 5 minutes?

10. What are two characteristics of denture adhesives that should be considered when recommending one to a patient?

ANSWERS

1. Heat, Chemical Reaction, Microwave Energy, Light

2. Approximately 0.3 to 0.5%

3. Absorption of water by the denture compensates for the shrinkage during polymerization making the final dimensions almost exactly the same as those of the mouth.

4. Better retention to the denture base, easier to adjust, less brittle, do not impart as much occlusal impact to the underlying tissues, and less likely to fracture.

5. The resulting polymer from this laboratory polymerization is much stronger, bonded more tenaciously, and is more resistant to fluid absorption and color change than are the ones polymerized directly in the patient's mouth: the chairside products.

6. If tissue conditioner is allowed to remain in the patient's mouth for too long, it may become hardened, resulting in recreation of the irritated state of the residual ridge seen prior to treatment.

7. The transverse strength of heat-polymerized repairs is approximately 80% of the unbroken material, whereas it is only 60% of the original strength for the chemically polymerized product.

8. An irreversible hydrocolloid (alginate) impression should be poured immediately. However, if the impression cannot be poured for several minutes, the set material should be wrapped in a wet paper towel, which provides a 100% humidity environment. The major component of alginate is water, and if not protected, fluid may evaporate prior to stone being poured into the impression. Even with good intentions, water may be lost from the impression and therefore, in all situations, an alginate impression should be poured within 10 minutes.

9. This waiting time is necessary to allow the volatile components of the adhesive to evaporate and to allow the adhesive to slightly soften the surface of the impression tray. This softening allows the adhesive to diffuse into the outer portions of the tray, allowing for a more tenacious bond.

10. Denture adhesives may cause problems to a limited number of patients. First, sodium may leach from some of these materials and potentially be detrimental to those patients on sodium-free or reduced-sodium diets. Powder-based adhesives allow more sodium to be released into the saliva because of the increased surface area of the powders; therefore a paste may be more appropriate for these patients. Second, some denture cleaners may allow a mild acid buildup in the saliva and could potentially etch (remove superficial enamel and dentin) the dentition in those patients with retained natural teeth.

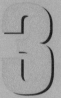

Anatomy of the Edentulous Ridges

Dr. Mohamed Sharawy

Although a thorough knowledge of all anatomical landmarks of the edentulous mouth is indispensable for the successful treatment of dental patients, certain structures are especially important when fabricating complete dentures. These structures, which affect the fabrication of complete dentures, and the structures that underlie those important landmarks will be discussed in this chapter.

Accurate impressions of the maxillary and mandibular arches should reproduce the landmarks that do not change their position with function (Ex: alveolar ridges and hard palate) and the landmarks that change their shape with function (Ex: frenula, vibrating line between soft and hard palate).

Identifying the anatomical landmarks in casts of the maxillary and mandibular arches and comparing them to the same structures in a patient's mouth should help to provide the clinician with the confidence that the impression procedure accurately reproduced the area to be covered with the denture.

Extraoral Features

The following extraoral anatomical features should be noted when the patient has his/her mouth closed (mandible in resting position) and his/her top and bottom lips lightly touching: philtrum, labial tubercle, vermillion borders, nasolabial groove, and labiomental groove (Figure 3–1). The philtrum is a midline shallow depression of the upper lip, which starts at the labial tubercle and ends at the nose. The labial tubercle is a little swelling in the midportion of the vermillion border of the upper lip. The lip is covered by the skin at its facial surface and the mucous membrane at its inner surface. The transitional area between the skin and the mucous membrane of the upper and lower lips is a pink or red zone of thinner epithelium, which is called the vermillion border. The nasolabial groove is a furrow of variable depth that extends from the wing (ala) of the nose to end at some distance from the corner of the mouth. The labiomen-

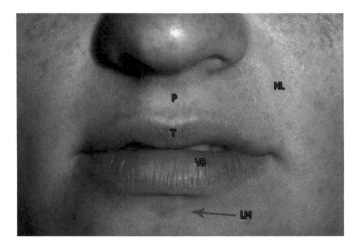

Figure 3–1 Note the Philtrum (P), Nasolabial groove (NL), Labial tubercle (T), Vermillion border (VB) and Labiomental groove (LM).

tal groove is a sharp or deep groove that lies between the lower lip and the chin. Obliteration or filling of one of the above-mentioned normal grooves can occur from a swelling caused by trauma, infection, cyst, or neoplastic growth.

Structures of the Facial Vestibules

The maxillary and mandibular dental arches separate the oral cavity into a facial vestibule and an oral cavity proper. With the patient in centric occlusion, the space that is bound by the lips and cheeks facially and the teeth and gingiva internally is called the labiobuccal, or facial, vestibule. The depth of the facial vestibule and fornices change with the way the cheek and lips are manipulated during impression making. Horizontal pull or functional movements of the lips and cheek should mold the soft impression materials and reproduce the position of the fornices.

The following facial vestibular anatomical landmarks should be identified on both arches: fornix of the vestibule; free gingiva; attached gingiva; unattached gingiva (alveolar mucosa); interdental papilla; median labial frenums; buccal frenums; and canine eminences.

The fornix of the vestibule is the site where the mucous membrane lining of the lips and cheeks reflects and joins the unattached gingiva, or alveolar mucosa. Some people call the fornix the mucobuccal fold—a term that is inaccurate. The depth of the vestibule in the upper and lower jaws is determined by the site of the fornix, which in turn is determined by the muscle attachments to the bony jaws. The muscle that limits the buccal vestibule in the upper and lower jaws is the buccinator. The muscle takes origin from the base of the alveolar process, at the upper first, second, and third molars and the external oblique ridge opposite the lower molars. It also takes origin from the pterygoid hamulus and the pterygomandibular raphé. The latter joins the buccinator with the superior constrictor muscle of the pharynx. The fibers of the buccinator have to cross the retromolar triangle (deep to retromolar pad) to join the pterygomandibular raphé medial to the medial pterygoid muscle.

The upper fornix is not supported by strong muscles but has small muscles opposite the region of lateral incisor called incisivus muscle. In addition to the latter, oblique fibers of nasalis muscle fix the ala of the nose to underlying bone and septal muscle, which attaches to the septum of the nose. These little muscles do not form a barrier to the subcutaneous tissue of the face. If, while taking an upper impression, the lips are pulled vertically instead of horizontally the action will artificially increase the depth of the vestibule, and the flange of the denture will extend into the subcutaneous space, causing irritation of the mucosa and alteration of the facial appearance.

Following extraction of teeth, the bone supporting the roots (alveolar process) undergoes resorption and therefore the depth of the vestibule become shallower. Surgical creation of a new fornix that would permit increase in the depth of the vestibule may be required before denture construction.

The free gingiva is the part of the gingiva that extends from the gingival margin to the attached gingiva (approximately the level of the gingival sulcus). The attached gingiva is the part of the gingiva that is held firmly to the underlying bone and cementum (hard tissue that covers the root of the tooth). The unattached gingiva is the part of the gingiva that is loosely attached to the underlying bone. It is continuous with the alveolar mucosa. The interdental papilla is the part of the gingiva located in the interdental

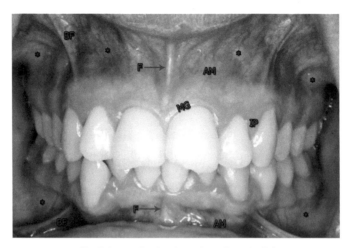

Figure 3–2   Facial vestibule showing: Fornix (*), upper median labial frenum and lower median labial frenum (F), buccal frenum (BF), alveolar mucosa (AM), interdental papillae (IP) and marginal gingiva (MG).

space. In some patients, the marginal, or free, gingiva is demarcated from the attached gingiva by the presence of a gingival groove (Figure 3–2).

The upper medial labial frenum, or frenulum, is a fold of mucous membrane that overlies dense connective tissue (Figures 3–2 and 3–4). It does not contain muscle fibers, in contrast to the buccal frenula. It anchors the upper lip to the gingiva. The frenum varies in size among individuals but it is usually more developed than other frenula found in the vestibule. When it is abnormally large, it extends to the interdental papilla between the two central incisors. An enlarged upper median labial frenum is frequently found in association with a diastema (large space between the two central incisors). In many edentulous patients, resorption of the alveolar bone brings the crest of the alveolar ridge closer to the frenum. Therefore, a normal frenum may need surgical excision before

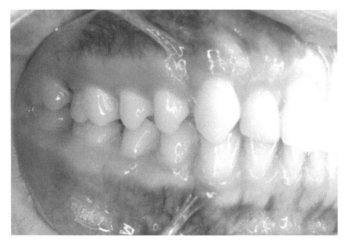

Figure 3–3   Buccal Vestibule. Note the prominent buccal frenums.

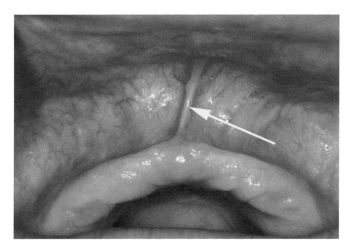

Figure 3–4 The upper medial labial frenum, or frenulum, is a fold of mucous membrane that overlies dense connective tissue.

successful denture construction can be initiated. In all cases, the dentures should be relieved away from the frenula, to avoid irritation of these folds and to prevent future instability of the dentures. The upper buccal frenum is a mucous membrane fold that overlies dense fibrous connective tissue and fibers of the caninus, or the levator anguli oris muscle (elevator of the angle of the mouth). The latter is one of the muscles of facial expression. The lower median labial frenum is morphologically similar to the upper median labial frenum but commonly less developed. The lower buccal labial frenum is also morphologically similar to the upper buccal labial frenum but again less developed. It contains muscle fibers from the depressor anguli oris, or triangularis (another muscle of facial expression) (Figure 3–3).

The canine eminence is a bony prominence in both the maxilla and mandible that denotes the roots of the canine teeth. The eminences of the upper jaw raise the upper lip; its loss leads to the sagging of the lip associated with aging.

Alveolar (Residual) Ridges

The roots of the teeth are supported by the alveolar process of the maxilla and the mandible. Following full mouth extractions, the alveolar ridges undergo significant boney changes, with the largest changes seen on the mandibular arch. Studies indicate that the mandibular ridge resorps approximately four times as much as the maxillary arch. The direction of mandibular resorption is downward and outward, while maxillary resorption is upward and inward. The results of this resorptive pattern often force a crossbite of the posterior dentures in order to maintain the dentures over the residual ridges (Figures 3–5, 3–6).

The maxillary tuberosity is the most posterior part of the alveolar ridge; it lies distal to the position of the last molar. It is a bulbous mass of mucous membrane that overlies a bony tuberosity. The maxillary tuberosity is important from a denture standpoint

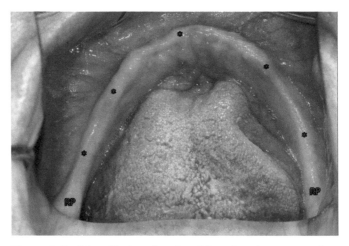

Figure 3-5   Mandibular alveolar ridge showing: crest of the ridge (*) and the retromolar pad areas (RP).

because it is considered a primary stress-bearing area and because surgery must be considered when the tuberosity is extremely large and compromises the clearance necessary for opposing dentures. The most distal structure in the mandibular residual ridge is the retromolar pad.

Maxillary Arch

The anatomical landmarks of the maxillary arch, which may affect denture fabrication, include the incisive papilla, palatine rugae, torus palatinus, mid-palatine raphe, uvula,

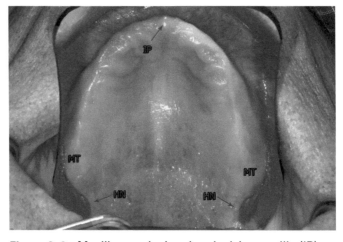

Figure 3-6   Maxillary arch showing: incisive papilla (IP), maxillary tuberosity (MT) and the hamular notch (HM).

fovea palatini, hamular notches, posterior palatal seal area, and vibrating line (Figure 3–6 through 3–8).

The incisive papilla is a small tubercle located on the palatal side between the two central incisors. It overlies the incisive foramen, through which the incisive nerve and blood vessels exit. Because of the sensitivity of this structure, care must be taken when inserting the maxillary denture to relieve almost all pressure in this area. The incisal papilla is a good landmark when contouring occlusion rims and positioning the dentures because studies indicate that the facial surfaces of the natural central incisors, when present, were approximately 8-10 mm anterior to the middle of the incisal papilla, and the tips of the canines were approximately in line with the middle of the incisal papilla (Figure 3–7).

The palatine rugae (Figure 3–7) are irregular mucous membranes that extend bilaterally from the midline of the hard palate in relation to the upper six anterior and sometimes bicuspid teeth. Many years ago it was felt that these structures could potentially play a large role is speech and in helping the patient position the tongue. Dentures were fabricated with artificial rugae in an attempt to aid patients in these areas, however current studies do not indicate that the rugae play a significant role in speech or tongue positioning, and they are no longer considered important when fabricating maxillary dentures.

When present, the torus palatinus (Figure 3–7) is a bony prominence of variable size and shape, which is located in the middle of the hard palate. Because the tissue overlying a palatal torus is usually very thin, and the torus is very rigid, any pressure caused by a maxillary denture during chewing and swallowing will often traumatize the tissue and lead to irritation and ulceration. Care must be taken during insertion to relieve any pressure to the torus caused by the denture. Additionally, an enlarged torus palatinus could act as a fulcrum that can lead to instability of a denture. Generally, any torus that has lateral undercuts or extends to the vibrating line should be considered for surgical removal.

The midpalatine raphé (Figure 3–8, A) is a line in the middle of the mucosa of the hard palate that overlies the mid-palatine bony suture. The tissue in this area is very thin, and any pressure from a denture will not be tolerated in most patients. Care must be taken when inserting the denture to provide necessary relief.

The uvula is a tongue-like projection extending from the distal extent of the soft palate. The uvula is muscular. Its exact function is unknown, however it helps in sealing

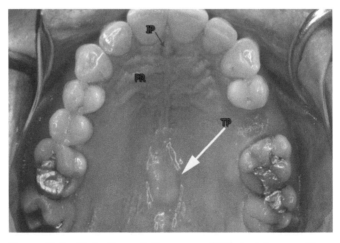

Figure 3–7 Note the palatine rugae (PR), incisive papilla (IP) and the torus palatines (T).

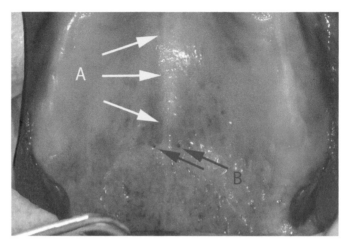

Figure 3–8 The midpalatine raphé (A) is a line in the middle of the mucosa of the hard palate, which overlies the midpalatine bony suture. The fovea palatini (B) are two depressions that lie bilateral to the midline of the palate, at the approximate junction between the soft and hard palate, and denote the sites of opening of ducts of small mucous glands of the palate.

the oral cavity from the nasal cavity during swallowing. Until recently, removing the uvula and part of the soft palate (uvulopalatopharyngoplasty, UPPP) in an attempt to relieve the symptoms of snoring and obstructive sleep apnea has been popular in the medical community. This procedure has lost favor, however, because of the reasonably low success rate, a certain amount of morbidity associated with the procedure, and the resultant difficulty in speech and swallowing in some patients. It is not involved in the construction of complete dentures.

The fovea palatini (Figure 3–8, B) are two depressions that lie bilateral to the midline of the palate, at the approximate junction between the soft and hard palate. They denote the sites of opening of ducts of small mucous glands of the palate. They are often useful in the identification of the vibrating line because they generally occur within 2 mm of the vibrating line.

The hamular process, or hamulus, is a bony projection of the medial plate of the pterygoid bone and is located distal to the maxillary tuberosity. Lying between the maxillary tuberosity and the hamulus is a groove called the hamular notch (Figure 3–9). This notch is a key clinical landmark in maxillary denture construction because the maximum posterior extent of the denture is the vibrating line that runs bilaterally through the hamular notches. The hamulus can be palpated clinically and it can be a possible site of irritation in denture wearing patients, if the denture touches this process. The tendon of the tensor velli palatini muscle runs across the hamulus to reach the soft palate. Under the tendon is a small bursa (membrane between the moving tendon and the hamulus). Inflammation and pain can result from mechanical irritation by unstable dentures.

Although not a truly anatomical feature, the vibrating line is very important to locate for proper construction of the maxillary complete denture (Figure 3–10). Although not precisely true, the vibrating line can be considered as the junction between the hard and soft palates and is important because it is the maximum posterior limit to the maxillary denture. This line runs from about 2 mm buccal to the center of the hamu-

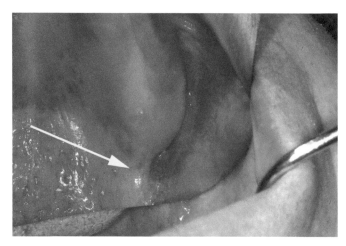

Figure 3–9 Lying between the maxillary tuberosity and the hamulus is a groove called the hamular notch. This notch is a key clinical landmark in maxillary denture construction because the maximum posterior extent of the denture is the vibrating line, which runs bilaterally through the hamular notches.

lar notch on one side of the arch, follows the junction of the hard and soft palates across the palate, and ends about 2 mm buccal to the center of the opposite hamular notch.

Additionally the vibrating line is the distal extent of the posterior palatal seal area (Figure 3–11). The posterior palatal seal area is very important in maxillary complete denture fabrication and must be identified and evaluated. It is the area of compressible tissue located anterior to the vibrating line and lateral to the midline in the posterior third of the hard palate. The distal extent of this area is the vibrating line, while the

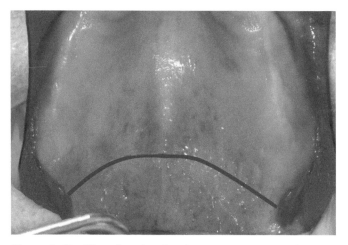

Figure 3–10 The vibrating line is a very important feature to be located in the construction of the maxillary complete denture. It can be considered as the junction between the hard and soft palates and is important because it is the maximum posterior limit to the maxillary denture.

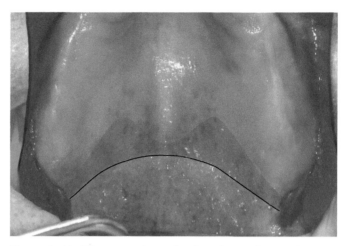

Figure 3–11 The posterior palatal seal area is very important in maxillary complete denture fabrication and must be
identified and evaluated. It is the area of compressible
tissue located lateral to the midline and in the posterior
third of the hard palate. The distal extent of this area is
the vibrating line, while the anterior border is indistinct.

anterior border is indistinct. The redundancy of the tissue in this area is caused by the
presence of mucous glands surrounded by abundant loose connective tissue. The depth
of compressible tissue is evaluated using palpation and noted for future reference. This
information will be used following master cast fabrication and is important in maxillary
denture retention.

Mandibular Arch

In the lower jaw, a triangular area of thick mucosa is found distal to the last molar, basically on the crest of the ridge, and is referred to as the retromolar pad (Figure 3–12). This
pad is extremely important in denture construction from both a denture extension and
plane of occlusion standpoint. The retromolar pads should be covered by the denture,
and the plane of occlusion is generally located at the level of the middle to upper-third
of this pad. Extending from the hamulus above to the area of the retromolar pad below
is the pterygomandibular raphé fold (Figure 3–13). The pterygomandibular raphé, which
underlies the fold, is the junction between the buccinator (cheek muscle) and the superior constrictor muscle of the pharynx. It is often visible in the maxillary impression and,
when present, is an excellent landmark for determining the distal extent of the maxillary
denture. It is usually insignificant when making the mandibular impression.

Just buccal to the crest of the mandibular ridge in the distal-buccal corner of the
arch is an area known as the masseter notch, or groove area (Figure 3–14). It is important in mandibular denture fabrication because of its influence on impression making. It
is a diagonal directed line that runs from the depth of the vestibule in the anterior to the

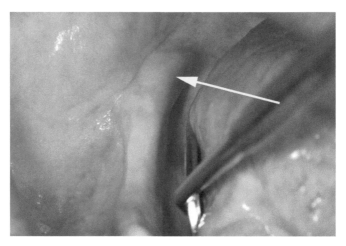

Figure 3-12 In the lower jaw, a triangular area of thick mucosa is found distal to the last molar, basically on the crest of the ridge, and is referred to as the retromolar pad. This pad is extremely important in denture construction from both a denture extension and plane of occlusion standpoint.

crest of the ridge in the posterior. It is formed by the actions of the masseter muscle. Because there is often a fatty roll of tissue overlying the buccinator muscle, medial to the masseter muscle, this cheek area must often be lifted to eliminate the fatty roll, particularly when making the final impression (Figure 3–15). If clinicians do not properly evaluate this area, the resultant completed mandibular denture is overextended. This overextension will cause significant discomfort to the patient and/or the mandibular denture will become dislodged on opening.

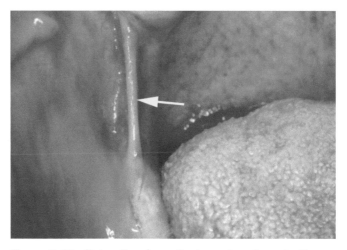

Figure 3-13 Extending from the hamulus above to the area of the retromolar pad below is the pterygomandibular raphé fold.

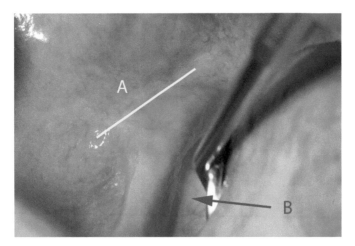

Figure 3–14 Just buccal to the crest of the mandibular ridge in the distal-buccal corner of the arch is an area known as the masseter notch, or groove area (A). The most distal extent of the inner surfaces of the mandibular ridges ends in an area called the retromylohyoid area, or fossa (B).

The buccal shelf (Figure 3–16) is located on the mandibular arch and is important to mandibular denture fabrication because it is the primary stress-bearing area of the mandibular arch. It is an area bounded on the medial side by the crest of the residual ridge, on the lateral side by the external oblique ridge, in the mesial area by the buccal frenulum, and on the distal side by the masseter muscle. It is just anterior to the pre-masseteric notch area. The buccal shelf consists primarily of thick cortical bone, in contrast to the crest of the ridge, which is fenestrated and consists of thin cortical bone overlying more cancellous bone.

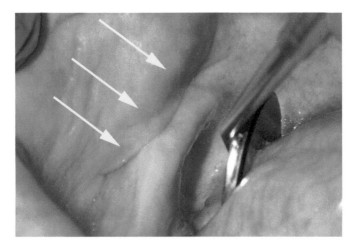

Figure 3–15 Because there is often a fatty roll of tissue overlying the buccinator muscle, this cheek area must often be lifted to eliminate the fatty roll, particularly when making the final impression.

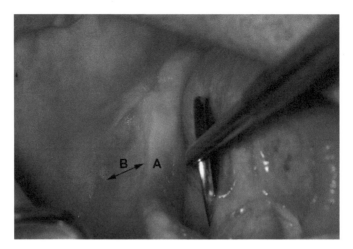

Figure 3–16   The buccal shelf (B) is located on the mandibular arch and is important to mandibular denture fabrication because it is the primary stress-bearing area of the mandibular arch. The residual ridge (A).

The tongue (Figure 3–17) is located in the floor of the mouth. It is important to become familiar with the normal features of the tongue because many systemic disease processes, such as iron deficiency anemia and pernicious anemia, for example, can cause changes in the tongue. Early recognition of these changes may help in the discovery of serious systemic illness. The tongue is important in denture construction because of its significant mobility and because of its involvement with deglutition and speech. Its activities must be accounted for when making impressions and when arranging the teeth on the mandibular denture. The dorsum of the anterior two-thirds of the tongue is rough because of the presence of projections known as lingual papillae. The junction between

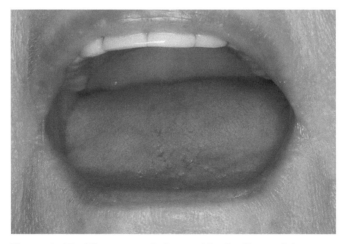

Figure 3–17   The tongue is located in the floor of the mouth. It is important to become familiar with the normal features of the tongue because many systemic disease processes can cause changes in the tongue.

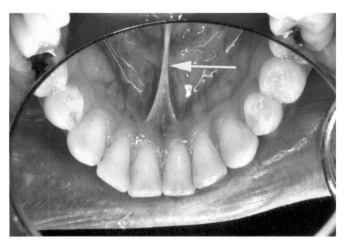

Figure 3–18 The ventral surface of the tongue is anchored to the floor by a mucous membrane fold known as the lingual frenulum.

the anterior two-thirds and the posterior one-third of the tongue is denoted by a V-shaped sulcus called the sulcus limitans. Along this sulcus are 10-13 larger papillae known as the circumvallate papillae. To observe these papillae, the tongue has to be pulled forward. In many patients, several normal fissures can be observed in the dorsum of the tongue. The ventral surface of the tongue (undersurface) is anchored to the floor by a mucous membrane fold known as the lingual frenulum (Figures 3–18 & 3–19). Along the sides of the lingual frenulum slightly tortuous vessels can be seen glistening through the thin and smooth mucous membrane of the tongue. These vessels are branches of the lingual artery (linguae profundus) and the lingual vein (ranine vein). Branches of the lingual nerve accompany these vessels. Careful handling of the dental instruments inside the mouth is advisable as injury to the vessels and nerves could occur.

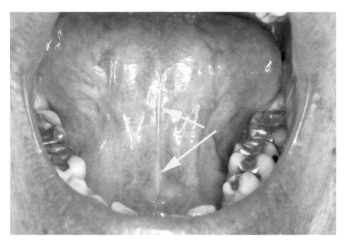

Figure 3–19 The ventral surface of the tongue showing veins on both sides of the lingual frenulum.

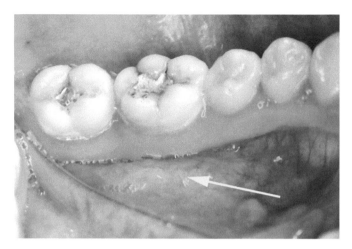

Figure 3–20 In the floor of the mouth, on both sides, prominent folds of mucous membrane called the sublingual folds are usually seen.

In the floor of the mouth, on both sides, prominent folds of mucous membrane called the sublingual folds are usually seen (Figure 3–20). At the medial end of each fold is a little swelling referred to as the sublingual caruncle, where the submandibular salivary gland duct opens into the oral cavity (Figure 3–21, A). Along the sublingual fold, one can see numerous tiny orifices for the ducts of the sublingual salivary glands. The orifice of the large parotid gland is found in the mucous membrane of the cheek opposite to the upper second molar. The parotid orifice is guarded by a mucous membrane swelling called the parotid papilla (Figure 3–22). The orifice of the parotid has been

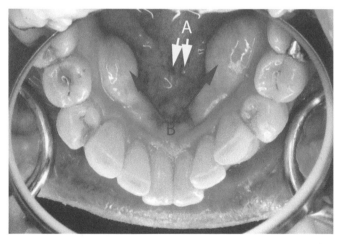

Figure 3–21 At the medial end of each fold is a little swelling referred to as the sublingual caruncle; this is where the submandibular salivary gland duct opens into the oral cavity (A). Some patients exhibit bilateral bony prominences of the inner surface of the mandible in the region of the premolar teeth called the torus mandibularis (B).

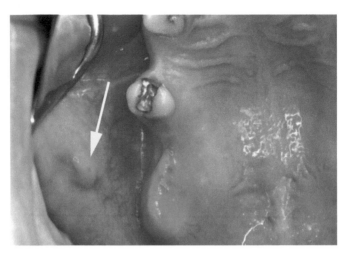

Figure 3–22 The parotid orifice is guarded by a mucous membrane swelling called the parotid papilla.

used as a landmark to help determine the level of the plane of occlusion. Because of its position, however, it is very difficult to visualize in many patients without moving the cheek to an unnatural position.

Along the inner surfaces of the middle to posterior one-third of the mandible, bony ridges known as the mylohyoid, or internal oblique ridges (site for attachment of the mylohyoid muscles) can be palpated. Occasionally prominent sharp, bony ridges must be surgically reduced prior to making complete dentures to minimize patient discomfort. These are important structures because of the attachment of the mylohyoid muscles and the influence of these muscles on the denture flanges.

Some patients will exhibit bilateral bony prominences of the inner surface of the mandible in the region of the premolar teeth called the torus mandibularis (Figure 3–21, B). These prominences must usually be removed prior to denture fabrication.

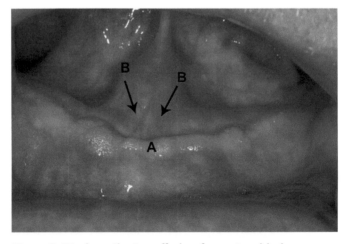

Figure 3–23 In patients suffering from atrophied mandibles, the residual ridge resorbs to the level of the genial tubercles, which can easily be palpated. (A) residual ridge, (B) genial tubercles

The most distal extent of the inner surfaces of the mandibular ridges ends in an area called the retromylohyoid area, or fossa (Figure 3–14, B). The fossa is bound laterally by the mandible and the most anterior border of the medial pterygoid muscle and medially by the tongue. The fossa is distal to the most posterior fibers of the mylohyoid muscle. The impression material may extend into the fossa. The opposing retromylohyoid areas are usually undercut, in relation to each other. One difficulty encountered when fabricating the mandibular denture is that these bilateral undercuts may greatly complicate the process of making preliminary and final impressions. The dentures may also require significant adjustments in these areas at the time of insertion.

In patients suffering from atrophied mandibles, the residual ridge resorbs to the level of the genial tubercles, which can be easily palpated (Figure 3–23). These bony midline lingual projections offer attachment to genioglossi and geniohyoid muscles. The dentures should be trimmed around the genial tubercles in those cases.

QUESTIONS

1. What is the name of the site where the mucous membrane lining of the lips and cheeks reflects and joins the unattached gingiva or alveolar mucosa? Some people call this the mucobuccal fold—a term that is inaccurate.

2. Besides location, what is one major difference between the upper medial labial frenum, or frenulum, and the buccal frenula?

3. Following full mouth extractions, the alveolar ridges undergo significant bone loss in most patients. Compare the amount of bone loss of the mandibular and maxillary arches.

4. Why is the incisal papilla a good landmark to note when contouring occlusion rims and positioning the denture teeth?

5. Why is the location of the fovea palatini important to note in the edentulous patient?

6. The maxillary complete denture should not cover the hamular process, or hamulus; why then is the location of the hamular process important?

7. What structure is located distal to the last mandibular molar and why is it important in the making of complete dentures?

8. Just buccal to the crest of the mandibular ridge in the distal-buccal corner of the arch is an area known as the masseter notch, or groove area. Why is this area of interest when fabricating a mandibular denture?

9. What and where is the buccal shelf and why is it important in the fabrication and wearing of mandibular complete dentures?

10. What is the area that determines the most distal lingual extent of a mandibular complete denture and what difficulties may the clinician have with this area?

ANSWERS

1. The fornix of the vestibule is the site where the mucous membrane lining of the lips and cheeks reflects and joins the unattached gingiva, or alveolar mucosa.

2. The upper medial labial frenum, or frenulum, does not contain muscle fibers, in contrast to the buccal frenula.

3. Studies indicate that the mandibular ridge resorps approximately four times as much as the maxillary arch.

4. The incisal papilla is a good landmark when contouring occlusion rims and positioning the dentures because studies indicate that the facial surfaces of the natural central incisors, when present, are approximately 8–10 mm anterior to the middle of the incisal papilla, and the tips of the canines are approximately in line with the middle of the incisal papilla.

5. The fovea palatini are two depressions that lie bilateral to the midline of the palate, at the approximate junction between the soft and hard palate, and denote the sites of opening of ducts of small mucous glands of the palate. They are often useful in the identification of the vibrating line because they generally occur within 2 mm of the vibrating line.

6. The hamular process, or hamulus, is a bony projection of the medial plate of the pterygoid bone and is located distal to the maxillary tuberosity. Lying between the maxillary tuberosity and the hamulus is a groove called the hamular notch. This notch is a key clinical landmark in maxillary denture construction because the maximum posterior extent of the denture is the vibrating line, which runs bilaterally through the hamular notches.

7. In the lower jaw, a triangular area of thick mucosa is found distal to the last molar, basically on the crest of the ridge, and is referred to as the retromolar pad. This pad is extremely important in denture construction from both a denture extension and plane of occlusion standpoint. This pad should be covered by the denture, and the plane of occlusion is generally located at the level of the middle to upper one-third of this pad.

8. This area is important in mandibular denture fabrication because of its influence on impression making. Because there is often a fatty roll of tissue overlying the masseter muscle, this cheek area must often be lifted to eliminate the fatty roll, particularly when making the final impression. Clinicians may not properly evaluate this area and the resultant completed mandibular denture is overextended, causing denture instability and tissue irritation.

9. The buccal shelf is located on the mandibular arch and is important to mandibular denture fabrication because it is the primary stress-bearing area of the mandibular arch. It is an area bounded on the medial side by the crest of the residual ridge, on the lateral side by the external oblique ridge, in the mesial area by the buccal frenulum, and on the distal side by the masseter muscle. It is just anterior to the masseter notch area.

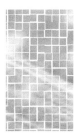

10. The most distal extent of the inner surfaces of the mandibular ridges ends in an area called the retromylohyoid area, or fossa. This area is the most distal extension of the mandibular denture, and the opposing retromylohyoid areas are usually undercut in relation to each other. One difficulty encountered when fabricating the mandibular denture is that these bilateral undercuts may greatly complicate the process of making the preliminary and final impressions. The dentures may also require significant adjustments in these areas at the time of insertion.

CHAPTER

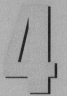

Diagnosis and Treatment Planning

Dr. Jack Morris

To have an excellent prognosis for any dental treatment requires proper preplanning, which will include at least a thorough examination, diagnosis, and a treatment plan. After the examination is complete and all diagnostic information has been evaluated, only then should a final diagnosis, treatment plan, and prognosis be formalized and discussed with the patient. Patients may require pre-prosthetic surgery, antifungal therapy, or soft relines to obtain better tissue health before definitive treatment can be initiated. Prior to forming a treatment plan, all reasonable patient treatment options should be discussed with the patient to include implant-retained or supported prostheses. The final treatment plan should be the best treatment for the patient based on his or her chief complaint, medical history, clinical exam, financial resources, and the time required to complete the planned treatment. Dentists must realize that, just as dentate patients vary in their dental treatment complexity, edentulous patients also vary in the difficulty of their treatment plan. This occasionally means that, based on the dentist's evaluation of the patient and the patient's desire to have a complex implant restoration, a patient should be referred to a specialist for treatment. To successfully treat edentulous patients, the clinician must develop good diagnosis and treatment planning skills to better identify the complexity of the patient. Once these skills are developed, both the success rate of the dentist when treating edentulous patients, and the number of referrals to a prosthodontist will rise.

A great deal of information is required to complete a proper diagnosis, including patient attitude, past and present medical conditions, past and present dental condition, and extraoral and intraoral examinations.

Diagnosis

M. M. Devan said "we must meet the mind of the patient before we meet the mouth of the patient." Edentulous patients come to us looking for solutions to their problems, and often these problems are both physical and psychological. A good initial interview is very critical to the diagnostic process. Clinicians must allow patients to communicate their chief complaint in their own words and take note of how patients present themselves. This might include how patients dress, their concern for their physical appearance, and their overall attitude and expectations concerning treatment. It is important as a health care provider never to treat a stranger. Taking time to allow the patients to voice their concerns and expectations will contribute to their trust and confidence in their dentist's ability to diagnose and successfully treat their oral condition.

Medical History

Acquiring a thorough medical history must be one of the very first steps in successfully treating any dental patient. A good medical history questionnaire combined with verbal qualification by the patient is essential to any dental treatment plan. Any medical or psychological condition that is a deviation from "the norm" must be noted and evaluated for its potential effect on patient treatment. Uncontrolled diabetics, patients with cardiovascular disease and subsequent treatment with blood thinners, and immunocompromised patients may be excellent denture patients but might not be considered good surgical risks and therefore, pre-prosthetic surgery may be contraindicated. The date of the patient's last physical exam is important because the medical condition of the patient may have changed dramatically if the last exam was several years ago. A history of movement disorders such as Parkinson's Disease could affect one's ability to treat the patient as well as the patient's ability to successfully wear the complete denture. Patients with a history of psychological and cognitive impairment diseases might have unreasonable expectations of complete denture treatment and may be unable to significantly cooperate in their own care. One condition that could alter routine treatment is a history of head and neck radiation which could complicate any need for pre-prosthetic surgery and also result in xerostomia for the patient.

Present Medical Condition

It is essential to update the patient's medical history at each follow-up appointment to ensure that the patient is truly being appropriately followed for their medical conditions and that they are correctly taking any prescribed medications. With the aging denture population, many patients are taking numerous medications, many times prescribed in an uncoordinated fashion by multiple physicians. If the clinician has any concerns about a particular medication or possible conflicting medications that a patient is taking, a referral to the patient's primary care provider is appropriate. Consults should be written to appropriate physicians to evaluate any questionable medical conditions. Many elderly patients must be accompanied to their appointments by friends or family members who also might be questioned concerning the patient's health.

Vital signs to include blood pressure and pulse are important to establish an initial base line; patients could require a referral if they are not within normal limits. Baseline vital signs may be critical information in any future medical emergency. Many of today's medications can cause xerostomia, which can affect the patient's oral health and ability to wear complete dentures successfully. Patients taking antihistamines as well as medications for depression, anxiety, high blood pressure, muscle relaxation, urinary incontinence and Parkinson's disease can have dry mouth as a side effect. Any allergies should be identified and noted in the patient's record. Knowing that a patient has allergies to antibiotics and pain medications is extremely important because it is occasionally necessary to treat dental infection and pain following any pre-prosthetic surgery.

A greater number of patients are being recognized as allergic to latex and metals, particularly nickel. These allergies must be considered for even routine care of the patient and when contemplating the metal to be used in a removable partial denture.

A medical history must include vital signs, medications being taken, allergies, past medical history, and present medical condition. Sufficient information is essential to allow the dentist to make an assessment of the patient's general overall health. Will the patient be able to tolerate long appointments or, due to their failing health, should appointments be as short as possible? A good written medical questionnaire and verbal interview is essential for the dentist to help determine the patient's diagnosis and subsequent treatment plan as well as the projected prognosis for the complete denture patient.

Dental History

A complete denture exam should include a thorough dental history of the patient, which includes at least the following: What is the patient's chief dental complaint? Were their teeth lost due to caries, periodontal disease, or trauma? Has periodontal disease or trauma compromised the residual ridges? How long has the patient been edentulous? If the patient has been edentulous for some time and has never worn dentures, why not? How long has the patient worn complete dentures, and were the dentures fabricated after some healing time or inserted immediately? A patient with recent extractions will be expected to experience more immediate changes to the residual ridge than a patient who has been missing teeth for many years. Has the patient had good follow-up care to include relines and remakes as needed? If not, why not? Are the dentures properly extended, stable, and retentive? Are the esthetics and phonetics of the present dentures acceptable? Can significant improvements be made? Are the patient's expectations reasonable? How much tooth display is visible at rest and when smiling? Is the occluding vertical dimension (OVD) acceptable with the existing prosthesis? Are the denture teeth porcelain or plastic, and what type occlusal scheme exists? Will the patient tolerate a change if indicated? Overall, is the patient pleased with his or her present prosthesis? What are the patient's likes and dislikes with any existing prostheses? What are the patient's expectations for the new dentures? Can you as the clinician meet those expectations? Are the patient's concerns with the present dentures justified? How many dentures has the patient had in the last five years? A patient presenting with two or more sets of recently fabricated dentures often indicates a patient who may have an exacting or unreasonable mental attitude.

Clinical Extraoral Examination

Good physical diagnostic skills involve observation, palpation, and auscultation and should be utilized when performing the clinical head and neck exam. When examining a patient, it is important to be thorough and sequential. A good clinical exam form is helpful in accomplishing this (Figure 4–1). The patient's range of mandibular movement should be observed for any type of irregular movement or deviation. The muscles of mastication and facial expression should be observed during movement and conversation as well as palpated to locate any muscle tenderness or dysfunction. Uncoordinated mandibular movement or temporomandibular disorder/pain could certainly complicate any attempt to obtain accurate interocclusal records and might help determine that a simple occlusal scheme should be selected for this patient. The temporomandibular joint should be palpated as well as auscultated and any pain, tenderness, popping, or clicking should be noted.

The neck should be palpated for any lumps, masses, or enlarged lymph nodes. The lips and skin should be evaluated for any type of nonhealing lesions or unusual nevi. The commissures of the lips should be examined and any evidence of angular cheilitis (Figure 4–2) noted. The lip length, thickness, and curvature should be noted with the patient's existing prosthesis in place. The face should be observed and noted in frontal and profile facial form. The patient's facial midline should be noted. Does the middle of the philtrum of the lip and the patient's midline on their existing maxillary prosthesis coincide?

Complete Denture Examination, Diagnosis and Treatment Planning Form

Patient:_____ Date:_____

1. **Chief complaint** (patient's own words):

2. **Past Dental History:**
   a. Date of last visit to dentist:
   b. Reason for last visit and treatment received:
   c. Date of last extraction:
   d. Previous prosthesis type(s):
   e. Number of previous complete dentures:
   f. Ability to adjust to previous dentures:
   g. Patient reaction to previous treatment:

3. **Evaluation of Present Dentures:**
   a. Esthetics:
   b. Phonetics:
   c. VDO:
   d. Base extension:
   e. Stability and retention:
   f. Occlusion:
   g. B-L tooth position:
   h. Occlusal plane height:
   i. Pattern of tooth wear:
   j. Denture hygiene:
   k. Evidence of self-adjustment:
   l. Patient criticism of previous denture (own words):
   m. Patient expectations of new denture:
   n. Compare your observations with the patient's comments:
   o. Problems noted:
   p. Can improvements be made?

4. **Soft Tissue Examination:** (note areas of potential pathology):

5. **Hard Tissue Examination (Radiographic exam):** pre-pros surgery required? ( )

6. **Saliva:**   amount: excessive ( )   scanty ( )   average ( )
   consistency: thick ( )   thin ( )   average ( )

7. **Facial Appearance:** frontal: square ( ) tapering ( ) ovoid ( )   combination ( )
   profile: straight ( ) curved( ) combination ( )
   muscle tone: good ( ) fair ( )   poor ( )

8. **Lip form:**   length: long ( )   short ( ) average ( )
   thickness: thick ( )   thin ( ) average ( )
   curvature: curved upward ( )   curved downward ( )

9. **Maxillary Ridge Form:**   Mandibular Ridge Form:
   a. shape _____   a. shape _____ shape: square, tapering, ovoid, combo.
   b. size _____   b. size _____ large, medium, small
   c. width _____   c. width _____ broad, narrow, average
   d. cross section _____   c. cross section _____ square, trapezoid, triangular, flat

(Continued)

10. **Ridge relationship:**
    a. Antero-posterior _____ CI I (normal), CI II (retro), CI III (prog)
    b. Medio-lateral _____ normal, unilat cross-bite, bilat cross-bite
    c. Parallelism _____ parallel, divergent, convergent

11. **Tuberosities**   R _____ (bone/soft tissue) large, medium, small, undercut
    L _____ (bone/soft tissue) large, medium, small, undercut

12. **Inter-ridge space:** large ( )   small ( )   average ( )

13. **Tongue:**   size: large ( )   small ( )   average
    position: retracted ( )   normal ( )
    control: can move to follow directions ( )   can not ( )

14. **Hard Palate Form:**   high vault ( )   shallow vault ( )   average( )   v-shaped ( )

15. **Soft Palate Form:**   CI I (gradual) ( )   CI II (moderate) ( )   CI III (steep) ( )

16. **Floor of mouth:**   location: high ( )   low ( )   average ( )
    mobility: mobile ( )   immobile ( )   average ( )

17. **Ability of patient to repeat CR position:**   easy ( )   hard ( )   may be impossible ( )

18. **Patients Mental Attitude:**
    philosophical ( )   exacting ( )   hysterical ( )   indifferent ( )   senile ( )

19. **Patients Adaptive Potential:**   good ( )   poor ( )

Treatment Prognosis: good ( )   fair ( )   poor ( )

Summary of Special Procedures Needed: Additional Radiographs ( )
Biopsy ( )
Pre-pros surgery ( )   Surgical template ( )
Tissue conditioning ( )   Anti-fungal therapy ( )

Treatment Plan and Sequence:

Figure 4–1   Complete denture examination, diagnosis, and treatment planning form.

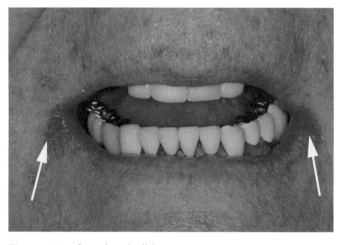

Figure 4–2   Angular chelitis

Intraoral Examination

The intraoral exam should begin first with a general evaluation of the patient's oral mucosa (Figure 4–3). Note the condition of the mucosa—specifically whether it is flabby or bound down, pink and healthy, or red and edematous. Excessively thick or thin areas of oral mucosa should also be noted. The mucosa should be evaluated as it relates to the ridge. For example, are there large areas of keratinized attached tissue on the ridge or is there mostly movable mucosa on the ridge? All areas of the oral cavity should be generally inspected for any type of pathology to include the soft palate and the lateral borders of the tongue.

Some complete denture patients refuse to remove or clean their prostheses for prolonged periods (Figure 4–4) and as a result might have extremely irritated and

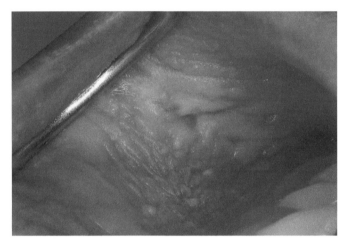

Figure 4–3   Hyperkeratotic lesion in cheek oral mucosa

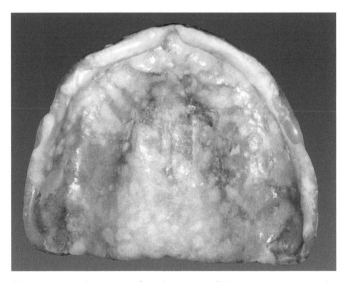

Figure 4–4   Denture of patient who failed to remove and clean denture

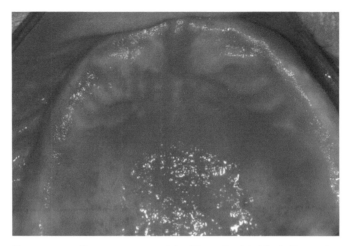

Figure 4–5   Denture stomatitis. Note the highly inflamed tissues of a patient who rarely removed the maxillary complete denture.

traumatized tissues (Figure 4–5). These patients are much more susceptible to fungal overgrowth and colonization of the prostheses and subsequent inflammatory papillary hyperplasia—especially in the palate (Figure 4–6). Areas of redundant tissue adjacent to denture borders, called epulis fissuratum (Figure 4–7), are usually quite painful and are caused by excessive denture flange length. These areas should also be noted and appointed for surgical excision if the condition does not resolve following the removal of the overextended denture border.

The saliva should be evaluated both in amount and consistency. A normal amount and thickness of saliva is paramount in the ability of most patients to comfortably wear dentures. The saliva acts as a lubricant and also serves as the interface between the denture base and the tissue allowing for denture retention. A patient with xerostomia or excessive saliva containing much mucous can have difficulty obtaining an adequate seal

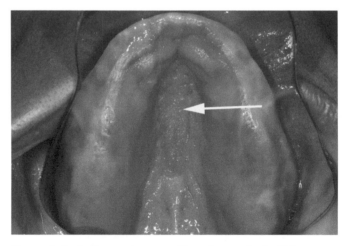

Figure 4–6   Inflammatory papillary hyperplasia. This condition must be addressed prior to fabrication of a new denture.

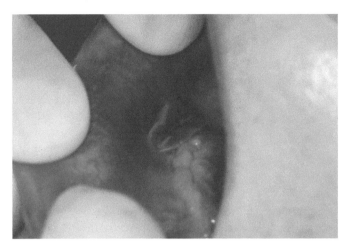

Figure 4–7   Epulis fissuratum. Usually caused by an overextended denture flange.

for their prosthesis. A patient with normal salivary flow will benefit from its adhesive and cohesive qualities. Patients with dry mouth not only have poor prosthesis retention but also a greater tendency for oral mucosa tenderness. During the oral exam, the salivary gland orifice should be inspected for proper opening and salivary flow. Ideally the saliva would be of a thin, serous type as compared to thick, ropy saliva.

During the course of the examination it is helpful to note whether the patient has a problem with gagging. A hypersensitive gag reflex can complicate successful fabrication of a complete denture. Often patients will volunteer their gagging problems while discussing their dental history or this could be detected while performing a routine hard and soft tissue exam with an intraoral mirror. Most of these patients can be successfully treated by the dentist using proper impression techniques. However, a very small percentage of patients have a truly hypersensitive gag reflex and might be best treated by a prosthodontist.

A current panoramic radiograph reflecting the patient's present condition must be evaluated. Conditions to especially note are the mandibular bone height, the position of the mental foramen, retained root tips, unerupted teeth, residual cysts, bony pathology, maxillary sinus position and health, and any unusual TMJ anatomy. Retained root tips and impacted teeth should be evaluated for any pathology and whether they are completely retained in bone. Teeth and root tips that are only covered by soft tissue or are exposed to the oral cavity should be considered for removal. The removal of deeply impacted teeth and root tips may cause excessive bone to be lost and cause more harm to the denture bearing surface by removing than just leaving and following them periodically with radiographs—especially in patients who are in poor health. In every case the patient should be informed of the risk and benefit of the removal of the impacted teeth and root tips, and a decision should be agreed upon by the dentist and the patient.

The maxillary ridge should be evaluated for size, shape, and cross-sectional form. Generally speaking, a larger ridge will have more surface area for better retention and stability as compared to a small ridge. The residual ridge shape is classified as square, tapering, or ovoid. The shape is probably most important as it relates to the opposing arch because mismatched arch shapes can make tooth arrangement challenging. Next cross-sectional form should be noted. Ridges are generally U-shaped, V-shaped, knife edged, or flat. The worst type of ridge is a knife edged or flat ridge, which does not provide a good foundation base for the denture. The most ideal ridge would be a u-shaped ridge—almost flat at the crest of the ridge with tall non-undercut approximating buccal and palatal walls. These ridges provide maximum retention, stability, and support. The ridge should also be evaluated for any exostoses or bilateral posterior undercut. Bulbous tuberosities can result in bilateral posterior undercuts and insufficient interocclusal space. In these situations, preprosthetic surgery is usually indicated.

The form of the hard palate should be determined. Any pedunculated torus (Figure 4–8) or a torus that extends into the posterior palatal seal area should be removed if possible. The hard palate is usually classified as a high, average, shallow, or V-shaped. An average U-shaped palate is ideal. A V-shaped palate or high vault can compromise the seal of the denture.

The soft palate is classified as Class I, Class II, or Class III depending upon the amount of movement or slope of the soft palate relative to the hard palate. Generally the more severe the angular change from the hard to the soft palate, the easier and yet more critical the exact location of the vibrating line becomes. A denture cannot extend onto the movable soft palate without significantly increasing the possibility of loss of denture retention and causing tissue irritation and discomfort to the patient. Generally, a soft palate that moves slightly and slopes little is considered a Class I palate. One that drops abruptly at the junction of the hard and soft palate is considered a Class III palate. A Class II palate would fall between the above mentioned examples.

Similar to the maxillary ridge, the mandibular ridge is evaluated for size, shape, and cross-sectional form. A larger ridge can provide more surface area for stability, support, and retention, and again the shape of the arch is most important in its relationship to the opposing arch. As with the maxilla, a U-shaped ridge in cross-section is much more favorable than a V-shaped, knife edged, or flat ridge. The ridge should be evaluated for any tori (Figure 4–9), exostoses, and bilateral undercuts. Diagnostic casts are often necessary to adequately evaluate the residual ridges.

Maxillary and mandibular ridges should be evaluated for how much space the border tissues allow for complete denture fabrication. If frenula attachments are close to the crest of the residual ridge then denture borders must necessarily be short, which

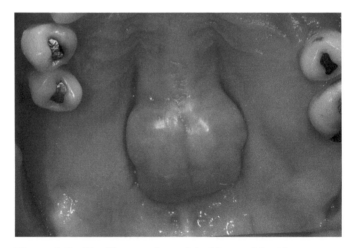

Figure 4–8 Maxillary pedunculated torus. Must be removed if it is so large that it will interfere with space for the tongue, is undercut, or extends so far posteriorly that it prevents the placement of a posterior palatal seal.

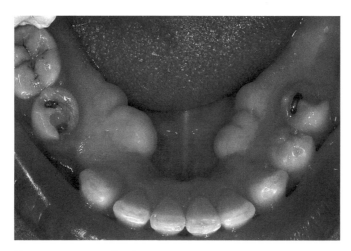

Figure 4–9   Mandibular tori. Must generally be removed.

could compromise the retention of the denture. As the lips and cheeks are simulating muscle movement, the dentist should note whether the attachments are near the crest of the ridge or whether the muscle and tissue attachments are away from the crest of the ridge to allow for a more substantial denture foundation. It is especially important to note the muscle attachments on the lingual side of the mandibular ridge. Is the anterior lingual flange of the mandibular denture going to be compromised because the genial tubercles are near the crest of the ridge? A patient with short lingual flanges because of high lingual attachments (often referred to as high floor of the mouth) can have compromised lateral stability of the denture. Palpate the mylohyoid ridge. Is it extremely large or sharp? Evaluate the retromylohyoid area, space, or fossa. As the patient touches his lips with the tongue is the retromylohyoid space obliterated or is there space that could be occupied by the lingual flanges of the denture base? Once again, for most patients, the longer the flanges of the dentures, the more support, stability, and retention will be obtained with the denture.

How do the opposing residual ridges relate to each other? The occluding vertical dimension can be approximated in most patients by having them lightly close on a finger placed between the anterior ridges; thereafter some statement can be made about the relationship of the residual ridges. Another method is to evaluate the ridges when the patient closes into a position where the ridges are approximately parallel to each other. In some patients this is almost impossible and these notations must be made after casts are mounted on an articulator at the appropriate occluding vertical dimension. The anterior-posterior relationship of the residual ridges of the complete denture patient can be misleading. As the residual ridge resorbs, the maxillary ridge resorbs upward and inward, and the mandibular ridge resorbs downward and outward. The crest of the anterior mandibular ridge resorbs four times more than the anterior crest of the maxilla in the first seven years after teeth are extracted, therefore significant changes should be expected particularly when contemplating immediate dentures. Essentially the maxilla is getting more narrow and shorter, and the mandible is getting longer and wider tending to make the patient appear prognathic in the anterior and to have a crossbite ridge relationship in the posterior. In observing the anterior posterior position of the ridges, it is important to note the location of the incisive papilla and realize that the incisal edges of the maxillary natural teeth were, on average, 7-8 mm anterior to that position. Many patients will exhibit significant bone loss in this area, with the incisive papilla literally being on the anterior slope of the ridge. Is the patient's antero-posterior relationship prognathic (Class III), retrognathic (Class II), or a normal (Class I) relationship? Generally speaking a Class I patient is an easier complete denture patient than a Class III patient, and a Class II patient is the most difficult of all. Severe Class II patients should be considered for referral to a prosthodontist.

The medio-lateral relationship of the opposing ridges should also be evaluated. Do the arches coordinate? Is one arch shaped differently than the other? Will teeth have to be set in a crossbite relationship? Are the ridges generally parallel at the proper occluding vertical dimension? Ridges tend to be parallel at the proper occluding vertical dimension unless there has been some type of irregular resorptive pattern (Figure 4–10). Ridges that are not parallel at the proper occluding vertical dimension can make the completed dentures quite unstable during function. Learning to use such dentures may present a significant challenge for the patient. Evaluation of the patient's inter-ridge space at the estimated OVD is necessary. Excessive inter-ridge space or too little inter-ridge space can greatly compromise proper denture fabrication. Tuberosities should also be evaluated at the estimated OVD. A mouth mirror, which is usually 2 to 2.5 mm thick, can be used to evaluate if enough space is available for each denture bases to be at least 1 mm thick.

The tongue size and position should be noted. A very large tongue can be seen in patients who have been edentulous with no replacement prosthesis for an extended period (Figure 4–11). An enlarged or oversized tongue can greatly compromise a patient's ability to successfully wear a complete denture. According to Dr. C. Wright, the position of the tongue greatly affects the ability of a patient to successfully wear complete dentures. He reported that 35% of people had a retracted tongue, which could compromise a denture patient's ability to seal the lingual border of the mandibular denture. Additionally he felt that the ideal position of the tongue was with the apex of the tongue slightly below the incisal edges of the mandibular incisors and with the dorsum of the tongue visible above the teeth in all parts of the mouth. The control or coordination of the tongue should also be noted. Is there any neuromuscular condition that affects the patient's speech, swallowing, or general muscle coordination? If so, this may compromise the ability of a patient who is a first time denture wearer, to satisfactorily adjust to the dentures.

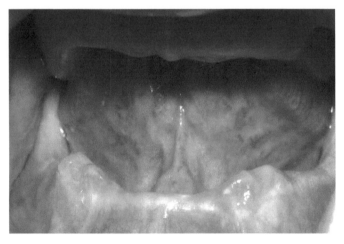

Figure 4–10   An irregular bony resorptive pattern may make complete dentures unstable.

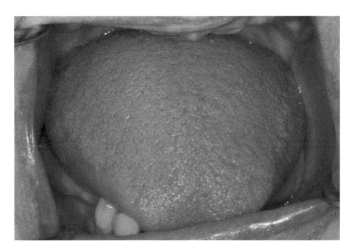

Figure 4–11 Example of a very large tongue, which may cause great difficulty in wearing a complete denture especially for a first time denture wearer.

Mental Attitude of Patient

Successfully wearing a complete denture is a learned skill for most patients and especially for new denture patients. Therefore, the mental attitude of the patient may play a very important role in the edentulous patient's ability to adapt and can be very valuable information for a dentist to help evaluate the ultimate prognosis of denture patients. Dr. House has classified complete denture patients into four mental attitude categories—philosophical, exacting, indifferent, and hysterical.

The philosophical patient exhibits an attitude that is optimistic, cooperative, rational, and sensible. The patient is willing to accept advice and desires the proper restoration to return himself/herself to an excellent state of oral health. This is the ideal patient type. The exacting patient is precise, meticulous, and could make extreme and unreasonable demands of the dentist. This type of patient often questions even minute details of the denture, including the alignment of a single posterior tooth, and whether the new dentures will ever look right or function well. These patients can often require excessive amounts of the practitioner's time to satisfy their demands. These patients can be far less than ideal. The hysterical patient is often excitable, nervous, excessively hypersensitive, and often very pessimistic. This patient might dread dentistry and feel that he or she may never be able to wear the new dentures. This patient may require professional psychological counseling in order to be treated successfully. Some have suggested that dentists are fully justified in charging increased fees to this patient because of the extra treatment time required. The indifferent patient is likely to lack motivation and might be unwilling to follow instructions regarding his or her oral health. Many times this patient is seeking treatment not because of concern for his or her dental health but because a spouse or family member has encouraged them to care about oral health. Patients in this category are less likely to persevere and learn to function with their complete dentures. These patients can be the most difficult category of patient to treat because of their lack of motivation.

Additional Diagnostic Information

Diagnostic casts are very helpful to further evaluate the anatomy and condition of the residual ridges. Generally diagnostic casts are made from preliminary impressions made with irreversible hydrocolloid (alginate) in stock trays (Figure 4–12). Good diagnostic casts should include the retromolar pads and border tissues as well as the pterygomaxillary notch and the posterior palatal seal area (Figure 4–13). See Chapter 6 on Preliminary Impressions and Custom Impression Trays for further information.

Another tool to help the dentist identify the complexity of their denture patient is called the Prosthodontic Diagnostic Index (PDI). The American College of Prosthodontists has recommended that practioners use the PDI to classify edentulous patients. This system is said to help better identify difficult denture patients and help

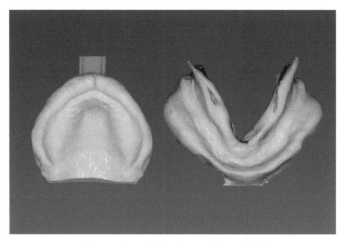

Figure 4–12   Examples of nicely made preliminary impressions

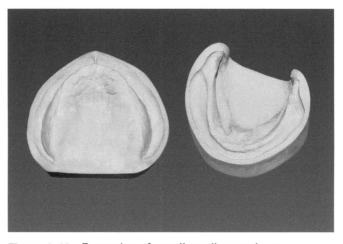

Figure 4–13   Examples of excellent diagnostic casts

dentists better understand when to refer a patient. The PDI could also help dentists with reimbursement if insurance companies are willing to qualify that all denture patients are not the same difficulty. This classification system uses four general diagnostic assessment criteria: mandibular bone height, maxillomandibular ridge relationship, residual ridge morphology, and muscle attachments. The system also identifies several other criteria and diagnostic modifiers that can be expected to increase complete denture difficulty. These modifiers include systemic considerations, psychosocial considerations, tongue anatomy/activity, temporomandibular disorders, conditions requiring preprosthetic surgery, interarch space, refractory patients, patients with a history of paresthesia or dysesthesia, maxillomandibular ataxia, and maxillofacial defects.

After all the PDI diagnostic criteria and modifiers have been identified, the patient is categorized from Class I to Class IV (Figure 4–14). A Class I patient is uncomplicated and should be able to be treated by a general dentist with limited complete denture experience. The prognosis for this patient should be good to excellent. A Class II patient has some moderately complicating factors, such as systemic disease or residual ridge anatomy, and should be successfully treated by a general dentist with experience treating patients with complete dentures. For the experienced general dentist or prosthodontist, the prognosis for this patient should be good. A Class III patient has additional complicating problems, such as TMD symptoms, limited or excessive interarch distance, and possibly a need for pre-prosthetic surgery. This type of patient is best treated by a prosthodontist or a general dentist with additional training in advanced prosthodontic techniques. The

Complete Edentulism Checklist

	Class I	Class II	Class III	Class IV
Bone Height-Mandibular				
21 mm or greater	X			
16-20 mm		X		
11-15 mm			X	
10 mm or less				X
Residual Ridge Morphology-Maxilla				
Type A-resists vertical & horizontal, hamular notch, no tori	X			
Type B-no buccal vest., poor hamular notch, no tori		X		
Type C-no ant vest, min support, mobile ant ridge			X	
Type D-no ant/post vest, tori, redundant tissue				X
Muscle Attachments-Mandibular				
Type A-adequate attached mucosa	X			
Type B-no b attach mucosa (22-27), +mentalis m		X		
Type C-no ant b&l vest (22-27), +genio & mentalis m			X	
Type D-att mucosa in post only			X	
Type E-no att mucosa, cheek/lip moves tongue				X
Maxillomandibular Relationships				
Class I	X			
Class II		X		
Class III			X	
Conditions Requiring Preprosthetic Surgery				
Minor soft tissue procedures		X		

(Continued)

Minor hard tissue procedures	▓	▓		▓
Implants - simple	▓	▓		▓
Implants with bone graft - complex	▓	▓	▓	
Correction of dentofacial deformities	▓	▓	▓	
Hard tissue augmentation	▓	▓	▓	
Major soft tissue revisions	▓	▓	▓	
Limited Interarch Space	▓	▓		▓
18-20 mm	▓	▓		▓
Surgical correction needed	▓	▓	▓	
Tongue Anatomy	▓	▓	▓	▓
Large (occludes interdental space)	▓	▓		▓
Hyperactive- with retracted position	▓	▓	▓	
Modifiers	▓	▓	▓	▓
Oral manifestation of systemic disease	▓	▓	▓	▓
mild	▓		▓	▓
moderate	▓	▓		▓
severe	▓	▓	▓	
Psychosocial	▓	▓	▓	▓
moderate	▓	▓		▓
major	▓	▓	▓	
TMD Symptoms	▓	▓		▓
Hx of paresthesia or dysesthesia	▓	▓	▓	
Maxillofacial defects	▓	▓	▓	
Ataxia	▓	▓	▓	
Refractory Patient	▓	▓	▓	

Figure 4–14   Prosthodontic Diagnostic Index (PDI)

prognosis for this patient is guarded to good for the experienced general dentist or prosthodontist. At the final end of the spectrum is the Class IV patient, the most complicated and debilitated patient. This patient might be characterized by very poor edentulous arches that are indicated for pre-prosthetic surgery but this may not be possible because of the patient's health, finances, or preference. This patient is best treated by a surgical specialist and a prosthodontist. The prognosis for this patient would be poor if being treated by an experienced general dentist and only guarded for the prosthodontist.

 Treatment Planning

The proper treatment planning for a patient requires that all information gathered on a patient be considered when determining the treatment to be completed and the sequence of this treatment. Lab test results and referral recommendations as well as results of any soft or hard tissue biopsies should be reviewed before a final diagnosis and treatment plan are formalized. Once all information has been obtained, a formal treatment plan should be discussed with the patient. This would include how treatment will be sequenced as well as an estimate of the length of time to complete the treatment. An estimate of cost for the treatment should also be discussed and approved by the patient.

Generally a patient should be free of dental pain to include TMD pain before definitive prostheses are fabricated. Any needed preprosthetic surgery should be accomplished early in the treatment plan to include extractions, alveoloplasty, tori removal, frenectomies, exostoses, and tuberosity reductions. If the patient has existing dentures, these will need to be modified after the surgery and managed during the healing period with soft reline material. If preprosthetic surgery will render the patient edentulous, immediate dentures may need to be fabricated. The patient's esthetic requirements during this healing period will need to be evaluated by the dentist and completely explained to the patient. Depending on the number of teeth being removed, this might require that two sets of complete dentures be fabricated—an immediate set and (after healing) a definitive set.

If a patient has TMD pain, every effort should be made to have the patient pain free before fabricating definitive prostheses. This might be as simple as modifying the existing worn prostheses with acrylic resin to a more a appropriate vertical dimension of occlusion or fabricating an acrylic TMD splint that fits over the existing prosthesis. If this does not resolve the problem then it might be necessary to refer the patient to an oral and facial pain specialist before definitive prostheses are fabricated.

Once the patient is pain free and appropriate healing has taken place, only then is the patient ready to have definitive prostheses fabricated. After the prostheses are fabricated and initially followed-up to ensure proper fit, function, and homecare, the patient should return for periodic exams at least annually to evaluate the prostheses as well as the patient's general oral health.

Prognosis

After reviewing the Complete Denture Evaluation, Diagnosis, and Treatment Planning Form as well as the Prosthodontic Diagnostic Index (PDI) the practitioner should be able to make some judgment about the prognosis of their patient. A patient who has a Class I antero-posterior ridge relationship, has proper size and function of the tongue, has normal quality and quantity of saliva, has U-shaped (cross-section) edentulous ridges that approximate the opposing arch, has successfully worn complete dentures in the past, and is a philosophical patient (PDI I) will have a good prognosis. A patient who is in very poor health, has a Class II antero-posterior ridge relationship, a retracted tongue, maxillary posterior bilateral undercuts in need of pre-prosthetic surgery, ropy saliva, and an indifferent attitude (PDI IV) will have a poor prognosis. Many times the greatest predictor of success for complete denture patients is whether they have successfully worn complete dentures in the past.

References

Appleby, R. C., Ludwig T. F.: Patient evaluation for complete denture therapy. J Prosthet Dent. 1970; 1:11-17.

Chaytor, D. V.: Diagnosis and treatment planning for edentulous or potentially edentulous patients. In Zarb, G. A., Bolender, C. L., editors. Prosthodontic treatment for edentulous patients. 12th ed. St. Louis, MO: Mosby; 2004. pp. 73-99.

DeVan, M.: Physical, biological, and psychological factors to be considered in the construction of dentures. J Am Dent Assoc. 1951; 42:290-3.

Heartwell, C. M.: Psychologic considerations in complete denture prosthodontics. J Prosthet Dent. 1970; 1:5-10.

House, M. M.: The relationship of oral examination to dental diagnosis. J Prosthet Dent. 1958; 2:208-219.

Ivanhoe, J. R., Cibirka, R. M., Parr, G.R.: Treating the modern denture patient: a review of the literature. J Prosthet Dent. 2002;6:631-635.

MacEntee, M. I.: The complete denture a clinical pathway. Carol Stream, IL: Quintessence Publishing Co. Inc.; 1999. p. 1-7.

McGarry, T. J., Nimmo, A., Skiba, J.: Classification system for complete edentulism. J Prosth 1999; 1:27-39.

Parr, G. R.: Complete denture examination, diagnosis and treatment planning form. In: Ivanhoe, J. R., Rahn, A. O., editors. Clinical Guide for Complete Dentures. 2006 ed. Medical College of Georgia School of Dentistry. 2006. p. 38.

Rahn, A. O.: Diagnosis. In: Rahn, A. O., Heartwell, C. M., editors. Textbook of complete dentures. 5th ed. Philadelphia: Lea & Febiger; 1993. pp. 131–67.

Winkler, S.: Essentials of complete denture prosthodontics. 2nd ed. Littleton, MA:PSG Publishing Co, Inc.; 1988. pp.1-7.

Wright, C.: A study of the tongue and its relation to denture stability. J Am Dent Assoc. 1949;39:269-75.

Zarb, G. A.: The edentulous milieu. J Prosthet Dent. 1983; 6:825-31.

QUESTIONS

1. List four classifications of patients' mental attitudes.

2. Name four classes, or categories, of medications that cause xerostomia.

3. What types of examination techniques should be utilized when performing a head and neck exam?

4. What type of soft palate, as classified by House, turns down abruptly as related to the hard palate and requires the most precision when determining the location of the vibrating line?

5. Name four anatomic structures that, when present, complicate the fabrication of a complete denture?

6. Which cross-sectional ridge form is the least desirable?

7. According to Tallgren, at what rate does the mandible resorb compared to the maxilla during the seven-year period following extraction of all remaining teeth?

8. Which antero-posterior ridge relationship is the easiest, or most ideal, for the fabrication of complete dentures?

9. Too little or excessive interarch space can complicate the construction of complete denture? True or False.

10. According to Wright, what percentage of the population has a retracted tongue?

ANSWERS

1. Hysterical, exacting, indifferent, and philosophical.

2. High blood pressure medication, antihistamines, muscle relaxants, and many drugs used to treat anxiety and depression.

3. Observation, auscultation, and palpation (look, listen, and feel).

4. Class III

5. Mandibular tori/maxillary torus, high frenula attachments, large bulbous tuberosities, and inflammatory papillary hyperplasia.

6. Knife edged or flat.

7. Mandible four times greater than the maxilla.

8. Class I

9. True

10. 35 %

CHAPTER

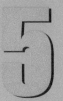

Pre-prosthetic Surgical Considerations

Dr. Henry Ferguson

Surgical goals for treatment of patients should address the following factors: providing the patient with the best possible tissue contours for prosthesis support, function, and comfort; maintaining as much bone and soft tissue as possible; and doing this in the safest, most predictable manner for the patient. With these goals in mind, we can then work backward, with a concept of the final result, sequencing the treatment(s) that will realize these goals. These goals can be reached through the achievement of specific objectives, which include creating a broad ridge form, providing an adequate amount of fixed tissue over the denture bearing areas, establishing adequate vestibular depth for prosthetic flange extension, establishing proper inter-arch relationships and spacing, supporting arch integrity, providing adequate palatal vault form, and when required, to provide proper ridge dimensions for implant placement.

 Patient Evaluation and Expectations

Prior to the performance of any procedure, several key steps must be performed. The objective of a thorough patient evaluation, review of the past medical history, and physical evaluation is to identify treatment-modifying factors required for the safe and uneventful treatment of the patient.

The physical examination includes thorough evaluation of the oral hard and soft tissues and radiographs. This examination will reveal the difficulty of performing the desired preprosthetic surgical procedures or even whether they are possible. For instance, the referring dentist may desire that the patient receive a reduction of the tuberosities but radiographic evaluation by the surgeon may reveal that this procedure is not possible because of the position of the maxillary sinus.

Radiographically, the panoramic radiograph is the workhorse image for preprosthetic surgery. With this radiograph one can visualize many of the important anatomic and structural relationships necessary to accurately create a treatment plan for preprosthetic procedures. For the mandible and maxilla in general, pathologic lesions, retained roots, impacted teeth, and overall ridge morphology can be seen. For the mandible, relationships between the inferior alveolar canal and the ridge crest, and position of the mental foramina to the ridge crest can be observed. For the maxilla, relationships between the floor of the maxillary sinus and the alveolar crest, anterior nasal spine, and the anterior maxillary alveolar crest can be determined. Additionally, the hard tissue contribution versus soft tissue component of hyperplasic tuberosities can be determined. Other radiographic images may be required when specific anatomic relationships need to be observed.

For preprosthetic procedures and treatment plans, which may include implant placement, more sophisticated, radiographic studies may be required. Tomographic studies and computerized tomography (CT scans) may be used. The CT scan can provide cross-sectional detail of the maxilla in both the axial and coronal views. This provides excellent information regarding such important planning factors as alveolar height and width, facial, lingual, and palatal alveolar contours, relationships between the maxillary crests and the sinus floor and nasal floor, and the mandibular inferior alveolar canal and mental foramina to the crestal bone.

Treatment Planning

With the desired preprosthetic surgery identified, and the physical evaluation and radiographic examinations completed, a problem list is made. Treatment planning now becomes the next critical step. No procedures should be performed without a treatment plan designed to sequence and address the patient's problem list. Based on state of health, complexity of treatment plan, and level of anxiety, referral may be made to place the patient in an environment where all of these important factors can be safely addressed.

Goals for treatment should address the following factors: providing the patient with the best possible tissue contours for prosthesis support, function, and comfort; maintaining as much bone and soft tissue as possible; and doing this in the safest most predictable manner for the patient. With these goals in mind we can sequence the treatment(s) that will achieve these goals.

Review of Flaps

Access to and exposure of the surgical site is critical. The clinician's tool for adequate exposure is the full thickness mucoperiosteal flap. This aggressive surgical approach with its greater visibility, protection of adjacent tissues, time efficiency, and more routine postoperative course is far more valuable and less traumatic to the patient than other less effective techniques. Diagnostic casts are excellent aids in outlining areas of surgical focus and for flap design.

For most of the procedures a midline crestal incision is recommended. In edentulous areas, there is usually a dense scar band on the crest of the ridge (Figure 5–1). This tissue is stronger, more resistant to tears, and holds sutures well. When teeth are present

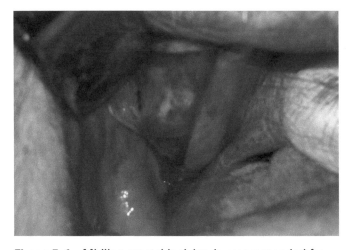

Figure 5–1   Midline crestal incision is recommended for most flap procedures.

and the surrounding soft tissues are to be included in the flap, a sulcular incision sharply to bone is recommended. The reflection should be subperiosteal and deliberate. When working around teeth, the papillae should be gently reflected, then the remaining attached tissues in a uniform plane before attempting to reflect more apically. Being deliberate, precise, and having patience will reward the clinician with a clean subperiosteal dissection. The dissection should proceed apically as far as needed to visualize the area of concern. Dissection antero-posteriorly should be made as necessary to allow for elevation of the flap and appropriate exposure without placing tension on the flap. Although envelope flaps are usually adequate for most procedures, if access is a problem, both anterior and posterior releasing incisions are recommended. The base of the flap must be wider than the crestal aspect so that blood supply to the flap will not be compromised.

When the procedure is completed and the flap is repositioned, the clinician must feel the underlying bony contours through the flap to ensure that the intended goal has been reached. Then the flap is reelevated and copiously irrigated along the entire length of the flap to remove all debris. Once the flap is anatomically repositioned, a suture is used to secure the flaps position. Sutures are placed to approximate and not strangulate the tissues.

Commonly Used Preprosthetic Procedures

Common preprosthetic procedures include ridge alveoloplasty with extraction(s); ridge alveoloplasty without extractions for recontouring of the knife edged ridge or other ridge deformity or contour problems; intraseptal alveoloplasty; maxillary tuberosity reductions; recontouring of palatal and lateral exostosis and contour problems; mandibular tori removal; maxillary tori removal; mylohyoid ridge reduction; and genial tubercle reduction. Soft tissue procedures might include maxillary tuberosity soft tissue reduction, maxillary labial frenectomy, mandibular lingual frenectomy, and excision of redundant tissue.

Ridge Alveoloplasty with Extraction

After extraction of a tooth or teeth, the clinician must make a determination about the appropriateness of the remaining ridge contour(s) to fit into the preprosthetic plan, and if the recontouring will be made at the time of the extraction(s) or at a later time. If more than finger compression is needed, a full thickness flap should be elevated to a point apical to the area in need of recontouring. Depending on the amount of recontouring needed, a bone file may be sufficient to produce the desired contours. For greater recontouring, a side cutting rongeur or handpiece and acrylic resin bur can be used (Figure 5–2). When using these burs, always use copious irrigation to avoid overheating the bone and subsequent bony necrosis. Irrigation also cleans the flutes of the bur and carries away debris. After bulk recontouring, a bone file is uses to "fine tune" the recontouring. Bone files or rasps give the clinician a great tactile sense and good control. When finished, the flap is repositioned, contours palpated to verify that a desired endpoint has been reached, and is approximated primarily (Figure 5–3). When soft tissue recontouring is needed, reposition the flap; observe where the adjustments are needed, and use a sharp

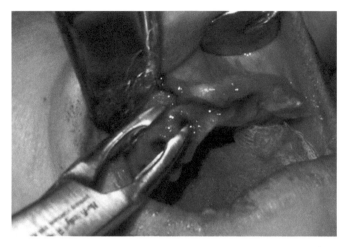

Figure 5–2 Bone rongeur used to accomplish bone reduction during a ridge alveoplasty along with extractions.

pair of scissors or surgical blade to make the cuts. It is usually more prudent to sequentially remove small amounts of tissue than to remove too much at one time. Consideration must also be given to maintenance of vestibular depth and form when trimming and approximating the flap.

Intraseptal Alveoloplasty

When the ridge has acceptable contour and height but presents an unacceptable undercut, which extends to the base of the labial vestibule, the intraseptal alveoloplasty might be considered. This procedure is best accomplished at the time of extraction or early in the postoperative healing period. After extraction of the teeth, the crestal tissue is slightly elevated to fully expose the extraction sockets. Using a small rongeur or handpiece and bur, the intraseptal bone is removed to the depth of the socket

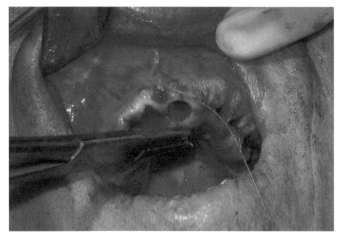

Figure 5–3 Primary closure of the flap following extractions and ridge alveoplasty.

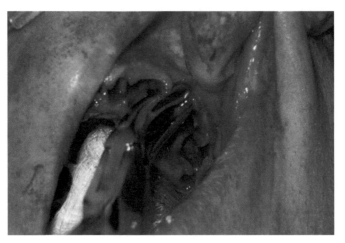

Figure 5–4   Interseptal alveoplasty during extraction procedures.

(Figure 5–4). After adequate removal of bone, finger pressure is applied in a constant, controlled manner until the labiocortical plate is greenstick fractured and can be positioned palatally, narrowing the crest and eliminating the undercut. If significant resistance is encountered, a vertical cut in the bone can be made using osteotome or bur from inside the most distal sockets outward, carefully scoring the bone. Periosteum and soft tissue should not be violated. Finger pressure should be applied to the area of the vertical bone cut to achieve mobility of the segment and guide its repositioning. A bone file can be used to smooth roughened edges, and the site can be irrigated. The crestal soft tissue can now be approximated and closed with interrupted or continuous sutures. Ideally, a surgical stent or soft-tissue-lined immediate denture can be inserted to maintain the repositioned bony segment until the initial stages of healing have taken place, at about two weeks after the procedure.

Edentulous Ridge Alveoloplasty

For routine elimination of sharp (knife-edged) ridges and removal of undesirable contours, undercuts, or prominences, direct vision and frequent palpation until the desired endpoint is reached will be sufficient. When the mandibular or maxillary edentulous ridges require multifocal, moderate, or greater amounts of recontouring, use of diagnostic casts to identify areas of concern, and fabrication of surgical guides, are recommended. In this way, the clinician has a model with the specific areas outlined to assist in the exact orientation once tissues are reflected and, if necessary, a surgical guide to assist with the detailed removal and recontouring of the bone.

The edentulous ridge alveoloplasty begins with identification of the areas of concern. A full thickness flap is designed and implemented to fully expose the targeted areas. Using bone files/rasps, rongeurs handpiece, and burs or combinations, the targeted areas are recontoured. Digital palpation with the flap in place is done until the desired endpoint is achieved. The site is irrigated and close primarily with an interrupted or continuous suture technique.

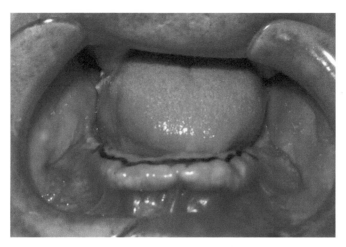

Figure 5–5 Marking the midline crestal incision to be used for access to remove buccal exostosis on the mandibular ridge.

Buccal Exostosis

This approach can be used on either arch and for irregularities on the palatal aspect of the maxillary alveolus. A crestal incision is made to extend beyond the margins of the areas requiring recontouring (Figure 5–5). A full thickness flap is elevated to completely expose the involved area (Figure 5–6). When an envelope flap will not provide the necessary exposure without placing tension on the flap, a releasing incision, as described earlier, may be incorporated into the flap design. For gaining assess to a palatal exostosis, make the incision longer and reflect more tissue to gain enough relaxation in the flap. Because of the greater palatine and incisive branch anastomosis, vertical releases in

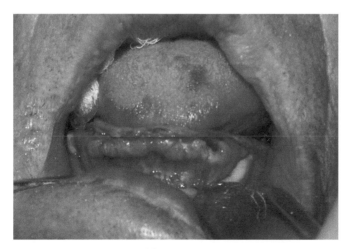

Figure 5–6 Elevation of full thickness flap to expose buccal exostosis, which will be recontoured prior to prosthodontic procedures.

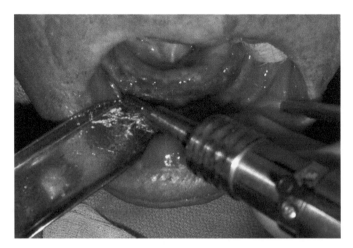

Figure 5–7   Exposed exostosis demonstrating the use of a rotary instrument for recontouring. Note retractor providing exposure of operating site and protecting adjacent soft tissue.

the palate area not recommended. Once the irregularity is exposed, the tissue is elevated and protected, and the appropriate instrument is used to recontour the bone to the desired endpoint (Figure 5–7). The area is palpated through the flap to confirm adequate reduction or recontouring. When completed, the area is irrigated and closed.

Maxillary Tuberosity Reductions

Maxillary hyperplasic tuberosities present real problems for gaining appropriate interarch distance posteriorly. The tuberosities can be hyperplastic in the horizontal or vertical planes, and may involve osseous hyperplasia, soft tissue hyperplasia, or both. To identify the hard tissue and soft tissue component that requires recontouring, a panoramic radiograph will usually suffice. This will provide information about the hard and soft tissue contributions and the overall contours of the tuberosity and proximity to the maxillary sinus. It is important to remember that maxillary sinuses may pneumatize into the tuberosity areas. A crestal incision is made from a point anterior to where the recontouring will start, over and up behind the tuberosity. Tissue must be elevated on both the buccal and palatal aspects to fully expose the tuberosity (Figure 5–8). After making sure that all soft tissue is protected, instrumentation can start (Figure 5–9). The tuberosity can be recontoured with bone file, rongeur, or bur (Figures 5–10 and 5–11). If a great deal of bone needs to be removed, again as in other procedures, a surgical guide may be necessary. If the maxillary sinus has pneumatized, care must be taken when removing the bone, and the sinus membrane may become exposed. However, this is not a problem as long as the membrane is intact.

Mandibular Tori

In the dentate arch, tori pose few, if any, problems. Occasionally tori can be large enough to interfere with tongue mobility and speech, and the thin mucosa overlying the tori may be chronically irritated or injured when eating certain foods. In the edentulous arch, tori may pose significant interference when wearing a removable prosthesis and often must be removed.

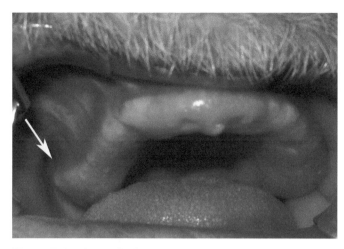

Figure 5–8 Arrow indicates a bony undercut on the lateral surface of the maxillary tuberosity.

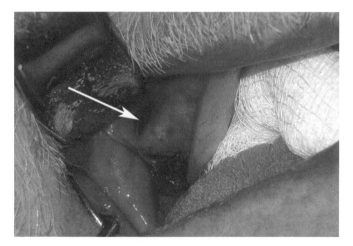

Figure 5–9 Tissue flap is elevated to expose bony undercut (arrow) that requires recontouring.

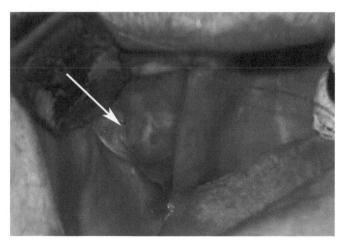

Figure 5–10 Arrow indicates recontoured buccal bone with the undercut eliminated.

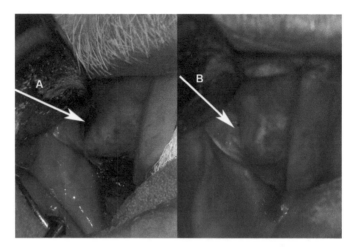

Figure 5–11   Before (A) and after (B) recontouring the buccal bone to eliminate an undercut on the lateral aspect of the maxillary tuberosity.

A midline crestal incision is made to extend about 1.0 -1.5 cm distal to the most posterior tori, to decrease tension and tearing of the flap. A full thickness lingual mucosal flap is slowly elevated. Because the tori may be pedunculated, dissection of the very thin mucosa located in the undercuts may be tenuous. However, like other procedures discussed, patience and a steady hand will prevail. After elevating all mucosa off of the tori(s) to a point below the tori where normal lingual cortical anatomy is found, a tissue retractor must be placed to maintain exposure and protect the flap. If an osteotome slips, it should hit the retractor and not perforate the floor of the mouth. Similarly, the tissue must be out of the way when using a rotary instrument and bur. For smaller tori, bone file and rongeur or rotary instrument and bur may be used for bone reduction (Figure 5–12).

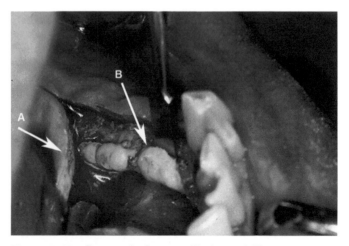

Figure 5–12   Removal of a mandibular tori. The arrow (A) indicates the reflected tissue flap and the arrow (B) indicates the bony projection to be removed with the osteotome.

After all tori have been removed and bone smoothed, the flap is repositioned and the lingual plate palpated to confirm achieving the desired contours. Use the suture technique of choice, but because of the length of the incision, a continuous suturing technique with good margin inversion is recommended. To minimize hematoma formation 4x4 gauze is rolled into the appearance of a cigar, the tongue is elevated to the roof of the mouth, and the gauzed is placed under the anterior aspect of the tongue over the repositioned sutured flap. Have the patient lower the tongue. The weight of the tongue will push the gauze down and forward, pushing the gauze against the flap and the flap against the bone. These will tamponade any small oozing and eliminate dead space.

Maxillary Tori

A maxillary tori may pose a significant problem in the fabrication and wearing of a maxillary complete denture. The tori may be especially problematic when it is positioned more posteriorly, creating problems with posterior palatal seal of the prosthesis (Figure 5–13). A midline incision is placed over the torus with oblique releasing incisions at each end. When the tori are multilobulated and pedunculated, elevation of the thin mucosa may be difficult. After the torus is exposed, adequate flap control for best visualization is important (Figure 5–14A). An excellent method of keeping the flaps open is to suture the margin of the flap to the crest of the ridge on the same side. For some larger pedunculated multilobulated tori, a midcrestal incision with elevation of the entire palatal mucosa is recommended. This dissection must stay subperiosteal to avoid injury to the palatal blood supply. The desirable end point is for the palatal vault to be smooth and confluent with no undercuts or elevations (Figure 5–14B).

The margins of the flap are digitally positioned and pressed against the bone. Removal of redundant tissue can now be performed, keeping in mind that all bone must be covered with tension-free closure. Also keep in mind that the thin mucosa overlying the torus does not hold a suture well, so margin trimming should be conservative or not at all (Figure 5–15). Hematoma formation in the palate under the flap is a great concern. Excellent methods of applying pressure are with the placement of a temporary denture

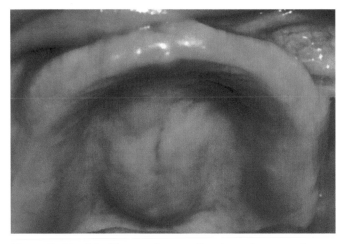

Figure 5–13 Maxillary tori extending into the posterior palatal seal area.

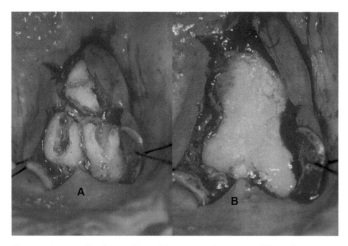

Figure 5-14 Pedunculated bony tori exposed by elevating subperiosteal flaps (A) Smooth palate created by the tori removal (B)

with soft reline material over the surgical site or with a well-fitting, surgical guide with soft reline placed over the area. The pressure should be maintained for several days. The patient can remove the appliances for local wound care and oral rinsing.

Mylohyoid Ridge Reduction

In the mandibular post-extraction ridge remodeling sequencing, the alveolar bone and external oblique ridge resorb because of lack of stressing and functional remodeling. The mylohyoid ridge, which supports the attachment of the mylohyoid muscle, remains relatively intact, and becomes a prominent feature in the posterior mandible.

After providing profound anesthesia, a midcrestal incision is made anterior to the site of ridge reduction and carried posteriorly gradually deviating toward the buccal, to

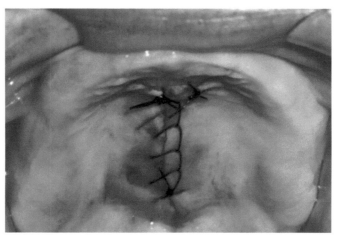

Figure 5-15 Primary closure achieved after bony recontouring is complete.

avoid potential injury to the lingual nerve. The flap is elevated to expose the mylohyoid ridge and attached muscle. Using sharp dissection, the tendenous attachments of the mylohyoid muscle are stripped. The muscle will retract into the floor of the mouth and reattach during healing. A bone bur can be used to reduce the ridge to the desired height. A bone file can be used to fine-tune the contouring. When completed, the area should be copiously irrigated and closed primarily with interrupted or continuous sutures. Once the flap has been closed, ideally a denture with a soft reline is placed to allow for the lingual flange to help with displacement of the detached mylohyoid muscle.

Genial Tubercle Reduction

In the post-extraction ridge remodeling of the anterior mandible, the alveolar ridge and tooth-bearing areas resorb because of lack of stressing and functional loading. The superior pair of genial tubercles provides insertion for the paired genioglossus muscles, while the lower paired tubercles provide insertion for the paired geniohyoid muscles. Because of the constant movement of the tongue and stressing of the tubercles once the alveolus has resorbed and remodeled, the genial tubercles can become very prominent structures in the anterior mandible and impede proper seating of the denture.

The clinician must be aware that this surgical site lies between two moving structures—the tongue and the lip. Therefore this is an area that may be prone to wound dehiscence, making this a very difficult surgery.

A full thickness flap is elevated to expose the genial tubercle and genioglossus muscle attachments. The tendenous muscular attachments are sharply detached from the bone to randomly reattach more inferiorly. With exposure of the bone and protection of the flap, the bone height can be reduced with the instrument of choice to the desired level. The wound is copiously irrigated and closed primarily.

Soft Tissue Procedures

With loss of teeth, bony resorption, and remodeling, soft tissue relationships that existed with teeth and were not problematic may become concerns. With reduction of ridge height and contour, soft tissue and muscular attachments change. These muscular and soft tissue changes are often deleterious to prosthesis stability and function, and require removal or alteration. Additionally, with the potential trauma and chronic irritation caused by ill-fitting prostheses, the development of hyperplastic tissues in the denture-bearing and peripheral tissue areas may occur. These hyperplastic tissues contribute to lack of denture fit and stability, and can contribute to patient discomfort.

Because it is very difficult to replace oral mucosa after it has been removed, the treatment plan must detail the sequence in which the soft tissue abnormalities will be addressed. Treatment will usually address the bony abnormalities first, to achieve normal bone healing with good soft tissue coverage. Additionally, if implant placement is part of the treatment plan, bone augmentation may be required. Preserving redundant soft tissue to provide coverage for bone augmentation should be considered. The soft tissue issues may be addressed after the grafting and or implants have healed. In general, excised, redundant hyperplastic soft tissues are the result of chronic irritation from an ill-fitting prosthesis. However, because of the chronic irritation, pathologic changes within the tissues can occur. Therefore, as a rule, a portion of all excised hyperplastic tissues should be submitted for histopathologic examination.

Maxillary Soft Tissue Tuberosity Reduction

Interarch distance is a critical element for proper fabrication of denture bases, and hyperplastic maxillary tuberosity tissues often impinge on adequate interarch distance. To determine if the reduction will be primarily bone or soft tissue, a panoramic radiograph that can discriminate the soft tissue shadow from bone is required. If not available, sounding of the soft tissue with the anesthesia needle after the region is anesthetized will provide the clinician with detail of the tissue thickness. If a great deal of tissue removal is anticipated, a surgical guide is recommended.

A midline elliptical incision is made sharply to bone with the widest part of the ellipse directly over the area where the most tissue is to be removed. The anterior and posterior portions of the ellipse should taper into the normal portions of the ridge anteriorly and to the posterior tuberosity posteriorly. The ellipsed portion is elevated and removed. The clinician can now look into the area made by the removed section of tissue and evaluate the tissue height above the bone. Directing attention to the buccal and palatal edges of the incision, the clinician will thin the tissue by removing a uniform thickness—staying an even distance from the surface and remembering to adjust the angle while thinning around the curve. Buccally, there are no structures of concern to the clinician as he/she makes contact with the bony lateral aspect of the ridge. Palatally, the clinician needs to be careful not to extend the thinning too deep into the palatal aspect of the ridge because of the greater palatine neurovascular bundle. Once the excess tissue has been removed and there is a uniform thickness of mucosa, digital pressure will approximate the buccal and palatal flap margins to evaluate the amount of vertical reduction that has been accomplished. Having the patient close down gently on the clinician's fingers will allow for evaluation of the change in interarch distance. If the vertical reduction is acceptable, the wound margins are approximated and trimmed to get a tension-free butt joint closure. The wound is closed with an interrupted, or continuous, suture technique.

If the tissue has been thinned and no additional vertical change is possible within the soft tissue, and yet more is needed, then the flaps will need to be reflected buccally and palatally. Bony reduction will need to be done to achieve the desired vertical change. (Refer back to bony tuberosity reduction).

Maxillary Labial Frenectomy

Labial frenal attachments are thin bands of fibrous tissue/muscle covered with mucosa that extend from the lip or cheek and attach into the periosteum on the sides of, or the crest of, the alveolar ridge. Except for frenal attachments, which attach at the incisive papillae and contribute to the midline diastema, most frenal attachments—like other soft tissue structures—are of little consequence when teeth are present. On the edentulous ridge, which has experienced resorption and remodeling, the muscular and soft tissue attachments may directly affect the seating, stabilization, and construction of the prosthesis, as well as subject the patient to reduced function and discomfort. Although this is a simple technique, it yields great benefit.

Although other techniques exist, the following is recommended for a simple frenectomy. Infiltration anesthesia to the lip around the frenum is usually adequate.

Injecting directly into the frenum may distort the anatomy. After achieving good anesthesia, two small, curved hemostats are placed with the curved sides against the tissues over the superior aspect of the frenum and the inferior aspect of the frenum. The tips of the hemostats will touch in the deep aspect near the vestibule. A surgical assistant should suction and retract the lip superiorly. Holding the top hemostat, the clinician will use a surgical blade and follow the curvature of the upper hemostat, cutting through the upper aspect of the frenum (Figure 5–16). This is repeated for the lower hemostat. The frenum will now be excised, leaving a diamond-shaped wound (Figure 5–17). Exploring the wound, any frenal remnants should be excised directly to periosteum. A suture is placed through the wound margin engaging the periosteum in the depth of the vestibule right below the anterior nasal spine. A knot is tied and the margins will be drawn together and pulled down to the periosteum in the depth of the vestibule. Additional sutures are placed in a similar manner so that the diamond-shaped wound now closes in a linear manner (Figure 5–18). If the frenum extended to the crest of the ridge and was

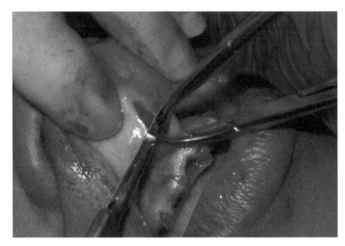

Figure 5–16 Maxillary labial frenectomy using two curved hemostats as guides for tissue excision.

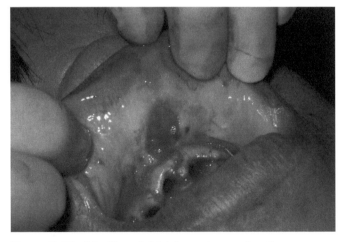

Figure 5–17 Maxillary labial frenectomy after tissue excision prior to primary closure.

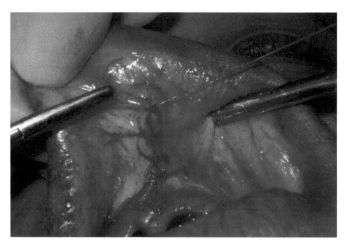

Figure 5–18   Maxillary labial frenectomy primary closure with sutures.

excised thorough attached tissue, all parts of the wound will close primarily except that part in the attached tissue. No attempt should be made to close that area and it should be left to granulate and heal by secondary intention.

Excision of Redundant/Hypermobile Tissue Overlying the Tuberosities

Redundant hypermobile tissue is often the result of ill-fitting dentures, ridge resorption, or both. After identifying the area to be excised, parallel incisions on the buccal and lingual or palatal aspects of the tissue are made sharply to bone. The incisions will taper into each other posterior to the area to be incised. The excised piece of tissue will be dissected from the bone and removed. Digital pressure is applied to check for primary closure of the wound margins. If additional tissue needs to be removed, tangential incisions on the buccal and palatal, or lingual, sides of the wound are made to remove and thin out additional tissue. This is done carefully until the wound margins approximate primarily. The wound is irrigated and closed primarily. Care should be taken to avoid significant undermining of the buccal/facial aspects of the flaps, and loss of vestibular depth when closing the wound.

Excision of Inflammatory Fibrous Hyperplasia (Epulis Fissuratum)

Inflammatory fibrous hyperplasia is a generalized hyperplastic enlargement of the mucosa and fibrous tissue in the alveolar ridge and vestibular area. The etiology is most closely associated with chronic trauma to the involved areas from ill-fitting prosthesis. Inflammatory fibrous hyperplasia progresses in stages, and the surgical procedure indicated varies with the stage. For those lesions in the early stages, there is not a significant degree of fibrosis of the involved tissues, and nonsurgical therapies may be effective. In the later stages where there is significant fibrosis and hyperplastic changes, excision of the hyperplastic mass of tissue is the treatment of choice (Figure 5–19).

Several treatment options exist based on the size of he hyperplastic mass of tissue to be removed. If the tissue mass is not extensive, use of lasers or electrosurgery

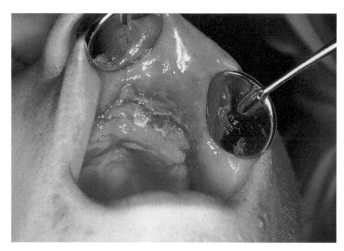

Figure 5–19 Inflammatory fiberous hyperplasia in the maxillary labial vestibule.

techniques provides good results for tissue excision. For more extensive tissue masses, the margins of the tissue mass are elevated using tissue forceps, and an incision is made at the base of the mass, but not through the periosteum. A supraperiosteal dissection is made under the entire mass of the hyperplastic tissue, and the mass is removed.

The normal mucosal margins are sutured in place, and the superior margins are sutured to the depth of the vestibule. In order to minimize soft tissue creeping and loss of vestibular height with secondary intension healing, a surgical stent with an extended anterior flange lined with soft tissue conditioner, or the existing denture with the flange extended to engage the height of the vestibule. A soft tissue conditioner should be placed, and the prosthesis should only be removed for wound care and rinsing, and cleansing of the intaglio surface of the prosthesis. Secondary epithelialization will take four to six weeks.

Inflammatory Papillary Hyperplasia of the Palate

Inflammatory papillary hyperplasia of the palate is a condition affecting the palatal mucosa, thought to be caused by ill-fitting prosthesis, poor hygiene, or fungal infections and the associated inflammation. Its clinical presentation appears as multiple nodular projections in the palatal mucosa. The lesions may be erythematous or may have normal palatal mucosal coloration (Figure 5–20).

Early treatment consists of prosthesis adjustments, tissue conditioner, and proper oral hygiene. In more advanced presentations, several treatment options have been suggested. Because this is primarily an inflammatory disorder, there is no need to excise the full thickness of the palatal tissue. In any of the described treatment options, the superficial inflamed layers of the palatal mucosa are removed leaving the palatal periosteum intact to heal by secondary intension. These techniques include removal of the inflamed mucosa with electrosurgery loops, laser ablation of the superficial layers, sharp dissection, use of coarse fluted burs, or dermabrasion brushes to bur or abrade this layer, and cryotherapy (Figure 5–21). As mentioned earlier, no matter which technique is used, care should be taken to ensure that the periosteum is not violated and the underlying bone is not involved. The palate is covered with a surgical stent or denture with a soft

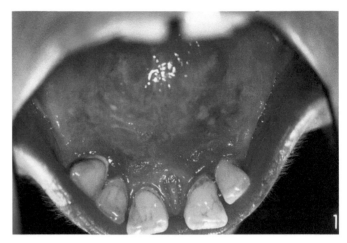

Figure 5–20   Inflammatory papillary hyperplasia of the palate.

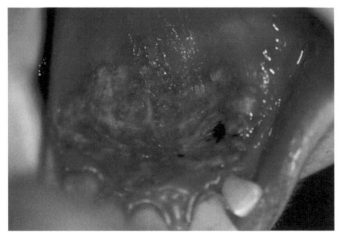

Figure 5–21   Inflammatory papillary hyperplasia removed using cryotherapy.

tissue conditioner to assist with patient comfort and provide coverage while secondary epithelialization takes place in the following four to six weeks.

 ## Surgical Guides (Templates)

When moderate amounts of bone recontouring are required and the treatment plan requires a degree of precision in the amount and location of bone to be removed, surgical guides are excellent adjuncts. Using a duplicated diagnostic cast, the areas of concern are modified to achieve the ideal ridge form. A clear rigid guide is then fabricated using a vacuum-formed technique. During the surgical procedure, after recontouring has been accomplished, the surgical guide is placed over the area with the flap repositioned, and areas of soft tissue blanching are observed. These blanching areas represent areas where additional removal of bone and recontouring are still required. This procedure is repeated until no blanching exists and the surgical guide is stable when seated. Soft tissue trimming, if necessary, can now be done.

References

Miloro, M., Ghali, G.E., Larsen, P.E., Waite, P.D.: Peter's Principles of Oral and Maxofillial Surgery, Hamilton, Ontario: BC Decker Inc., pp. 157-188.

Ochs, M.W., Tucker, M.R.: Preprosthetic Surgery In: Contemporary Oral and Maxillofacial Surgery, 4th Ed, St. Louis, MO: Mosby Publishing pp. 248-304.

Peterson, L. J., Indresano, A.T., Marciani, R.L., Roser, S.M.: Principles of Oral and Maxillofacial Surgery, Volume 2, Philadelphia, PA: Lippencott Company, pp. 1103-1132.

Spagnoli, D.B., Gollehon, S.G., Misiek, D.J.: Preprosthetic and Reconstructive Surgery In: Principles of Oral and Maxillofacial Surgery 2ed., Hamilton, Ontario: B.C. Decker, Inc., pp. 157-187

Tucker, M.R.: Ambulatory Preprosthetic Reconstructive Surgery In: Oral and Maxillofacial Surgery Volume 3, St Louis, MO.: Mosby Publishing, pp. 1103-1132.

QUESTIONS

1. What other diagnostic imaging might be used for preprosthetic surgery treatment planning besides typical panographic radiographs?

2. Surgical access is often gained through the use of full thickness mucoperiosteal flaps. What are the advantages to this surgical approach over other flap techniques?

3. What three instruments are commonly used for recontouring bone during preprosthetic surgery?

4. True or False: Maxillary tori may present more of a problem for a complete denture patient if it extends past the vibrating line where the posterior palatal seal is usually placed.

5. What techniques can be used to remove inflammatory papillary hyperplasia after controlling the causative factors?

ANSWERS

1. Tomographic studies and computerized tomography (CT Scans) may be used. The CT scan can provide cross-sectional detail of the maxilla in both the axial and coronal views.

2. This aggressive surgical approach with its greater visibility, protection of adjacent tissues, time efficiency, and more routine post-operative course is far more valuable and less traumatic to the patient than other less effective techniques.

3. a. bone file   b. side-cutting rongeur   c. handpiece and bur

4. TRUE

5. a. electrosurgery loops   b. laser ablation   c. sharp dissection to periosteum
   d. dermabrasion brushes   e. cryotherapy

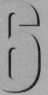

Preliminary Impressions, Diagnostic Casts, and Custom (Final) Impression Trays

Dr. John R. Ivanhoe
Dr. Kevin D. Plummer

Dental patients require a thorough examination, diagnosis, and treatment plan prior to initiating any definitive treatment—which, for most patients, requires the use of maxillary and mandibular diagnostic casts (Figure 6–1). Diagnostic casts allow for the evaluation of hard and soft tissue anatomy without the presence of the patient. They also allow for determination of necessary preprosthetic surgery, can be mounted on an articulator, and the interocclusal space can be evaluated. Perhaps most important, for a complete denture patient, diagnostic casts provide the base from which custom impression trays are fabricated.

Diagnostic casts are made from preliminary impressions and are often very accurate representations of the hard and soft tissues of the ridges, but with poor detail of the depth and width of the vestibules and surrounding muscular attachments. This lack of detail is often the result of the impression trays and materials required when making the impressions rather than poor clinical techniques. Because custom impression trays cannot yet be fabricated for the patient, stock impression trays must be used. These trays are made to fit the average patient and therefore lack the accuracy required for making detailed master casts. Because of low cost and ease of use, irreversible hydrocolloid impression materials are the materials of choice for making the preliminary impressions. Because of their high viscosities, however, these impression materials will often displace the soft tissues of the vestibules, resulting in an overextended impression and resulting cast. This vestibular inaccuracy in the diagnostic cast is not important for diagnosing and creating treatment plans for most patients, but is unacceptable in either the diagnostic or master cast for a complete denture patient. Fabricating complete dentures requires master casts with extreme accuracy of the vestibules and therefore requires the use of accurate custom impression trays and specific lower viscosity impression materials.

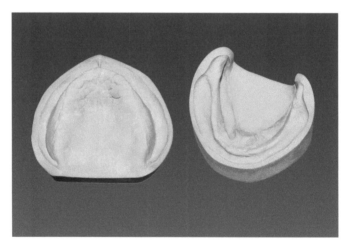

Figure 6–1 Examples of well-made diagnostic casts. Note that the casts demonstrate all desirable anatomical features of the patient, including the vestibules, yet the impressions were not overextended onto movable muscle and frenulum attachments.

Making the Preliminary Impressions

Stock impression trays are selected for both the maxillary and mandibular arches. Because of the limited selection of stock tray sizes, shapes, and extensions, the clinician must examine the trays intraorally and select the most accurately fitting tray (Figures 6–2 and 6–3). When available, a tray is selected that will provide about 5–6 mm (1/4 inch) even spacing between the tray and the tissues. For the right-handed dentist, the correct

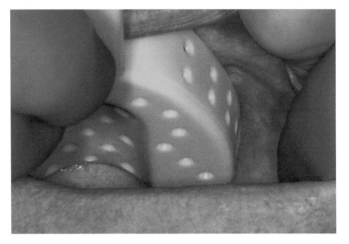

Figure 6–2   The clinician must examine the tray intraorally to ensure that adequate space exists between the impression tray and the tissues, and that the tray flanges are adequately extended.

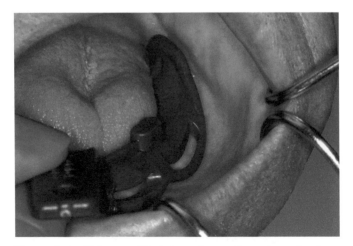

Figure 6–3   This mandibular stock tray fits appropriately and provides adequate space for the impression material. Note that, although the flanges of the tray extend into the vestibules, the surrounding soft tissues are not being displaced.

body position is to the right and in front of the patient, and the tray is inserted by distending the left corner of the patient's mouth with the left index finger or a mouth mirror, placing the posterior two-thirds of the right side of the tray into the right corner of the mouth, and rotating the tray into position inside of the mouth.

The clinician should place the posterior border of the tray slightly beyond the hamular notches for the maxillary arch and over the retromolar pads for the mandibular arch. With the lips being held outward, the front part of the tray is rotated into position while retaining the proper posterior alignment of the trays over the hamular notches or retromolar pads. The impression tray is the correct size if it provides coverage of all desired tissues and provides a uniform space of approximately 5–6 mm (1/4 inch) between the tissues and impression tray. The buccal flanges of the tray, in relation to buccal slopes of the residual ridges, are also evaluated to ensure that adequate space exists for the impression material (Figure 6–4).

The clinician should note the position of the tray when it is correctly located in the mouth. The relation of the handle of the tray should be aligned with the middle of the patient's face; this will be the desired alignment when the preliminary impression is being made.

The tray is refined, as necessary, with "periphery wax" to reshape the tray to assure proper spacing between the tray and the tissues and gain additional flange extension (Figure 6–5). For example, periphery wax is often necessary in the palatal area of the tray for those patients with a high palatal vaults. The purpose of the periphery wax is to create 5–6 mm (1/4 inch) spacing between the tray and the tissues, which will support the impression material and minimize slumping of the material away from the tissues. A film of impression material adhesive should be sprayed or painted to the tissue side of the tray and to any periphery wax that was placed on the tray. It should be allowed to dry as per the manufacturer's recommendations.

Prior to making the impression, the patient is instructed to rinse his or her mouth with water to reduce the viscosity of the saliva. Using the proper water/powder ratio, the irreversible hydrocolloid material is mixed according to the manufacturer's instructions, and the impression tray is loaded approximately one-half to three-quarters full. Do not

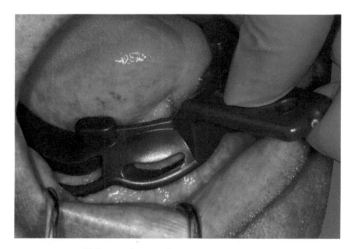

Figure 6–4 This stock tray fits well in the anterior area. It extends into the vestibule but it is not overextended and will not distort the soft tissues during the impression-making procedure.

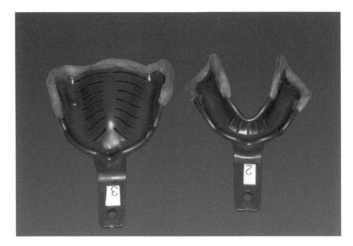

Figure 6–5 Periphery wax has been added to these trays to gain additional extension. Periphery wax may also be necessary to minimize large voids between the stock tray and the underlying tissues. A well-fitting tray should exhibit approximately 6 mm (1/4 inch) of space between the tray and the tissues. This proper fit will adequately support the impression material and minimize potential slumping of the material away from the tissues.

overfill the tray because excess material will be expelled as the tray is seated and often lead to severe gagging, which will often compromise the patient's ability to breath.

Prior to inserting the impression tray, the patient should be asked to swallow to eliminate excess saliva. Impression material should be placed, by finger, into any areas that the clinician feels may not be adequately reached by the impression tray. These areas often include the palatal vault, retromylohyoid spaces, and/or buccal vestibules (Figure 6–6).

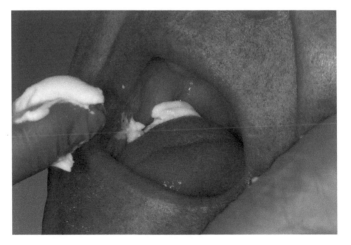

Figure 6–6 Prior to inserting a tray with the impression material loaded, additional material may be placed in areas that may be difficult to record. In this example, reversible hydrocolloid material has been placed in the retromylohyoid area prior to inserting the tray.

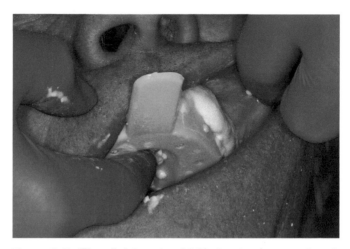

Figure 6–7 The clinician should lift the cheek upward and away from the ridge to ensure that the impression tray has been adequately seated and to allow impression material to record this area. This procedure also allows trapped air bubbles to be expelled so as not to be captured in the impression.

To minimize gagging, continually remind the patient to take short breaths through the nose and not to swallow. The loaded tray is placed in the mouth and centered over the residual ridges, hamular notches, and/or retromolar pads. When making the mandibular impression, instruct the patient to raise the tongue while the impression is being seated. While seating the tray, the cheeks should be lifted beyond their normal relaxed position to allow impression material to completed fill the vestibules and to allow air bubbles to be expressed (Figure 6–7). It is important to lift the cheeks outward in the mandibular notch areas so that the commonly seen roll of fatty tissue will not be trapped in the impression (Figures 6–8 and 6–9).

The tray is seated from the posterior to the anterior so that the material flows toward the anterior rather than toward the posterior. It is important to note the position of the anterior flange of the impression tray. It should be seated in the middle of the labial vestibule. In many instances, an impression will be unacceptable because either the tongue forced the impression tray too far forward and important posterior anatomy was not captured in the impression or the vestibule was not captured because the tray was not fully seated. Seat with the index finger of both hands on each side of the tray in approximately the region of the first molar. The tray is positioned as during practicing by noting the location of the handle in relation to the middle of the face. The clinician must continuously monitor the patient and ensure that excess impression material is not permitted to flow posteriorly, which would compromise the patient's ability to breath. If this happens, the excess can often be removed with a mouth mirror. The clinician may never leave an impression in a patient's mouth and turn away from the patient. The clinician must always have control of the impression tray in case of a sudden complication.

Once seated, all soft tissues surrounding the vestibular borders should be manipulated (border molded) to minimize overextension of the impression material (Figure 6–10). (See Chapter 7 on Final Impressions for the proper border molding technique.) This tissue manipulation is accomplished while the impression material is still very flowable.

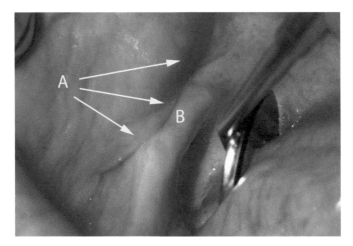

Figure 6–8 Note that a "fatty" pad of tissue (A) is often present in the distobuccal area of the mandibular arch and may fold over the retromolar pad (B) and become trapped in an impression. This fold can be minimized by lifting this tissue upward and away from the retromolar pad while seating the impression.

The tray is held steadily in position until the impression material has set, as determined by the manufacturer. Although the tray must be held securely in the mouth with the fingers, the clinician should be able to direct only minimal pressure to the trays. The purpose of the fingers is to maintain the position of the impression tray and prevent it from dislodging vertically away from the ridge and distorting the impression.

The patient is instructed to relax the lips while the clinician removes the impression. This allows air under the impression, which breaks the seal and releases the impression from the arch. Because irreversible hydrocolloid impression material may tear if exposed to continuous slow stretching forces, a sudden snapping movement is used to remove the impression.

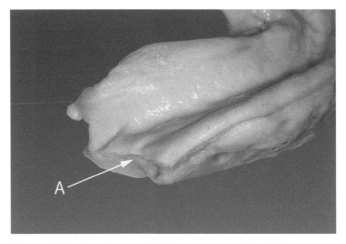

Figure 6–9 The fatty pad (A) was trapped in this impression. This impression must be remade.

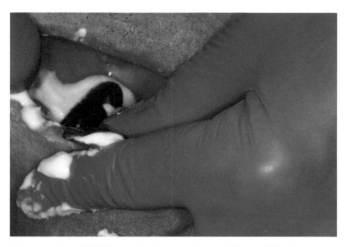

Figure 6–10 While maintaining the position of the impression tray, the soft tissues beyond the vestibular areas should be manipulated (border molded) to prevent gross overextension of the impression. Grossly overextended borders in preliminary impressions will cause inaccurate, overextended vestibules in the diagnostic casts, resulting in overextended custom impression trays. An inordinate amount of time is often wasted correcting the flange length of custom impression trays because the preliminary impression was not properly formed. The more closely a preliminary impression resembles a final impression, the easier almost all following clinical procedures will be.

The impression is examined to assure acceptability (Figures 6–11 and 6–12). At a minimum, preliminary impressions and diagnostic casts for complete denture patients must include all hard and soft tissues of the ridges, the entire vestibules, retromylohyoid areas, entire hard and initial 3–4 mm (1/4 inch) of the soft palate, and hamular notches. If the decision is made to remake an impression, the initial impression should be carefully evaluated to determine the cause of the initial problem in order to minimize the likelihood of having the same problem occur a second time. An impression must be remade for many reasons including:

1. Incorrect tray position in the mouth, which has caused one or more anatomical areas not to be captured in the impression.
2. Excessive areas of the impression tray showing through the impression material indicating pressure that may have resulted in a distorted impression.
3. Any void or discrepancy too large to accurately correct on the cast.
4. Incorrect border formation as a result of incorrect border length of the tray. A sharp border usually indicates that the impression is underextended in that area.
5. Obviously distorted impression because of movement of the tray during the setting of the final impression material.
6. Poor detail in the impression because of a poor mixing technique or because the material had begun to set before the impression was fully seated.

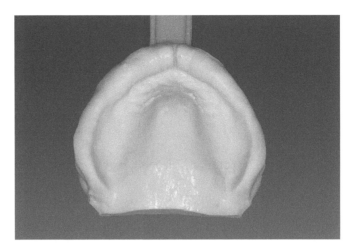

Figure 6–11   A well-made maxillary preliminary impression. Note that all anatomical areas of the ridge have been accurately recorded and, even though the border thickness is a little excessive, the border length is excellent. This impression closely resembles a final impression and as such will allow the fabrication of an excellent diagnostic cast and eventual custom impression tray.

Once deemed acceptable, the impression is thoroughly rinsed to remove excess saliva, disinfected, and immediately taken to the laboratory and poured. If any delay is encountered in pouring the impression, the impression must be wrapped in wet paper towels or placed in a humidor to minimize the loss of water from the impression. Loss of water will cause the impression to unacceptably and irreversibly become distorted. An irreversible hydrocolloid impression should be poured in dental stone within 10 minutes.

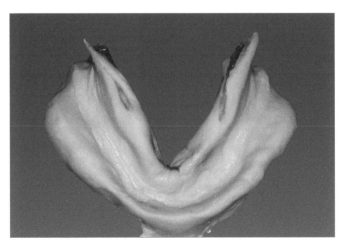

Figure 6–12   This mandibular preliminary impression not only records all desired anatomical areas but also exhibits excellent border extensions.

Pouring the Diagnostic Casts

A mix of dental stone is prepared using the water/powder ratio provided by the manufacturer's instructions. A clean mixing bowl and spatula should be used, and the powder is gently added to the water to minimize the trapping of air within the mixture. A mechanical spatula and vacuum mix are generally not necessary when mixing the dental stone for a diagnostic cast, although a more dense stone will be formed if this technique is used. All excess water is carefully removed from the impression by gently blowing with an air pressure hose. However, the impression material must not be allowed to become dried. Mix the material thoroughly assuring that all dry stone is wet, and a smooth mixture with minimal bubbles is achieved.

A vibrator set to a medium to low speed should be used when pouring the impression. High speed vibration will often trap air bubbles in the cast in critical areas. The stone is carefully and slowly vibrated into the anatomical areas of the impression in small increments until the impression is completely filled and borders covered (Figure 6–13). Avoid locking stone around any portion of exposed impression tray. This problem could make removal of the cast difficult after the stone is set if it is locked onto the tray. After the stone has reached its initial set and is hard enough to handle, a second mix of artificial stone is made and a base of approximately 15–17 mm (3/4 inch) in height and slightly wider than the initial pour of the impression is formed. Allowing the initial pour of stone to achieve its preliminary set before inverting the impression will help minimize the slumping of stone away from the impression, which would result in an inaccurate impression. Inverting the poured impression before the initial set also lets air and water rise to the critical tissue detail area resulting in a weaker and possibly distorted cast. The cast is inverted onto this mound of stone and the width of the future land areas are extended to 5 - 6 mm (1/4 inch) beyond the impression (Figure 6–14). Although the ridge crests cannot be visualized at this time, an attempt should be made

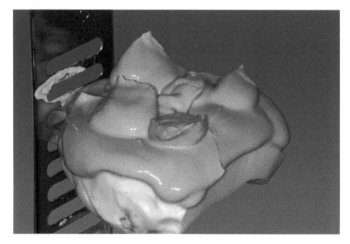

Figure 6–13 The initial pour of a preliminary impression. Note that small nodules have been placed on the surface of the material. Once this initial pour of stone has achieved its initial set, it is inverted into a second pour of stone to form the completed diagnostic cast. These nodules will help provide additional strength to the two-pour cast.

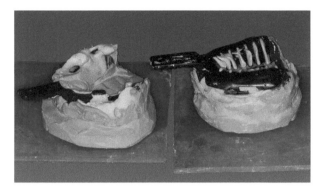

Figure 6–14A   These maxillary and mandibular preliminary impressions have been inverted into a second pour of stone to form a base for the diagnostic cast. Note that the stone on the maxillary cast has been allowed to harden while in direct contact with the impression tray. This is incorrect, and this tray will be difficult to separate from the cast.

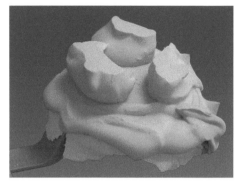

Figure 6–14B   Trimming the retention nodules flat will stabilize the initial pour when inverted into the second pour of stone.

to make the ridge crests parallel to the table top. Trimming the retention nodules flat and as parallel to the ridge crests as possible will give a stabile platform to rest the initial pour on while forming the base (Figure 6-14B). This will aid in shaping the cast at the next laboratory step. The stone should be allowed to set undisturbed as per the manufacturer's recommendation, generally for about 45 minutes.

 ## Shaping the Diagnostic Casts

The impression tray and material should be carefully removed from the casts; breakage of the cast at this step may necessitate the remaking of the impression. All debris and impression material is removed from the cast. The cast should be carefully examined to ensure that all desired tissues have been captured. A successfully formed diagnostic cast should exhibit all ridge and vestibular areas and all desired anatomical structures. When properly shaped, the cast should also exhibit land areas around the vestibules and a base of approximately 12–13 mm (1/2 inch) in thickness. This base thickness provides for sufficient strength while minimizing excessive thickness.

Excess stone is removed from the casts with a cast or model trimmers and running water. A slurry mixture of water and stone will be formed by the model trimmer as the cast is being trimmed. The slurry mixture should not be allowed to touch a dry cast surface because it will quickly stick to the dry surface and become almost impossible to remove. Therefore, prior to trimming, always wet all cast surfaces. All slurry and residue should be continuously and thoroughly rinsed off casts immediately as trimming proceeds; if allowed to dry, the slurry mixture will compromise the accuracy of the diagnostic cast. While the slurry must be removed with clean water, the casts should not be left under running water for extended periods because the stone surface can be unacceptably dissolved. Dry trimmers eliminate this potential problem.

The bottom of the base of the cast is initially trimmed so that the crests of the ridges are parallel to the base, and the thinnest areas of the casts are approximately 12–13 mm

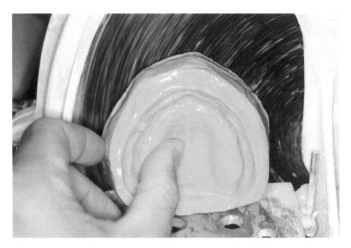

Figure 6–15   The bottom of the cast is the initial surface trimmed using a model trimmer. The bottom should be trimmed so that the ridge crests are parallel to the bottom, or bench top, and the thinnest portion of the base of the cast is approximately 12 mm (1/2 inch) thick.

in thickness (Figure 6–15). The sides of the cast are not trimmed until the ridges are parallel to the bottom of the cast and the base is the proper thickness. The sides of the base of the cast can now be trimmed and will be perpendicular to the ridges. When trimming the sides, enough excess is left to provide the land area beyond the anatomical surface of the cast. The land area should be approximately 2–3 mm (1/8 inch) wide on the buccal and labial sides and 5–6 mm (1/4 inch) wide in the posterior (Figure 6–16). The vestibular depths should be approximately 2–3 mm in depth where possible and a knife, arbor band, or acrylic bur may be used to flatten the land area on the cast and

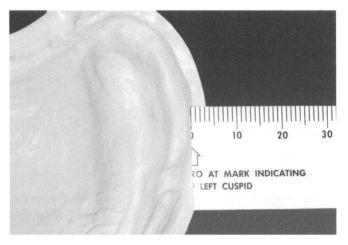

Figure 6–16   Once the base of the cast is properly formed, the sides of the cast can be trimmed to create land areas approximately 3 mm (1/8 inch) in width in the labial and buccal areas and 6 mm (1/4 inch) posterior to the retromolar pads and hamular notches. The land areas will later be trimmed vertically to create vestibules no deeper than 3 mm (1/8 inch).

reduce the depth of the vestibule as necessary. It is important to reduce the depths of the vestibules of the casts so that the entire vestibules are easily accessible for adaptation of custom tray material in future procedures. The trimmed casts can be finished with wet-or-dry fine sandpaper, 320 grit. The casts are allowed to thoroughly dry before proceeding to the fabrication of custom impression trays.

Custom (Final) Impression Trays

There is general agreement among dentists that an impression made using a custom tray is necessary to achieve the desired goals of a final impression and master cast. This is because, for most patients, it is difficult to make an acceptable master cast with the proper extension and tissue detail from an impression made using an irreversible hydrocolloid impression material and a stock impression tray.

When making a final impression, the goal is to make as exact a replica of the soft and hard tissues as possible, with maximum coverage of supporting tissues and minimal extension onto movable tissues and muscle attachments. The impression must be able to be used to create a master cast that will exhibit these same characteristics. An exact replica of the tissues is necessary to create a denture/tissue interface with intimate contact throughout, which will result in excellent retention, stability, and support of the denture. When completed and inserted, an acceptable denture base should cover basically all immovable tissues on an arch. The base will also lightly contact the surrounding soft displaceable tissues but not be allowed to restrict the movement of underlying muscles and frenulum. Restricting these movements could adversely affect the function of the patient and will usually result in tissue irritation and pain to the patient.

A correctly formed tray must be fabricated so that the clinician's desired impression philosophy and technique can be achieved. It must be fabricated of a material that is rigid and stable, and easily adjusted as necessary, while not bulky. This tray material is often some type of autopolymerizing or light-activated acrylic resin.

Custom Impression Tray Extensions

The ideal coverage of a maxillary final impression tray, when evaluated intraorally, is that the tray extends to the vibrating line in the posterior and ends 2 mm away from the depth of the vestibule in the buccal and labial flange areas of the tray (Figure 6–17). A mandibular tray ends 2 mm above the depth of the vestibules in the buccal, labial, and lingual areas, and a 2 mm horizontal space would separate the tray from the tissues in the masseter notch area. It would also end 2 mm short of the extent of the retromylohyoid area. Having trays fabricated to these measurements is important because they will minimize the amount of "chair time" lost by the clinician due to tray adjustments.

Creating impression trays with these characteristics requires acceptable diagnostic casts made from excellent preliminary irreversible hydrocolloid impressions (Figure 6–18) Because the technician only has the diagnostic casts to work from, he/she must assume that the vestibular depths and extensions present on the diagnostic casts are accurate, and fabricate the trays using these measurements. Overextended or underextended preliminary impressions lead to diagnostic casts with overextended or underextended

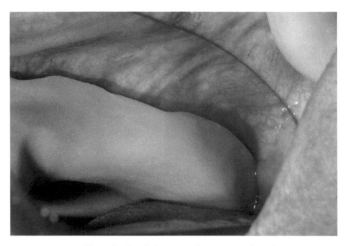

Figure 6–17   The desired 2 mm of space exists between the custom impression tray and the depth of the vestibules on this maxillary arch.

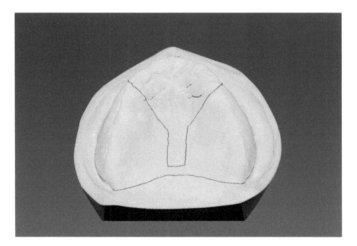

Figure 6–18   The mushroom-shaped nonstress-bearing area of the maxillary arch has been outlined. Note that the area also includes the median palatal suture area.

vestibular extensions. This results in overextended or underextended final impression trays, which often cause significant clinical delays during the final impressions appointment because of the need to excessively reduce or add to the impression trays.

Impression Philosophies as Related to Tray Fabrication

Impression philosophies differ concerning the amount and placement of pressure applied to the underlying hard and soft tissues during the impression-making procedure. Generally a clinician's impression philosophy will be "mucostatic," "functional," or "selective pressure." With the mucostatic philosophy, the clinician attempts to make the impression with minimal to no pressure to any of the underlying structures. With the selective pressure philosophy, an attempt is made to place light to moderate pressure on specific areas of the arches and minimal to no pressure on other areas.

With the functional philosophy, the clinician attempts to place mild to moderate pressure over the entire usable ridges when making the impression. This technique is generally limited to those patients with an existing denture, and the denture becomes the impression tray. The denture is lined with some type of soft flowable impression material, and the patient is allowed to wear the denture for a specific period of time. The soft lining material adapts to the underlying tissues and is used as the final impression.

Obviously the impression trays for the differing philosophies must vary in design. Therefore, the laboratory technician must know the technique to be used by the clinician when making the custom impression tray! Because it is probably the most common philosophy used, the selective pressure impression tray will be described here.

The Selective Pressure Impression Tray and Stress-Bearing Areas

This philosophy requires that the impression tray be fabricated so that, during the making of the impression, light pressure is applied to those areas of the arch that can best tolerate the anticipated functional loads, and yet minimal to no pressure is applied to those areas of the arch that are not suited to accept these loads. Those areas of the arches that can best tolerate the functional loads are called "primary" and "secondary" stress-bearing areas, while those that do not tolerate functional loads are called nonstress-bearing areas.

While opinion of the exact position of these areas may vary slightly with the individual clinician, they are reasonably well described. Generally the crest and slopes of the maxillary arch are described as "primary" and "secondary" stress-bearing areas, while the rugae and incisive foramen areas are considered nonstress bearing. The buccal shelves and slopes of the mandibular arch are generally considered to be primary and secondary areas. Because of the degree of bone loss on the mandibular arch and the resultant knife-edged ridge, the crest of the ridge on the mandibular arch will not accept functional loads on many patients and is therefore generally considered a nonstress-bearing area.

Block Out and Relief Wax

To minimize tray and cast breakage and to allow the clinician to make the impression using his/her impression philosophy, the diagnostic cast must be modified with wax prior to fabrication of the custom impression tray.

To achieve an acceptable selective pressure impression, the impression tray must be fabricated so that only those areas of the tray that overlie primary and secondary stress-bearing areas are in physical contact with those tissues during the impression procedure. The primary and secondary stress-bearing areas should be outlined on the diagnostic casts as an aid to the laboratory technician (Figures 6–18 and 6–19). Ideally,

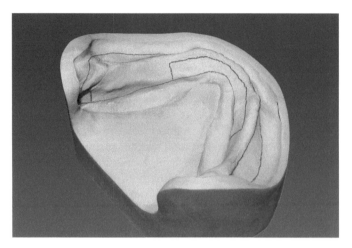

Figure 6–19   The nonstress-bearing area of the mandibular arch, primarily the crest of the residual ridge, has been outlined.

when making the impression, there should be no tray/tissue contact in those areas that overlie nonstress-bearing tissues. To create this effect, a relief chamber should be present in the tray in these areas. The relief chamber is created by applying one thickness of baseplate wax over all nonstress-bearing areas of the diagnostic cast prior to fabricating the impression tray (Figures 6–20 and 6–21). This wax is commonly called "relief wax."

Additionally, to allow tray removal from the diagnostic cast, all excessive undercuts and tissue irregularities present on the diagnostic cast are minimally relieved or blocked out using a baseplate wax. This is often referred to as "block out" wax.

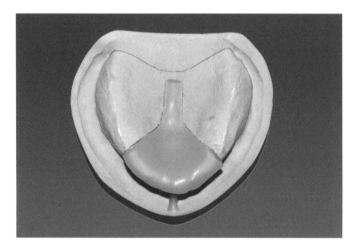

Figure 6–20   Relief wax has been properly positioned over the nonstress-bearing areas and attached to the maxillary arch. It is one thickness of baseplate wax that is attached to the cast with melted wax approximately every 12–16 mm (1/2 inch).

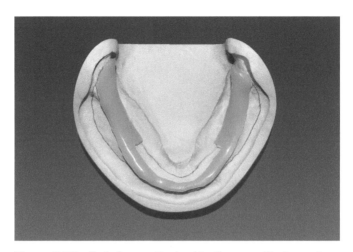

Figure 6–21   Relief wax attached to the mandibular arch over the nonstress-bearing areas.

Fabrication of the Impression Tray

The impression tray is usually fabricated of autopolymerizing or light-activated acrylic resin. When using light-activated resin, a sheet of resin is simply adapted to the diagnostic cast, which has been modified with relief and block out wax. Tray handles are formed using excess material, and the tray is polymerized following the manufacturer's recommendations. If autopolymerizing resin is used, generally a 3 to 1 ratio of polymer to

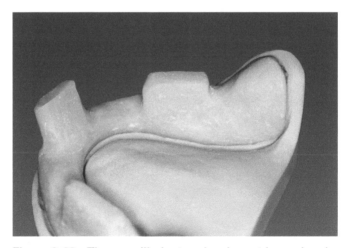

Figure 6–22   The mandibular tray has been trimmed and finished by the laboratory technician. A 2 mm space has been created between the depth of the vestibule and the flange of the tray. This same spacing should exist intraorally if the preliminary impression and diagnostic casts were not over- or underextended.

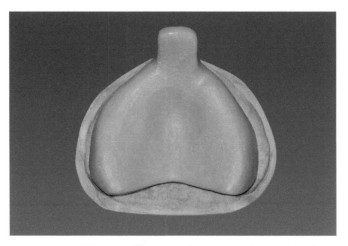

Figure 6–23   The maxillary tray has been trimmed and finished and its posterior extension ends at the vibrating line. Note that the handle projects from the tray at approximately the angulation of the natural central incisors.

monomer is mixed, formed into a resin paddy, adapted to the diagnostic cast, and allowed to polymerize. Handles can be added as desired by using additional material. The polymerized impression trays are then trimmed to the desired extent—as marked on the diagnostic cast—smoothed, and finished (Figures 6–22 & 6–23).

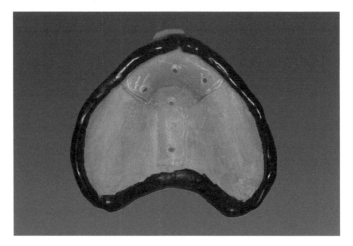

Figure 6–24   Following the border molding procedure, the relief wax is removed from the impression tray. This will provide a void (relief chamber) between the impression tray and the nonstress-bearing tissues. This spacing minimizes the possibility of physical contact between the tray and underlying tissues during the impression-making procedure. Note that multiple holes have been created in the tray to aid in the escape of the impression material and reduction of hydraulic pressure during the impression-making procedure. Although these holes may provide some retention of the impression material, that is not their primary purpose.

Clinically, following the border molding procedure, the relief wax is removed immediately prior to making the final impression, which creates a pressure-free relief chamber over the nonstress-bearing tissues (Figure 6–24) and results in pressure being primarily applied only to the primary and secondary stress-bearing areas.

References

Davis, D. M.: Developing an analogue/substitute for the maxillary denture-bearing area. In Zarb, G. A., Bolander, C. L., eds., Prosthodontic Treatment for Edentulous Patients. 12 th ed. St. Louis: Mosby Inc; 2004. pp. 221-225, pp. 243-246.

Felton, D. A., Cooper, L. F., Scurria, M. S.: Predictable impression procedures for complete dentures. In Engelmeier, R. L., ed., Complete Dentures. Dent Clin North Am. Philadelphia: W. B., Saunders, 1996; 40:43-46.

Hayakawa, I.: Principles and Practice of Complete Dentrues. Tokyo: Quintessence Publishing Co; 2001. pp. 41-42.

Rahn, A. O.: Developing complete denture impressions. In Rahn, A. O., Heartwell, C. M., editors.: Textbook of complete dentures. 5th ed. Philadelphia: Lea & Febiger; 1993. pp. 236–37.

Sowter, J. B.: Custom impression trays. In Barton R. E., ed. Removable Prosthodontic Techniques. Revised edition. Chapel Hill: University of North Carolina Press; 1986. pp. 16-22.

QUESTIONS

1. What is the primary difference in requirements between an acceptable diagnostic cast used for treatment planning for the average patient and one used for complete denture patients?

2. How does the clinician know if a particular stock impression tray is the correct size for a patient?

3. What is the purpose of periphery wax?

4. In what situation can a clinician leave an impression unattended in a patient's mouth?

5. How quickly should an irreversible hydrocolloid impression be poured?

6. What are the goals when making a final impression?

7. What are the physical characteristics of a correctly formed impression tray?

8. What are three final impressions techniques?

9. How does the selective pressure technique differ from the other two techniques?

10. What are primary, secondary, and nonstress-bearing areas?

ANSWERS

1. Diagnostic casts with inaccurate or partially missing vestibules are often acceptable when creating a treatment plan for the routine dental patient. Diagnostic casts for the complete denture patient should have all vestibules present and have accurate extensions. Accurate vestibular extensions are necessary for the creation of acceptable custom impression trays.

2. The impression tray is the correct size if it provides coverage of all desired tissues without being overextended and provides a uniform space of approximately 5–6 mm (1/4 inch) between the tissues and impression tray.

3. Periphery wax is used to change the internal contour of an impression tray as necessary to ensure proper spacing between the tray and the tissues and also to gain additional flange extension. Occasionally it may be placed on the borders of a stock tray if the flanges have sharp edges. Periphery wax should not automatically be placed on all stock trays; it should be used only when necessary.

4. Never.

5. Within 10 minutes. Once removed from the mouth, the impression is quickly rinsed, disinfected, and wrapped in wet paper towels until it can be poured.

6. The goal when making a final impression is to make as exact a replica of the soft and hard tissues as possible, have maximum acceptable coverage of supporting tissues, and have minimal extension onto the surrounding movable tissues and muscle attachments.

7. It must be fabricated of a material that is rigid and stable, easily adjusted as necessary, and not bulky.

8. Mucostatic, functional, and selective pressure.

9. With the selective pressure technique, the clinician attempts to place light-to-moderate pressure on specific areas of the arches and minimal-to-no pressure on other areas. With the mucostatic technique, an attempt is made to place minimal-to-no pressure on the supporting structures. With the functional technique, pressure to the supporting structures is desirable.

10. The primary and secondary stress-bearing areas of the arches are those areas that are best able to withstand the functional forces that are applied to a denture. The nonstress-bearing areas are those that are least able to withstand those forces. With the selective pressure technique, an effort is made to direct these functional forces to the primary and secondary stress-bearing areas and eliminate them from the nonstress-bearing areas.

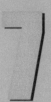

Final Impressions and Creating the Master Casts

Dr. John Ivanhoe

While the final impression appointment is important, it is essentially no more important than any other appointments. Inattention to detail on any visit will usually lead to an unsatisfactory completed denture and an unhappy patient. The goals of the clinician when making a final impression are to capture an exact likeness of the hard and soft tissues of the arches, have maximum possible extension of the impression over all tissue capable of supporting the denture, especially during function, and not to impinge on movable tissues that will be irritated by the denture during normal functional movements. Additional goals include not having pressure areas or voids within the impression (Figure 7–1). Several acceptable techniques exist for making final impressions for complete dentures that will meet these goals.

Factors that affect denture retention have been listed as atmospheric pressure, adhesion, cohesion, mechanical locks, muscle control, and patient tolerance. Additionally, intimate contact of the denture with the supporting tissues is a major factor of retention, which also dramatically improves the stability and support of the denture. Almost all of these factors are improved by maximum tissue coverage of the completed denture. However, overextension of the denture base onto movable tissue and muscle attachments will adversely affect the fit, comfort, and ability of the patient to wear the denture and therefore should be avoided.

A necessity that is often ignored or overlooked is that of the patient removing any existing dentures for a minimum of 24 hours, with 48 or 72 hours being more desirable, prior to making final impressions. Removing existing dentures prior to making final impressions is necessary to allow the underlying tissues to assume their most healthy and normal physiologic shape. Additionally, tissue irritation or indication that the patient has been wearing dentures (tissue abuse, inflamed papillary hyperplasia, or imprint of the old denture in tissue) must be eliminated prior to making the impression. This is often completed by adjusting the existing dentures, educating the patient about proper hygiene, having the patient leave the existing dentures out for at least eight hours a day, and/or relining the dentures with a tissue conditioner or interim soft liner. Once the patient has allowed tissue recovery, by leaving the dentures out for at least 24 hours, if the patient inserts a denture for even five minutes the tissues may be quickly distorted, and proper tissue recovery may require two or more additional hours of not wearing the

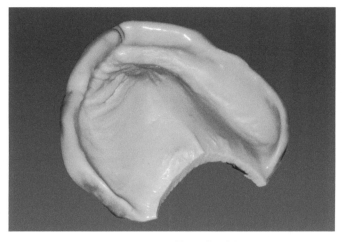

Figure 7–1   A completed maxillary final impression showing minimal pressure areas and voids

denture. Therefore patient should not "just wear their dentures into the dentist's office." When possible, impressions appointments should be scheduled early in the morning so patients do not have to go throughout the day without their dentures.

Proper Custom Impression Tray Extension

Because it is difficult to make an acceptable master cast with the proper extensions using a stock impression tray, custom impression trays become necessary. It is the responsibility of the clinician to determine which impression technique is to be used— functional, mucostatic, or selective pressure—and to outline the desired extent of the impression tray on the diagnostic cast. The desired extent of the tray should be drawn as an outline approximately 2 mm above the depth of the vestibules or obvious muscle or frenulum attachments on the labial, buccal, and lingual, and should extend posteriorly to the vibrating line on the maxillary arch and to the full extend to the retromylohyoid space on the mandibular arch. For casts indicating high muscle attachments, the tray outline may be several millimeters above the depth of the vestibule (Figure 7–2).

The laboratory technician should fabricate the custom tray so that the flanges follow the outline on the diagnostic cast (Figure 7–3). It would seem that having the impression tray 2–3 mm above the depth of the vestibule or obvious tissue attachments on the diagnostic cast would result in the tray being 2–3 mm above these areas intraorally, however this is usually not the case. Why would correctly fabricated trays on the diagnostic casts be excessively long when checked intraorally? This results from the use of an irreversible hydrocolloid impression material and stock impression tray. Because the stock trays were not properly extended custom trays, and it is difficult to properly border mold irreversible hydrocolloid impression material, the soft tissues around the borders of the impression were displaced in multiple areas. Displacement of the soft

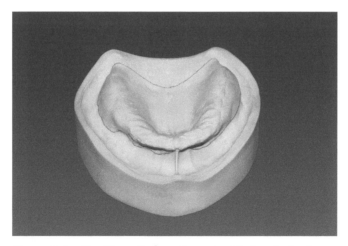

Figure 7–2 Maxillary diagnostic cast with the desired tray outline marked. Note the outline indicating the border of the tray is several millimeters above the depth of the vestibule in the anterior area because of very high frenulum and tissue attachments.

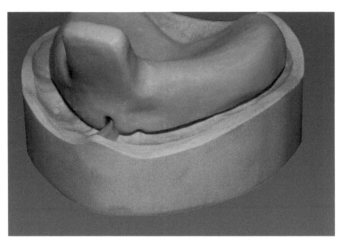

Figure 7–3 Custom impression tray fabricated with the labial and buccal borders of the tray approximately 2 mm above the depth of the vestibule. Although not visible, the posterior extent of the tray is the vibrating line.

tissues is usually in the form of the depth and width of the impression being deeper and wider than the actual useable vestibules, and the distal extent of the impression being excessively long. Hence the depth and width of the vestibules of the diagnostic cast are excessively deep and wide and often called "overextended." This would usually apply to the distal extension of the diagnostic cast as well. Therefore, even if the laboratory technician fabricates a tray that is 2–3 mm short of the depth of the vestibules, it will often impinge on the movable tissues intraorally (Figure 7–4). One of the goals in making a custom tray is to have the flanges of the tray 2–3 mm short of the actual vestibules and tissue attachments, and only visual examination intraorally by the clinician

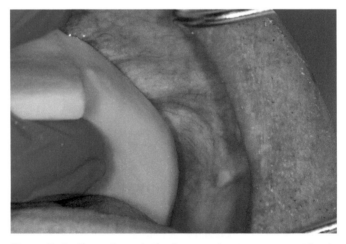

Figure 7–4 Even though the impression tray was cut back by 2 mm from the depth of the vestibule on the diagnostic cast, the borders of the tray are impinging on the movable tissues intraorally and must be shortened.

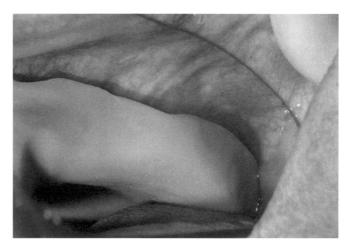

Figure 7–5   The buccal and labial flanges of the impression tray have been shortened sufficiently to create adequate space for the border molding material.

can determine if that goal was achieved. Careful attention should be paid to muscle and frenal attachment areas because the tray may require significant correction in those areas. The clinician is responsible for properly evaluating and adjusting the borders of the custom impression tray prior to initiating the border molding procedure (Figure 7–5).

In correcting the distal extension of the maxillary custom tray, one important feature to locate is the vibrating line (Figure 7–6). Although not exactly true, for clinical purposes it may be thought of as the junction between the more stable, almost immovable, hard palatal tissue and the movable tissues of the soft palate. This imaginary line

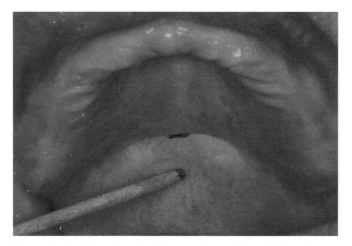

Figure 7–6   The vibrating line has been identified at the midline and is marked with an indelible marker. Note the obvious angular difference between the rather flat, hard palate and significant slope of the soft palate at the vibrating line. A noticeable change in tissue color is also present at that point.

crosses the palate, generally with an anterior curvature, and extends through the hamular notches bilaterally. Exact location of this line is important because it is the distal limit of the maxillary denture and also the distal limit of the posterior palatal seal area, which will be discussed later. Several techniques, or features, will aid the clinician in locating the vibrating line. The clinician will often visualize the position of this line by having the patient say "Ahh" and noting that the soft palatal tissues will usually lift while the hard palatal tissues remain immobile. Another technique to help locate the line is called the Valsalva maneuver in which the patient is asked attempt to blow air through their nose while the nostrils are gently pinched closed. While gently holding the tongue down with a mouth mirror, the clinician will often easily visualize the line because the soft palate will drop dramatically at the vibrating line using this technique. Other features indicating the position of this line may include a rather sharp color change between the hard and soft palatal tissues at the vibrating line and/or the presence of the fovea near the line. Lastly, and often the easiest to visualize, may be the rather significant angular change between the rather flat hard palate and the moderately to severely sloping soft palate. This junction indicates the vibrating line. Extension of the denture beyond the vibrating line will result in the denture terminating on excessively movable tissue and often cause lack of retention or irritation to the tissue. The vibrating line is located and marked using an indelible pencil or marker, and the impression tray is trimmed to this line (Figure 7–7).

The same general procedures are followed for the mandibular impression tray with the exception being that there is no vibrating line to be located. Unique difficulties associated with correcting the flange length of the mandibular tray include difficulty in visualizing the lingual border of the impression tray and the presence of a fatty roll of tissue often present in the masseter muscle areas (Figure 7–8). Extra care is necessary when reducing the tray in the masseter/buccinator muscles area because impinging on these tissues will cause irritation and discomfort to the patient and dislodgement of the completed denture when the patient opens his or her mouth. A properly shaped mandibular impression tray will most often exhibit the following three features: First the

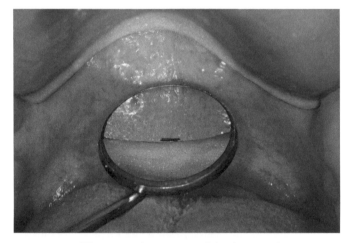

Figure 7–7 The posterior extent of the impression tray is shortened to coincide with the vibrating line. The tray is shortened to the proper length at the midline area and then a smooth curve is created, in most patients, which flows through the hamular notches.

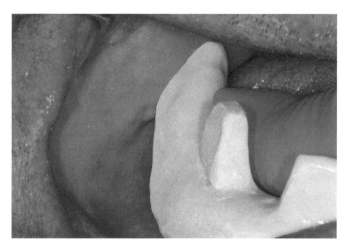

Figure 7–8   The fatty roll of tissue in the masseter muscle area must be removed from beneath the impression tray when evaluating the extension of the tray. Note the smooth slope of the impression tray from the vestibular area to the retromolar pad area. See Figure 10. Patients do not exhibit any sharp corners in the tissues in this area.

labial and lingual flanges in the anterior area will be approximately the same length unless the patient has had some type vestibular extension surgical procedure or severe loss of the residual ridge (Figure 7–9). Second, the distal-buccal flange will gradually taper from the vestibule to the crest of the residual ridge, often at approximately a 45 to 60⁰ angle, (Figure 7–10) and continuously flow into the retromylohyoid area (Figure 7–11). The longest part of the tray should be just lingual to the crest of the ridge with a smooth curvature mimicking the shape of the retromylohyoid curtain. And lastly,

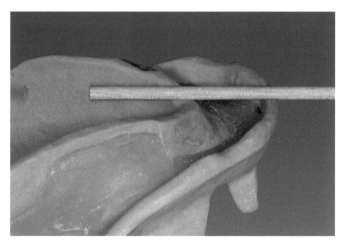

Figure 7–9   For most patients, the labial and lingual flange lengths will be of equal length unless the patient has had a surgical extension of the vestibular notch or severe bone loss resulting in the genial tubercle being elevated.

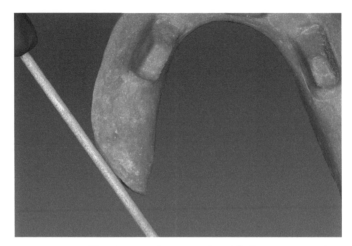

Figure 7–10 The impression tray should show a smooth continuous decrease in flange length as it continues from the buccal shelf area to the crest of the ridge. Patients do not exhibit sharp corners in this area intraorally.

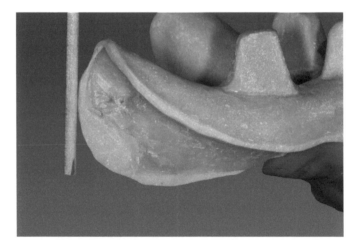

Figure 7–11 The border of the impression tray should continue as a smooth, continuous line from the masseter muscle area to the retromylohyoid area with the longest part of the tray located just lingual to the retromolar pad. This flange area should be gently rounded to mimic the shape of the retromylohyoid curtain.

the lingual flange will begin at the level of the labial flange in the anterior area and gradually become longer than the buccal flange as it approaches the retromylohyoid area (Figure 7–12). It generally exhibits a smooth continuous form, not an irregular shape, as it progresses from the anterior to the posterior. Once all extensions have been corrected, the impression trays are ready for border molding.

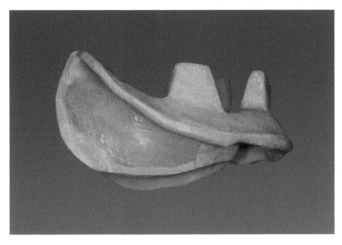

Figure 7–12 The lingual flange of the tray should resemble a smooth continuous line beginning at the level of the labial flange in the anterior and gradually increasing in length, as compared to the buccal flange, as it approaches and enters the retromylohyoid area.

Border Molding

Border molding is the technique for correctly extending the flanges of a custom impression tray. The flanges were intentionally adjusted intraorally to be 2–3 mm short of the actual desired final extent of the final impression to allow room for the border-molding material. The correction is completed using a soft but slightly viscous impression material that becomes at least semi-rigid as it cools, or polymerizes. This material is slightly overextended on the tray beyond the 3–4 mm the tray was shortened, thereby assuring at least complete coverage of all usable tissues (Figure 7–13). Once inserted and prior to the impression material becoming rigid, the soft tissues are manipulated until the desired extensions are recorded in this soft material (Figure 7–14). The technique is continued until the correct extension of the entire impression tray is captured (Figure 7–15).

Several materials have been used to border mold an impression tray, including modeling compound, heavy bodied vinyl polysiloxane and polyether materials. Green modeling compound is an excellent material with advantages and disadvantages. One advantage of modeling compound is that, if the final impression must be remade, often the impression material can be removed from the impression tray and the modeling compound border molding can be reused. Another advantage is that, because of its rigidity, it can be used to extend custom impression trays whose borders have become excessively short, more than 3–4 mm, of the desired final extension. Once chilled in ice water, this rigidity also allows the trimming of the material without fear of distortion. Another advantage is that, even when acceptably soft for border molding purposes, it is generally sufficiently viscous to retain its form. This often provides an ideal width (2–3 mm) to the tray flange. A disadvantage of modeling compound is that the need for planned

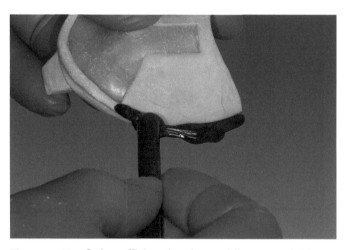

Figure 7–13 Only sufficient border molding material is added to the impression tray to slightly overfill the space created when the tray was shortened 2 mm from the depth of the vestibule. Therefore only approximately 3 mm of border molding material is required to assure complete fill of the vestibule. Excess material will overextend the flange length.

preparation and the use of several pieces of equipment and materials, including a water bath, a Bunsen burner, petrolatum jelly, sharp trimming knife, and an alcohol torch. Modeling compound is acceptably soft and yet not uncomfortably hot, between approximately 49^0C (120^0 F) and 60^0 C (140^0 F). Setting the hot water bath to the upper limit of this range provides an acceptable but minimal working time. Therefore only reasonably small areas of the borders can be corrected before the material cools and becomes

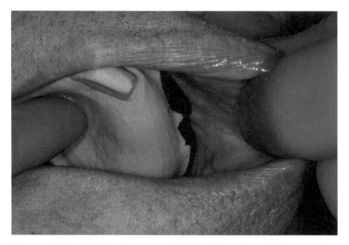

Figure 7–14 While the material is still softened, the border molding movements are completed. When removed from the mouth, if the impression tray shows through the border molding material, the tray was insufficiently reduced. Any border molding material should be removed, the tray further reduced, and the border molding procedure repeated.

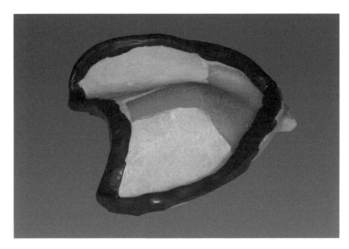

Figure 7–15   The border molding is completed, and all excess material has been removed. The material should be no more than 2–3 mm in height above the tray flange and only as thick as the desired flanges of the completed denture (2–3 mm). Additionally there should be no areas in which the impression tray has shown through the material.

too rigid to be useful. The material must be very soft to be used effectively and therefore must remain in the mouth for approximately 15 seconds to be sufficiently rigid not to distort when being removed from the mouth. It must immediately be immersed in ice water and become rigid before attempting to trim any excess material. A sharp knife blade must be used to allow for trimming of the material rather than breakage. Another disadvantage is that, once cooled, because of its rigidity it is often difficult to place and remove from bilateral undercut areas, particularly the retromylohyoid areas, without causing trauma to the tissues and discomfort to the patient.

Heavy bodied vinyl polysiloxane (VPS) is another excellent material for border molding. An advantage of this material is that it is a simple material to work with that requires minimal equipment. Additionally, because the working times of varieties of VPS vary, from approximately two to eight minutes, the clinician can select the one that best fits his/her impression technique. Generally a material with a working time of about two or three minutes in the mouth provides plenty of time to border mold and is ideal. Another advantage to using VPS is that, even when polymerized, it remains reasonably soft and yet acceptably rigid, and can be removed from undercut areas with minimal discomfort to the patient. An additional advantage of VPS is that, because of the extended working time as compared to modeling compound, it is often possible to border mold an extended border of an impression tray at one time as opposed to having to complete it one smaller section at a time, as is necessary with modeling compound. If an area of the border molding must be redone, it is quite simple to add additional material and repeat the procedure. A disadvantage to border molding and making the final impression with VPS is that the border molding and impression materials bond during polymerization and cannot be separated when desired. Therefore, if the final impression is not acceptable and must be remade, the border molding material will often be lost during the process of removing the impression material from the tray, resulting in the necessity of repeating the border molding procedure. Another disadvantage is that VPS adhesive must be used to bond the material to the impression tray requiring several minutes to set. This time may simply be lost to the clinician if the impression procedures are not properly planned. VPS does not have the viscosity or rigidity of modeling compound and therefore cannot be used to correct borders that are underextended by more than 4–5 mm. Also if not supported by the impression tray, VPS cannot be depended on to form tray flanges 2–3 mm in thickness. This is especially noticeable in the retromylohyoid areas, where the distal extent of the border molding and final impression is often thinned by the tongue to a "knife edge." This may result in a master cast with an indistinct shape in this area, which could result in a completed denture with an inaccurate border length and thickness.

Border Molding with Modeling Compound

Because of its minimal working time, border molding using modeling compound must be completed in multiple reasonably small areas (Figures 7–16 and 7–17). Once the compound is added to a flange area of the impression tray, the material is tempered in the hot water bath for approximately 5 to 8 seconds, placed in the mouth, border molded, and allowed to stay in the mouth for approximately 15 seconds following the border molding procedure. The impression tray is removed and immediately placed in ice water until rigid. It then must be examined and trimmed as necessary. The material has a dull, matte, surface when properly formed. The completed border should be approximately 2–3 mm in width in order to approximate the desired thickness of the flange of the completed denture. The material is then rechecked intraorally to ensure complete fill of the border and yet show no evidence of overextension. If the soft tissues are being displaced more than a slight amount, the material is overextended and the border molding technique must be repeated. If the impression tray is showing

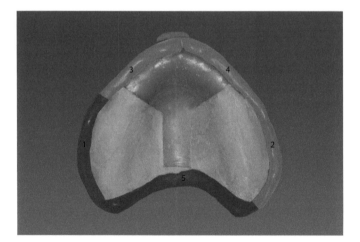

Figure 7–16   Because of the limited working time when using modeling compound to border mold, the border molding must be done in reasonably small sections. This is not necessary when using vinyl polysiloxane. The suggested sequence for border molding the maxillary arch, when using modeling compound, is illustrated.

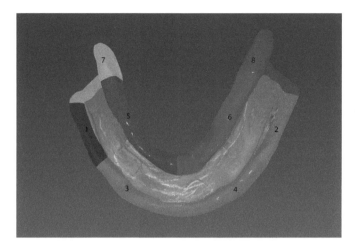

Figure 7-17 The suggested sequence for border molding the mandibular arch when using modeling compound. It is possible to border mold the longer segments of the mandibular tray with VPS, however, the material in the retromylohyoid area will almost always be "knife-edge" thin, if not manipulated correctly.

through the material, the material must be removed, the tray shortened, and the border molding repeated. Once one section is totally completed, a second section can be border molded. When completed, the material should smoothly flow from one area to the next without visible lines of demarcation. Each area must be totally completed prior to starting another area. Remember, once completed, the height of the border molding material above the tray should be no more than 2–3 mm because that was the amount of space created between the soft tissue and the impression tray prior to border molding.

Border Molding the Maxillary Arch

The initial border molding of the maxillary arch should begin with either the left or right buccal flange area. The modeling compound is added, and this area and border are molded by grasping the cheek between the thumb and fingers and manipulating the tissue outward, downward, and inward. The opposite area is then completed.

Observe the attachment of the buccal frenum. When border molding the frenulum area, move the cheek out, down, in, backward, and forward. This movement is necessary as the tissue in the region of the buccal frenum moves anteroposteriorly. Repeat for the opposite side.

Next, observe the space in the labial vestibule and the size of the labial frenum. During border molding of this region, the contour of the impression must be adjusted so that the lip is not over-supported. The labial flange should not be thinner than 2 mm at the completion of the border molding procedure, or it will not adequately support the final impression material. It should also not be more than 4 mm thick. Modeling compound is placed from the canine region on one side around to the midline, and this area is border molded by pulling the upper lip outward, downward, and inward. A side-to-side movement is not indicated because the labial frenum does not function in this manner. Repeat for the opposite side.

The final area to be border molded is the posterior extent of the tray. Impression compound is placed across the posterior portion of the tray from just buccal to the hamular notch on one side to the same position on the other side. Because the tray has been trimmed to the proper length, to the vibrating line, the compound should be placed within the tray and not extended beyond the posterior extent of the tray. The compound should be no more than 1–2 mm in thickness and 3–4 mm in width. Have the patient open his or her mouth wide, then protrude and move the mandible to the right and to the left. This action develops the distal extent of the denture in the hamular notch and also develops the space between the anterior border of the ramus coronoid process and the tuberosity. When using VPS, the entire border may be completed in one step using the same border-molding techniques as listed previously. Many clinicians find border molding half the tray at one time a much more controllable procedure. Depending on the complexity of the impression and the experience of the clinician, even smaller segments may be done with the VPS material.

 ## Border Molding the Mandibular Arch

When border molding with modeling compound, have the tongue slightly elevated whenever the heated compound impression is placed in the patient's mouth. This will facilitate the placing of the impression and will minimize distortion of the impression compound.

The buccal shelf areas are initially border molded and must be completed individually. Do not attempt to complete them simultaneously because the useful softness of the compound is only approximately 10 seconds. Add modeling compound to the right or left buccal shelf areas of the tray from the distal of the buccal frenum to the anterior part of the retromolar pad regions. Place the tray in the patient's mouth and border mold by manipulating the cheek outward, upward, and inward. Remove and chill. Repeat for the opposite side.

Border molding of the buccal and labial borders and frenulum are completed in a manner similar to what is done on the maxillary arch, with the exception of the lips or cheeks being manipulated outward, upward, and inward. The buccal notches will almost always be shorter and narrower than the adjacent borders.

Next add compound through the retromolar pad regions (doing each separately) and while inserting making sure to pull any fatty roll of tissue in the masseter area from beneath the impression material prior to final placement. The patient is asked to close onto the clinician's fingers while the clinician resists the closure movement and gently presses downward on the tray. This procedure forces the masseter muscle into action; the masseter, in turn, forces the buccinator in the direction of the distal buccal corner of the retromolar pad, creating the masseter groove.

The distolingual and postmylohyoid areas should be developed next by having the patient forcefully protrude the tongue and move it from side to side. This procedure develops the slope of the lingual flange in the molar region as well as the remaining length of the flange. If modeling compound excessively builds up inside of the lingual flange, it should be reduced, the material should be reheated, and the border molding procedure repeated.

Add modeling compound to the anterior region of the lingual flange if necessary and instruct the patient to push the tongue against the front part of the hard palate. This procedure develops the width of and length of the anterior lingual flange.

Border molding of the retromylohyoid areas are left until last because of the areas being bilaterally undercut in relation to each other. When using modeling compound, especially once chilled, it is often physically difficult to get an impression tray into and out of these areas. Also, if these areas are completed early on in the border molding sequence, it may make the remainder of the border molding quite uncomfortable to the patient. Add modeling compound to one distal-lingual flange area and instruct the patient to "open and protrude the tongue" to activate the retromylohyoid curtain and then to "close down on my fingers" to activate the medial pterygoid muscles, which function posteriorly to the curtain and tend to displace it forward. As the patient closes, resist the closure by downward pressure of the fingers to cause the medial pterygoid muscles to contract. If a formed border is not present or if the border is knife edged, the flange is usually too short. This procedure may have to be repeated several times to achieve the desired results. These areas are difficult to properly form and take skill to complete.

Lastly, heat the compound in the retromolar pad areas, temper, place the impression tray in the mouth, and instruct the patient to "open wide." This procedure reduces pressure over the retromolar pad areas. If the border is too long, a notch will be formed at the posterior medial border indicating the upward passage of the pterygomandibular raphe. Border molding of the mandibular impression is completed.

It is not possible to border mold the entire mandibular arch at one time using VPS material. The tray should be stabilized by border molding the buccal shelf areas and then completed as the clinician's experience level dictates. The retromylohyoid areas may require more than one insertion to develop the proper border thickness. On subsequent insertions with additional border molding material added, the area can be more easily thickened if the patient closes slightly as the tray is positioned and asked to moisten their lips gently to accomplish the border molding.

Preparing the Tray for the Impression

Any "relief wax" is removed from the tray. For the selective pressure technique, this creates a void or chamber between the nonprimary stress-bearing tissues of the arches and impression trays. This chamber minimizes the possibility of physical pressure from the tray to the tissues during the impression-making procedure. Any sharp ridges at the resin/wax interface are smoothed with an acrylic bur. Additionally, approximately five #8 round bur sized holes are cut through the tray in the chamber areas (Figure 7–18). These holes allow the relief of hydraulic pressures that will build because of the viscous impression material being squeezed between the tissues and the impression tray. No relief of the border molding material is normally required because most impression materials will be minimally viscous and therefore no extra space is required for the material. If a viscous impression material is selected, then approximately 0.5 millimeter of the border molding material should be removed. Adhesive specific to the particular impression material

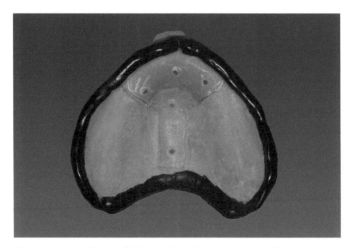

Figure 7-18   The relief wax has been removed from the impression tray creating a relief chamber in the area. All sharp edges have been rounded, and five relief holes have been prepared using a #8 round bur.

being used is applied to the entire tissue side of the tray and extends onto the labial and buccal surfaces approximately 4 mm. All impression compound border molding material should be coated with the adhesive.

Making the Final Impression

The final impression is made using the desired impression material. Some of the characteristics of an ideal material include being minimally viscous, polymerizing (setting) intraorally within 2–3 minutes, being hydrophyllic, being thixotropic, not flowing once removed from the mouth, not being excessively rigid, not being excessively expensive, being well tolerated by the tissues, being exacting in recording and maintaining tissue details, and the ability to be poured in a dental stone more than once.

The selected impression material is mixed according to the manufacturer's directions and applied evenly to the tray to a thickness of approximately 3 mm, being careful to avoid capturing air bubbles within the material. Only this minimal thickness of impression material is needed because a custom impression tray, rather than a stock tray, is being used and was fabricated to closely fit the underlying tissues. Because most impression materials are hydrophobic, while the impression tray is being loaded, the tissues to be captured in the impression should be freed of moisture. The patient should swallow all excess saliva, and the tissues should be carefully dried with 2 x 2 sponge gauze.

When inserting the impression tray, the clinician must carefully observe the seating of the tray onto the tissues. Before completely seating the impression, the clinician must properly position the impression tray over the ridge so that the anterior flange of the tray will seat properly and completely into the labial vestibule. When seating the mandibular impression tray, the clinician must take special care to not capture any fatty roll of tissue in the masseter muscle area as part of the impression. This can be accomplished by pulling this roll of tissue from beneath the tray on one side of the arch, slightly seating that side of the tray, pulling the opposing roll of tissue from beneath that side of the tray, and then partially seating this side of the tray. For the final seating, the patient should be asked to lift the tongue and, as the impression is being seated. the patient should be directed to relax the tongue. This procedure will minimize capturing the tongue, salivary glands, and other nondesirable areas within the impression. A similar procedure is accomplished when making the maxillary impression with the addition of having the patient move the mandible in extreme lateral motions as part of the impression procedure. This movement will cause the coronoid processes to help contour the lateral borders of the impression in the tuberosity areas.

Border molding of the impression must be initiated before the impression material begins to polymerize and must continue until the material begins to polymerize. If tissue manipulation is stopped prior to the initial polymerization, the material may again flow beyond the desired extensions, causing excessive thinning of the borders and overextension of the impression. Manufacturer's directions are followed for mixing and setting times of all materials.

Care is often required to minimize patient discomfort when removing an impression. On the maxillary arch this discomfort may be caused by excessive retention of the impression within the mouth. Generally an index finger can be used to lift the tissues away from one of the flange areas, which breaks the border seal by allowing air under the impression. On the mandibular arch this discomfort may be caused by the impression extending into bilateral undercuts in the retromylohyoid areas.

The impressions should be rinsed and then disinfected before further handling. The maxillary impression is trimmed back to within 1 mm of the vibrating line. Every impression must be objectively evaluated by the clinician to assure its accuracy and remade when necessary. (Table 7–1).

Table 7–1	REASONS FOR REMAKING IMPRESSIONS

1. Incorrect tray position in the mouth. A thick border on one side with a corresponding thin border on the opposite side is a good indication that the tray was out of position in the direction of the thick border. Pressure spots on the lingual surface of the maxillary labial flange usually indicate that the tray was not fully seated. Pressure spots on the anterior part of the mandibular lingual flange indicate that the mandibular tray is too far forward in the mouth, in many instances as a result of action of the tongue.
2. Pressure areas in secondary stress bearing areas, e.g., the region of the crest of the ridge of the mandibular tray or the rugae region of the maxillary tray.
3. Any void or discrepancy too large to accurately correct. Some voids may be corrected by adding new impression material to the impression and reinserting however any impression with a void this large generally should be remade in its entirety. Small voids may be correctable on the master cast since they will result in positive bubbles that can be removed with a cleoid/discoid instrument.
4. Incorrect border formation as a result of incorrect border length of the tray—a sharp border may indicate that the impression is too short in that area.
5. Incorrect consistency of the final impression material when the tray was positioned in the mouth.
6. Distortion of the impression material because of movement of the tray during the setting of the final impression material.

Posterior Palatal Seal Area

Probably the most critical of the retention factors listed earlier is that of atmospheric pressure. When the pressure of the air between the denture base and the underlying tissues is less that that of the atmospheric air pressure, excellent retention of the denture is expected, and patients often refer to this retention as suction. This retention is lost, most noticeably from the maxillary arch, if the denture/tissue contact (seal) around the denture borders has been lost and air is freely allowed between the denture and the underlying tissues. A loss of this seal is often caused by resin shrinkage during polymerization. Acrylic resin shrinks toward the area of greatest bulk of the denture, which is generally around the denture teeth. On the maxillary arch, this shrinkage usually results in the creation of a good seal around the labial and buccal sides of the denture and loss of seal at distal extent of the denture as it crosses the palate. In this area, as the resin shrinks toward the denture teeth, it tends to lift away from the cast resulting in a future loss of the seal and hence loss of denture retention. This shrinkage must be anticipated and steps taken to help ensure that resin/tissue contact will exist following processing. Some newer injection molding techniques minimize this problem. Be sure to check with the material manufacturer regarding recommendations concerning palatal seal areas.

This technique is called the placement of a posterior palatal seal within the denture. The procedure consists of an initial identification of compressible tissue in the posterior of the hard palate and the determination of the depth to which this tissue could be comfortably compressed by the denture base. The posterior limit of the posterior palatal seal area is the vibrating line, which extends from just buccal (2 mm) to one hamular notch area across the palate to just buccal to the opposite hamular notch (Figure 7–19). At the vibrating line, the tissue in the posterior palatal seal area can be compressed approximately 0.5 mm deep in the hamular notches and midline areas and 1 mm deep in other areas however the exact depth for a specific patient is determined by palpation. Intraoral identification of this area is eventually followed by a laboratory procedure, which consists of the removal of an area of stone from the master cast that corresponds to the amount of displaceable tissue palpated intraorally. The depth of stone to be removed from the cast is generally deepest toward the vibrating line and feathers to an indistinct anterior border.

When acceptable, the impression should be disinfected, prior to removing it from the operatory, and the posterior palatal seal area should be drawn on the impression with an indelible pencil (Figure 7–20), It can then be taken to the laboratory, beaded, boxed, and poured using an ADA-approved dental cast stone of choice following manufacturer's directions.

Creating the Master Cast

Acceptable master casts should be of the proper thickness, bubble and void free, and include an accurate representation of all impressed tissue surfaces and surrounding finished borders, often called land areas.

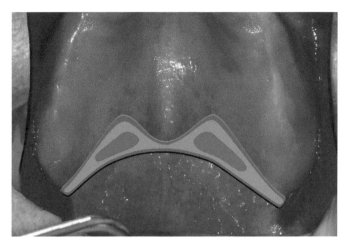

Figure 7-19   The shape of the average posterior palatal seal area is indicated in blue. Note that the black line, indicating the vibrating line, is the most distal extent of both the posterior palatal seal area and the completed denture. The green area represents an area of the hard palate that often has soft tissue than can be compressed approximately .5 mm. The orange area indicates the tissue that can generally be compressed approximately 1 mm. This degree of compressible tissue varies with each patient and must be determined intraorally. Stone will be removed from the master cast in this shape and depth as a laboratory procedure ending in a "feather edge" in the anterior.

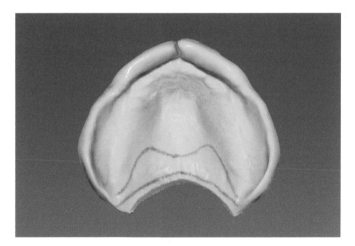

Figure 7-20   The completed maxillary final impression with the outline of the posterior palatal seal drawn on the impression with an indelible marker. Note that, even though not indicated on the impression, the posterior palatal seal will extend approximately 2 mm through the hamular notch areas.

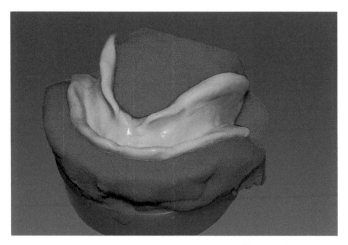

Figure 7–21 Play-doh ™ is used to form the beading/base for this mandibular impression. Note that the borders of the impression are at least 2 mm above the Play-doh™.

Prior to attempting to pour the final impressions, a form should be created around the impressions to simplify the procedure and to give the proper size and shape to the master casts by confining the dental stone while the impressions are poured. The procedure for developing this form is called "beading and boxing" the impressions. The purpose of beading impressions is to define the impression surfaces and also to aid in supporting the impressions during pouring. The impression surface is defined by creating shoulders outside the impressed tissue surfaces of the impression (Figure 7–21). Boxing is the process of enclosing the impression and beading material to confine the dental stone to both the desired shape and thickness, to minimize trimming the cast and excess use of the dental stone (Figure 7–22). Boxing is routinely completed with a wax made especially for this purpose, while beading is often done with a rope-type wax, Play-

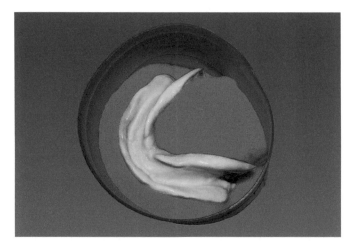

Figure 7–22 Boxing wax has been positioned around the beading/base material and is sealed to minimize loss of dental stone during the pouring of the impression.

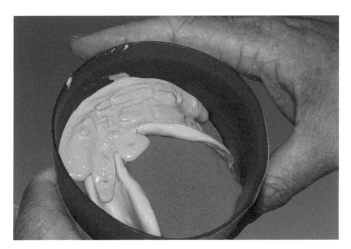

Figure 7–23 The initial pour of the stone into the impression is shown here. The stone is added in small increments and is slowly moved posteriorly using a vibrator set to a moderate to low vibration rate. Note the position of the thumbs and fingers. They are positioned to minimize the possibility of collapsing the boxing wax during the pouring of the impression.

doh™, irreversible hydrocolloid, or a mixture of stone and pumice. Both the beading and boxing materials must be inexpensive, easily handled by the technician, and sufficiently strong to retain size and shape while the impressions are poured (Figure 7–23). When the stone sets, it should then be reasonably easy to remove from both the master casts and impressions.

Once the stone has set and the beading and boxing materials have been separated from the master casts, the casts are trimmed to the final size and shape using model trimmer, acrylic burs, and laboratory knives. The bottom and sides of the base of the cast should be trimmed in a specific sequence to ensure an acceptable final result. When completed, the casts should be trimmed so that the ridges are parallel to the bottom of the base, and the base is of the proper thickness. Because most casts are often not poured with the proper thickness and ridge/bottom parallelism (Figure 7–24), the bottom of the cast should be trimmed first (Figure 7–25) until the crests of the residual ridges are parallel to the bottom of the cast and the cast is approximately the correct thickness. The thinnest portion of the master cast should be approximately 12–15 mm in thickness, which results in the cast being thick enough to resist breakage and yet thin enough to eventually fit into a processing flask (Figure 7–26). Remember, the thinnest portion of a cast is generally going to be between the depth of the vestibule and the bottom of the cast. The sides of the base of the cast can then be trimmed on a model trimmer until the width of the land areas is approximately 2–3 mm on the buccal and labial (Figure 7–27), and approximately 5–6 mm distal to the hamular notches and retromolar pads. Once the cast is dry, the level of the land areas and tongue area can be contoured and smoothed with an arbor band or acrylic bur until the vestibules are approximately 2–3 mm in depth and the land areas are parallel with the bottom of the cast (Figure 7–28). An excellent finish can be placed on the cast using silicon carbide wet/dry 320 sandpaper. When completed the master casts (Figures 7–28 and 7–29) are ready for the fabrication of record bases and occlusion rims.

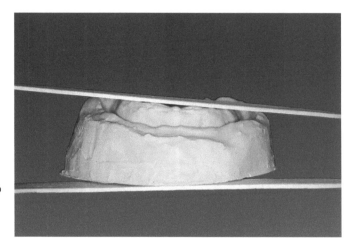

Figure 7–24 Note that the crests of the residual ridges are not parallel to the bottom of the base of the cast following the initial pour of the master cast.

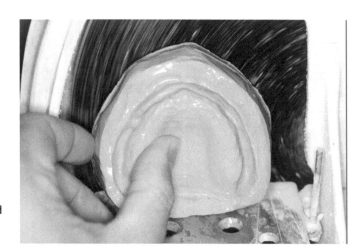

Figure 7–25 Prior to trimming the sides of the base of the cast, the bottom is trimmed in order to achieve an acceptable thickness and to make the ridges parallel to the bottom of the base.

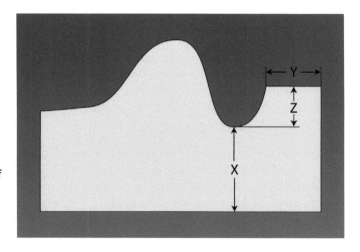

Figure 7–26 The thinnest portion of this cast is in the vestibule. (X) The minimum thickness of a master cast should be 12–15 mm in the thinnest area.

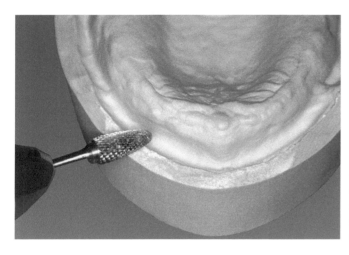

Figure 7–27   Once all trimming has been completed on the model trimmer and the cast has been allowed to dry, the land areas can be properly trimmed. The land areas should be trimmed so that the vestibules are no more than 3 mm in depth. Also see Z in Figure 7–26.

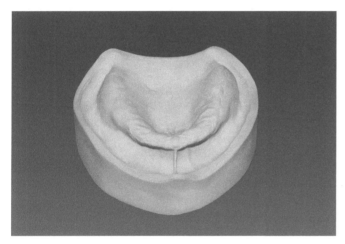

Figure 7–28   An example of a well-shaped and finished maxillary master cast.

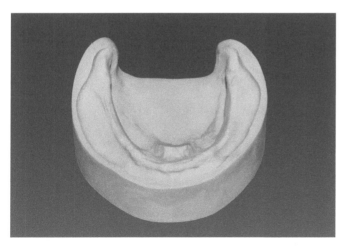

Figure 7–29   An example of a well-shaped and finished mandibular master cast.

References

Avant, W.: A comparison of the retention of complete denture bases having different types of posterior palatal seal. J Prosthet Dent. 1973;484-93.

Duncan, J. P., Taylor, T. D.: Simplified complete dentures. Dent Clin North Am. 2004;48:625-40.

Felton, D. A., Cooper, L. F., Scurria, M. S.: Predictable impression procedures for complete dentures. In Engelmeier, R.L., ed. Complete Dentures. Dent Clin North Am. Philadelphia: W.B. Saunders, 1996;40:39-51.

Kolb, H.: Variable denture-limiting structures of the edentulous mouth. Part I: Maxillary border areas. J Prosthet Dent. 1966;16:194-201, pp. 202-212.

Petrie, C. S., Walker, M. P., Williams, K.: A survey of U.S. prosthodontists and dental schools on the current materials and methods for final impressions for complete denture prosthodontics. J Prosthodont. 2005;14:253-262.

Petropoulos, V. C., Rashedi, B.: Complete denture education in U.S. dental schools. J Prosthodont. 2005;14:191-7.

Rahn, A. O.: Developing Complete denture impressions. In: Rahn, A. O., Heartwell, C. M., editors. Textbook of complete dentures. 5th ed. Philadelphia: Lea & Febiger; 1993. pp. 221–247.

QUESTIONS

1. What feature of a completed denture routinely increases the factors of retention?

2. What is the distal extent of a maxillary complete denture?

3. What is border molding?

4. Why is the "relief wax" removed from an impression tray just before making the final impression?

5. Why are multiple #6 or #8 round burr-sized holes cut into the impression tray just prior to making the final impression?

6. What is the location of the posterior palatal seal area, and what is its anterior and posterior limits?

7. How does the clinician minimize the capturing of the roll of tissue, seen in many patients in the masseter muscle areas, within the impression?

8. What are some of the characteristics of a good impression material?

9. What are some of the disadvantages of using modeling compound as a border-molding material?

10. Why should a maxillary denture not be extended onto the movable soft palate?

ANSWERS

1. Maximum tissue coverage

2. Vibrating line

3. Border molding is the technique of properly extending the flange length of an impression tray prior to making the final impression.

4. Removal of the relief wax creates a chamber, or relief area, within the impression tray that reduces the chance of physical pressure from the impression tray to the underlying nonstress-bearing tissues.

5. To reduce the hydraulic pressure that builds up within the impression caused by the viscous impression material being trapped between the impression tray and the underlying tissues.

6. Anterior limit is nonspecific and depends upon the available displaceable tissue. The posterior limit is the vibrating line.

7. By pulling the tissue from beneath the impression tray while seating the tray.

8. Is minimally viscous, polymerized intraorally within 2–3 minutes, is hydrophyllic, is thixotropic, will not flow once removed from the mouth, is not excessively rigid, is not excessively expensive, is well tolerated by the tissues, is very exacting in recording and maintaining tissue details, and can be poured in a dental stone more than once.

9. Planned preparation and the usage of several pieces of equipment and materials are required. Only reasonably small areas of the borders can be corrected at a time before the material cools and becomes too rigid to be used properly. Once cooled, because of its rigidity, it is very difficult to place and remove from bilateral undercut areas—particularly the retromylohyoid areas—without causing trauma to the tissues and discomfort to the patient.

10. Retention of the denture may be compromised, and the denture may cause irritation and trauma to the soft movable tissues.

CHAPTER

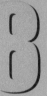

Record Bases and Occlusion Rims

Dr. Arthur O. Rahn
Dr. John R. Ivanhoe

At this time the clinician has completed making the final impression and fabrication of the master casts for the maxillary and mandibular arches. These casts will be used throughout the remainder of the denture construction, and the dentures will be processed on them. Prior to that time, jaw relation records will be made, the casts will be placed on an articulator, and denture teeth will be arranged on these casts. Therefore a method becomes necessary to accurately attach the opposing maxillary and mandibular casts to an articulator. This requires the use of record bases and occlusion rims (Figures 8–1 and 8–2).

The record base and occlusion rim are necessary for (1) establishing facial contours, (2) an aid in tooth selection, (3) establishing and maintaining the vertical dimension of occlusion during records making, (4) making interocclusal records, (5) the arrangement of the denture teeth, (6) the verification of the correct master cast mounting on the articulator, at the esthetic trial insertion appointment, and (7) a waxed-up mold for the external surface of the complete denture.

Record Base Fabrication

A satisfactory record base must be stable on both the master casts and intraorally. It should be rigid, accurately adapted to the casts, fully cover the entire supporting tissues of the arches, and also esthetic and comfortable to the patient. For strength, rigidity, and good adaptation of the bases on the cast and intraorally, autopolymerizing acrylic resin is generally the material of choice for their construction.

To protect the master casts, tissue undercuts and irregularities are blocked out with baseplate wax (Figures 8–3). This blocking out of the undercuts is particularly important when initially separating the record base from the master cast, which may result in a broken cast and the need for new final impressions and casts to be made. The common locations for undercuts or irregularities on the maxillary casts are on the labial of the

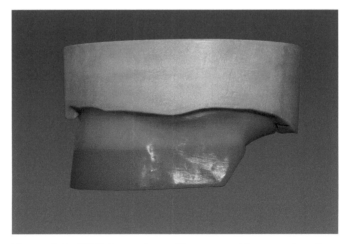

Figure 8–1   Well-formed maxillary record base and occlusion rim.

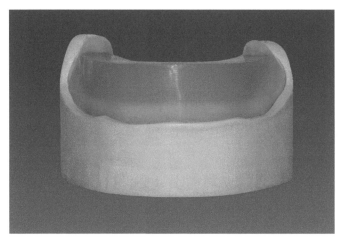

Figure 8–2   Well-formed mandibular record base and occlusion rim.

anterior ridge, in the rugae areas, and sometimes in the tuberosity areas laterally. On the mandibular cast, the retromylohyoid areas often must be rather heavily blocked out, and in many situations the posterior inferior portion of the record base is not ever extended into these areas. This is because these areas are often severely undercut in relation to each other, and the master cast may be damaged or the record base broken during its placement and removal from the cast.

Wax used in blocking out buccal and lingual undercuts should be applied in sufficient thickness to almost completely block out most undercuts. An exception is the

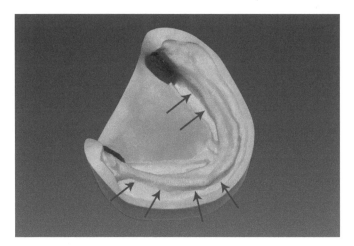

Figure 8–3   On this mandibular cast, note that undercuts on the labial and lingual side of the thin ridge have been blocked out with thin layers of baseplate wax (arrows), whereas in the more severely undercut retromylohyoid areas, the area has been entirely blocked out with red utility wax. The record base will not completely extend into the retromylohyoid area.

undercut on the labial or anterior portion of the maxillary cast, which need not be completely eliminated; the completed record base and occlusion rim can be placed and removed in an anterior direction. The adequacy of the block out may be evaluated by looking down on the cast from the direction that the record base will be placed and removed from the cast.

Following the block out of the master cast, the cast is soaked in room-temperature water for five minutes in order to expel air from within the stone, which will help minimize the formation of bubble-like defects in the completed record base. Air bubbles frequently will rise to the surface from within the master casts when separating medium and/or monomer is applied to the casts unless they have been soaked. The soaking of the cast must be completed after the cast has been blocked out with wax because the wax will not stick to a wet surface.

A tinfoil substitute is then used as a separating medium to protect the cast and allow the separation of the record base from the cast following the application of the monomer and polymer. The tinfoil substitute is applied twice, allowing the first application to dry prior to applying a second coat. Each application is applied as a thin film to all surfaces of the cast, including land areas and the sides of base that may come in contact with the resin (Figures 8–4). No pooling of the tinfoil substitute on the casts should remain. Brush only long enough to distribute the tinfoil evenly. Excess brushing causes the material to "ball up." Allow the second application of the tinfoil substitute to dry completely. When dry, the tinfoil substitute will have the appearance of a thin layer of cellophane. Therefore, do not attempt to expedite the drying time by blowing it dry with air under pressure. Doing so may cause the separating medium to be blown off the cast.

The record base is fabricated with autopolymerizing acrylic resin using a "spinkle-on" technique (Figures 8–5). This technique uses a material that can be completed quickly and provides an accurate and rigid final product.

When carrying out this technique, a small area of the vestibule is initially wetted with monomer (liquid). Then a thin layer of polymer (powder) is sprinkled onto the monomer until there is no visible liquid remaining and the mixture is reasonably

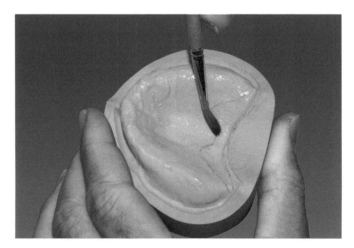

Figure 8–4   Tinfoil substitute is applied in two thin layers, allowing the first layer to dry prior to adding the second.

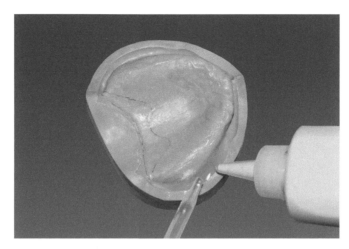

Figure 8–5 The initial placement of the monomer followed by the polymer. Although both the eyedropper with the monomer and the container with the polymer are shown together, the monomer is always placed first, followed by the polymer.

dense while having no dry polymer remaining. Continue the sprinkling and saturating process until the reflections of the casts are filled and the palatal portion of the maxillary and lingual, labial, and buccal slopes of both rims are approximately 2–3 mm in thickness.

The record base should be thinner on the crest of the ridges and buccal to the crest of the ridges because space may be limited when the denture teeth are being arranged at a future date. Once this sprinkle-on procedure is started, it must be totally completed. The application of the polymer just to the stone cast followed by the monomer, or allowing the resin to begin to polymerize, if more thickness of the record base is required, should be avoided. Either one of these situations will create porosity within the record base. Also, in order to prevent porosity caused by the rapid evaporation of the monomer, the casts and record bases should be placed into a humidifier or covered with a damp paper towel and a rubber plaster bowl inverted over the top until the resin has polymerized.

The resin should be allowed to polymerize for 15 minutes. Then the resin base can be carefully removed from the cast. Be careful removing the record base because excessive force may fracture the master cast. Also, do not remove the wax relief from inside of the baseplate unless it prevents the proper seating of the record base back on the cast. If left in place, it will enhance stability both on the cast and within the mouth.

On a lathe or with a handpiece, trim away any excess resin at the borders of the base and in the areas where artificial teeth will be set with an arbor band or acrylic bur. Smooth the base and recontour any areas that are too thick (more than 3 mm) (Figures 8–6). Because the record base may warp if heated, care must be taken not to apply excessive pressure when trimming the resin. The finished resin base must be sufficiently thick for strength and accuracy, yet it should not interfere with the arrangement of artificial teeth or in making interocclusal records. Replace the resin base back onto the cast. If there is a rocking of the base on the cast, the base must be remade.

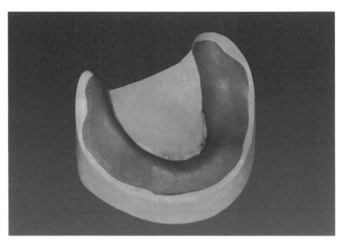

Figure 8–6   Note that the record base is rigid and accurately fits the master cast. The record base should fill the vestibules, which were border molded during the impression procedure in the mouth.

Occlusion Rim Fabrication

The occlusion rim is generally fabricated from pink baseplate or set-up wax, which is easily manipulated in the laboratory, easily contoured intraorally for proper shape, is esthetically pleasing, and can be shaped to the approximate size and shape of the teeth along with being comfortable to the patient. Although the occlusion rim can be completely fabricated from a sheet of baseplate wax, a "preformed" wax occlusion rim is often used (Figures 8–7). If a sheet of baseplate wax is used, it is warmed and rolled into

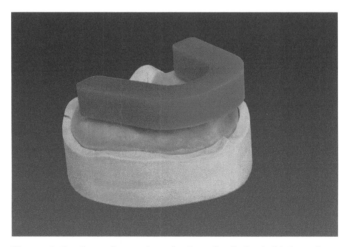

Figure 8–7   A preformed occlusion rim in its initial position before being properly aligned and attached to the record base.

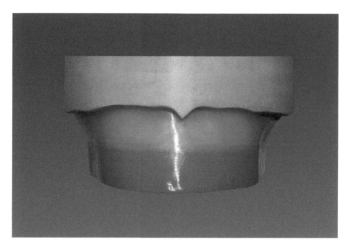

Figure 8–8 The maxillary occlusion rim, as viewed from the anterior, has been completed.

a cigar shape that is shaped to mimic the crest of the ridge of the cast before the teeth were extracted.

The occlusion rim is placed over the ridges of the previously made record base and gently pressed down until the occlusion rim is parallel to the base of the correctly trimmed master cast. The rim is sealed to the base, and all labial and lingual voids are eliminated with additional wax. The occlusion rim is smoothed (Figures 8–8).

The external size and shape of the occlusion rims is of utmost importance. The occlusion rims should be approximately the same size and shape as the natural teeth being replaced. When completed, the plane of occlusion on the maxillary arch should be approximately 22 mm in height, as measured from the bottom of the notch created by the labial frenulum, and approximately 18 mm in height on the mandibular arch. It should gradually taper toward the occlusal plane and be approximately 8–10 mm in width in the posterior, and 6–8 mm in width in the anterior region. The maxillary occlusion rim should be approximately 12 mm in height from the record base at the crest of the ridge in the tuberosity areas. The mandibular occlusion rim should be at the height of the top of the retromolar pad. Studies indicate that the labial surface of the natural central incisors averages 6–8 mm anterior to the middle of the incisal papilla. This should be kept in mind when forming the maxillary occlusion rim. Therefore, from canine to canine, the rims incline at approximately a 15^0 angle labially to provide adequate support for the lip (Figures 8–9 & 8–10).

The record bases and occlusion rims must be neatly constructed because patients often begin to form opinions about their new dentures based on the appearance and feel of the record bases and occlusion rims. In fact, may patients assume the record bases and occlusion rims are part of the completed dentures and become concerned about the appearance and fit. For these patients, it becomes important to continuously inform them that the record bases and occlusion rims are not part of the completed dentures, and that they may feel a little loose because of the required blocked-out undercuts. Speech difficulties are caused primarily because the occlusion rims are not completely contoured, and may be a little thick.

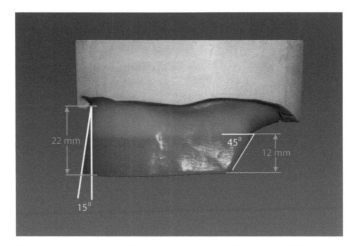

Figure 8–9 A properly contoured maxillary record base and occlusion rim along with the desired dimensions. Note that the plane of occlusion is parallel with the base of the cast, and the labial inclination of the anterior portion of the occlusion rim is at approximately a 15⁰ angle to offer lip support. The numbers provided (22 mm and 12 mm) are averages that will generally provide slightly more wax than necessary. This rim will be contoured intraorally to establish the final plane of occlusion and lip support. The posterior of the maxillary occlusion rim should slope occlusally at approximately a 45 degree angle from the record base, beginning approximately 8 mm from the posterior extent of the record base. This will generally provide space for the mandibular record base once placed intraorally.

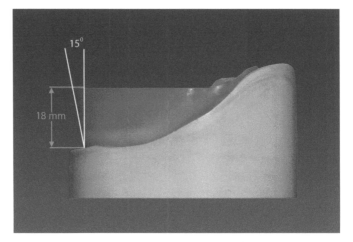

Figure 8–10 A properly contoured mandibular record base and occlusion rim along with desired dimensions. Note that the plane of occlusion runs parallel with the base of the cast, which was trimmed to be parallel with the residual ridges. Also the plane of occlusion is approximately at the level of the middle-to upper-third of the retromolar pad.

References

Rahn, A. O.: Record bases and occlusion rims. In: Rahn, A. O., Heartwell, C. M., editors: Textbook of complete dentures. 5th ed. Philadelphia: Lea & Febiger; 1993. pp. 265–268.

Sowter, J. B., Baseplates. In Barton, R. E., ed.: Removable Prosthodontic Techniques. Revised edition. Chapel Hill: University of North Carolina Press; 1986. pp. 32-39.

Zarb, G. A., Finer, Y.: Identification of shape and location of arch form: The occlusion rim and recording of trial denture base. In: Zarb, G. A., Bolander, C. L., eds. Prosthodontic Treatment for Edentulous Patients. 12th ed. St. Louis: Mosby Inc; 2004. pp. 252-261.

QUESTIONS

1. What are some of the procedures that require the use of a record base and an occlusion rim?

2. List some of the characteristics of a satisfactory record base.

3. Why is it important to properly block out undercuts on the master cast prior to fabricating the record base?

4. What area is a possible exception to complete block out of an undercut prior to record base fabrication, and why is this area an exception?

5. Why is the blocked-out master cast soaked in water for five minutes prior to fabricating the record base?

6. Can the drying time of the tinfoil substitute be expedited by drying with air under pressure?

7. What material and laboratory technique is used to create the record base?

8. Other than over-reduction, why must care be taken when trimming the polymerized record base with an arbor band or acrylic burr?

9. Can any average position of the natural central incisor be used as a guide in fabricating the maxillary occlusion rim?

10. The record bases and occlusion rims will eventually be destroyed. So, why should the laboratory technician spend time properly shaping them and making them neat and clean?

ANSWERS

1. The record base and occlusion rim are necessary for establishing facial contours; as an aid in tooth selection, in establishing and maintaining the vertical dimension of occlusion during record making; for making interocclusal records; for the arrangement of the denture teeth; for the verification of the correct master cast mounting on the articulator; at the esthetic trial insertion appointment; and as a wax-up mold for the external surface of the complete denture.

2. A satisfactory record base must be stable on both the master casts and intraorally, be rigid; be accurately adapted to the casts; be comfortable to the patient and esthetic; and fully cover the entire supporting tissues of the arches.

3. Because of the possibility of cast breakage when initially separating the record base from the master cast, which usually necessitates making a new final impression and creating a new master cast.

4. An exception is the undercut on the labial or anterior portion of the maxillary cast. It need not be completely eliminated because the completed record base and occlusion rim can be placed and removed at an angle from an anterior direction.

5. The cast is soaked in room temperature water for five minutes to minimize the formation of bubbles in the completed record base.

6. Do not attempt to expedite the drying time by blowing it dry with air under pressure because the separating medium may be blown off the cast.

7. The record base is fabricated with an autopolymerizing acrylic resin using a "spinkle-on" technique.

8. Because the record base may warp if excessively heated, care must be taken when trimming the resin.

9. Studies indicate that the labial surface of the natural central incisors average 6–8 mm anterior to the middle of the incisal papilla. This should be kept in mind when forming the occlusion rim.

10. The record bases and occlusion rims must be neatly constructed because patients often begin to form opinions about their new dentures based on the appearance and feel of these record bases and occlusion rims.

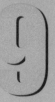

Occlusal Concepts

Dr. John R. Ivanhoe

The concept of denture occlusion is confusing to many clinicians. This confusion may result from the myriad of occlusal decisions that the clinician must make for each patient. Questions that must be addressed include but are not limited to the following: What type of posterior denture teeth are indicated? What type of articulator is required?, Is a balanced occlusion necessary for this patient?, and is a protrusive record necessary?

To simplify occlusal concepts, the following principles of occlusion for complete dentures are generally accepted:

1. Complete denture patients must make initial and complete occlusal contact while in centric relation. This is called centric occlusion.
2. All anterior and posterior denture teeth inclines and surfaces must function as a "unit" during excursive movements.
3. Any prematurity preventing the movements described in principles 1 and/or 2 must be eliminated.
4. Significant disclusion of the posterior denture teeth when a patient protrudes is contraindicated.
5. Anterior tooth contact is contraindicated in centric occlusion.

Posterior Occlusal Schemes

Posterior occlusion can be classified as either nonbalanced (monoplane) or balanced. Differing tooth morphologies are used, depending upon the type of occlusion being developed (Figures 9–1 and 9–2). A monoplane occlusion is considered one in which nonanatomic denture teeth are used at least on the mandibular arch and are arranged so that the occlusal surfaces lay on a flat (mono) plane (Figure 9–3). This flat plane is not necessarily parallel to the upper and lower members of the articulator. A balanced occlusion generally has anatomic or semi-anatomic denture teeth on both the maxillary and mandibular arches (Figure 9–4). Both occlusal schemes have simultaneous bilateral posterior occlusal contacts when the patient is in the centric relation position. In complete denture patients, this is called centric occlusion. It is desirable to have

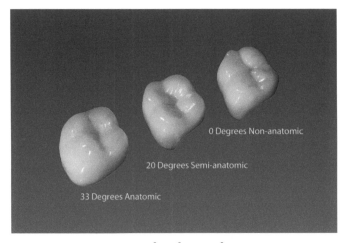

0 Degrees Non-anatomic

20 Degrees Semi-anatomic

33 Degrees Anatomic

Figure 9–1   Teeth with 33^0, 20^0, and 0^0 tooth morphologies.

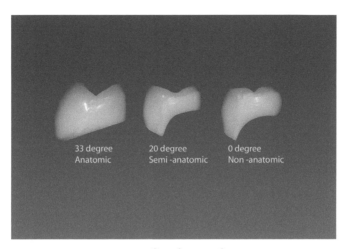

Figure 9–2   Teeth with 33^0, 20^0, and 0^0 tooth morphologies as viewed from the mesial.

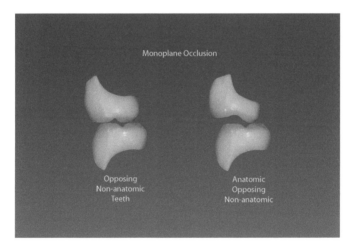

Figure 9–3   Two different monoplane occlusions. On the left are opposing 0^0 teeth set for a traditional monoplane occlusion. Imagine the potential poor esthetics, especially of the monoplane maxillary first premolar. On the right is a nonbalanced lingualized occlusion tooth arrangement. A maxillary anatomic tooth was selected to improve esthetics and possibly masticatory efficiency. Note there are no cuspal inclines to direct lateral forces to the residual ridges during excursive movements. This is one of the advantages to a monoplane occlusion.

simultaneous anterior and posterior bilateral contacts in all excursive movements, although this is often not achievable in a monoplane type occlusion. This will be discussed in further detail later.

As stated in Principle #5, anterior tooth contact is not indicated in centric occlusion for either type of occlusal scheme. Loss of the occluding vertical dimension because of surface wear of the posterior teeth may result in excessive force on the anterior denture

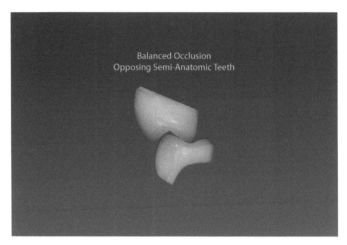

Figure 9–4 Opposing semi-anatomic (20⁰) denture teeth arranged for a traditional balanced occlusion.

teeth and hence the residual ridges. This is especially true if the dentures were fabricated with contact of the anterior teeth. It must be remembered that the anterior bone in edentulous patients is not usually cortical bone that can withstand strong occlusal forces. Therefore every attempt should be made to eliminate vertical and horizontal stresses on these ridges, including the elimination of anterior contacts while the patient is in centric occlusion.

As stated in Principle #1, to prevent denture instability and potential tissue abuse with either occlusion, a patient must make initial and complete occlusal contact while in centric occlusion. Therefore, per Principle #3, premature deflective occlusal contacts on inclined surfaces during closure, with either occlusal scheme, must be eliminated. Ideally all centric occlusion contacts would occur on horizontal surfaces. However, contacts on inclined surfaces are usually caused by tooth morphology and cannot always be avoided. Therefore, the clinician must assure that those occlusal contacts that occur on inclined surfaces are not prematurities. Because nonanatomic denture teeth are used on at least the mandibular arch for a monoplane occlusion and are cuspless, there is minimal chance that a patient will make initial contact on any inclined surface with this type of occlusion. The reverse is true for a balanced occlusion because there are many opposing inclined surfaces that may make deflective occlusal contacts during closure. This is especially significant if it was not possible for the clinician to make accurate interocclusal records.

 Traditional Balanced Occlusion

Although several methods of achieving a balanced occlusion have been used in the past, the most common and traditional method is to use anatomic or semi-anatomic denture teeth on both the maxillary and mandibular arches and arrange the teeth to a compensating curve.

The denture teeth must be arranged and/or adjusted to eliminate prematurities so that all anterior and posterior inclined surfaces act as a "unit" in centric occlusion and during excursive movements. This is discussed in greater detail later in this chapter. The steepness of these movements is dictated by the incisal guidance and the condylar inclination. This is a complex occlusion that provides multiple "cross tooth" and "cross arch" contacts on most if not all the posterior teeth (Figure 9–5). Although a balanced occlusal scheme may be desired or required for several reasons, it is a difficult occlusion to achieve and maintain from both a laboratory and clinical standpoint.

To accurately mimic the mandibular movements of the patient and create an occlusion in which all anterior and posterior inclines can be arranged or adjusted to act as a unit in excursive movements, a Class III (semi-adjustable) articulator with the maxillary cast positioned using a facebow is required. Additionally, to accurately match the excursive movements of the patient, the horizontal condylar inclinations on the articulator must closely mimic the movement of the heads of the condyles down the articular eminencies. Therefore accurate protrusive and/or lateral records must be made to program the condylar inclinations. This is an additional procedure that is not required when a monoplane occlusion is selected.

It is important that the clinician make an accurate repeatable centric relation recording when articulating the mandibular master cast. This is imperative for a patient receiving a balanced occlusion. Therefore, clinicians must carefully evaluate the repeatability of centric relation on all patients prior to selecting posterior denture teeth and the occlusal scheme. If the centric relation position cannot be accurately repeated, interocclusal records cannot be accurately made, the alignment of the opposing denture teeth will be inaccurate. Therefore, it may be almost impossible for the clinician to eliminate occlusal prematurities at insertion. This is a minimal problem with a monoplane occlusion because there are no opposing occlusal inclines to become prematurities. Almost all occlusal contacts occur on flat surfaces. Therefore, because being able to repeat centric

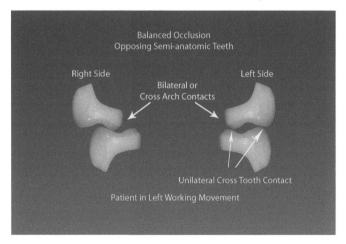

Figure 9–5 Opposing semi-anatomic denture teeth set in a traditional balanced occlusion and moved into the left working movement. Note the cross-arch occlusal contacts and cross-tooth contacts that occur on the left side. This cross-tooth contact is not seen in a lingualized occlusion, which is one of the advantages of a lingualized occlusion.

relation for many patients is difficult if not impossible, a balanced occlusion requiring opposing anatomic denture teeth is often contraindicated. For these patients, it will be difficult to make accurate the protrusive or lateral recordings necessary to properly program the articulator.

A balanced occlusion is primarily indicated for patients having good anterior and posterior residual ridge alignment. This is important because of the necessity for achieving good occlusion of the opposing anatomic or semi-anatomic posterior teeth while still arranging the teeth over the ridges. For patients with a normal buccal-lingual alignment of the posterior ridge or a total cross-bite ridge alignment, arranging the posterior tooth arrangement is reasonably easy. The difficulty arises when a patient has a normal buccolingual ridge alignment in the premolar areas and a complete reverse articulation (crossbite) alignment in the second molar area. For these patients, to maintain the teeth over the ridges, the first premolars must be in a normal buccolingual alignment and yet the second molars must be in a reverse articulation (crossbite). One or more teeth, usually in the first molar area, become the cross-over teeth. To have the teeth remain over the ridges means that the opposing buccal and lingual cusps cannot be set in a cusp-fossa alignment. The opposing cusp tips become end-to-end. It becomes impossible to position the teeth, while retaining good occlusion and reasonable esthetics. When arranged to the best occlusion possible, equilibration to eliminate excursive prematurities often destroys all semblances of normal tooth morphology. Therefore, from both a laboratory and clinical standpoint, the use of opposing anatomic denture teeth may not be realistic for patients without good ridge alignments. This includes those requiring a unilateral or bilateral posterior reverse articulation (crossbite) and prognathic and retrognathic patients. Once again, this is a minimal problem with a monoplane occlusion.

It must be remembered that creating a balanced occlusion requires a fairly significant commitment for both the technician and clinician, and therefore must provide sufficient benefits to be selected over a monoplane occlusion. One potential benefit may be the reduction of lateral forces during functional and parafunctional movements. One study indicated that a balanced occlusion might offer the benefits of improved lateral denture stability because of the bilateral posterior contacts. However Kydd found that the use of anatomic teeth, necessary for a balanced occlusion, actually increased the lateral forces to the ridges. Therefore some still question whether a balanced occlusion actually reduces the lateral forces on ridges.

Creating a balanced occlusion while the teeth are in actual functional contact? It was once believed that when food or anything else was placed between any of the opposing teeth, all opposing tooth contact (balance) was lost, so any potential advantage of a balanced occlusion would also be lost. The following question arises: Are functional contacts a significant issue, and what is the amount of time that the opposing teeth will actually contact in a 24-hour period? Functional contact of the opposing teeth has been estimated at only 17.5 minutes per day, therefore many clinicians believe that the effort necessary to create a balanced occlusion is not justified by this minimal daily occlusal contact time. However parafunctional, potentially destructive, occlusal contact time has been estimated at 2–4 hours per day. Therefore, even though the maximum occlusal force of complete denture patients only averages 35 pounds, functional and parafuntional contacts should be considered when selecting a posterior occlusal scheme.

Others believe that the opposing anatomic denture teeth used in a balanced occlusion may offer improved masticatory efficiency over the non-anatomic denture teeth used in a monoplane occlusion. However studies in this area have also been inconclusive. Esthetics are certainly improved for many patients with anatomic denture teeth.

More recently a simplified occlusion called a lingualized occlusion, which will be discussed later, has become popular and successful. It may be used to replace both conventional balanced and monoplane occlusions.

Conventional Monoplane Occlusion

For most clinicians and laboratory technicians, a satisfactory monoplane occlusion is a much simpler occlusion to achieve and maintain intraorally. Many clinicians successfully use a fixed or nonadjustable articulator and arbitrarily position the maxillary cast onto the articulator when creating a monoplane occlusion. This technique is not recommended. It may be determined at the trial insertion appointment that, for phonetic or esthetic reasons, a vertical overlap of the anterior teeth and hence balanced occlusion is necessary. Then a semi-adjustable articulator with the maxillary cast positioned using a facebow and the condylar inclination set with protrusive or lateral records is necessary. A fixed articulator does not allow the altering of the condylar inclination. Therefore the use of at least a semi-adjustable articulator with the maxillary cast positioned using a facebow is recommended for all patients.

Since there are few, if any, cuspal inclines to be concerned with, achieving an exact centric relation recording, while desirable for all patients and required for patients receiving a balanced occlusion, may not be a necessity for all monoplane occlusion patients. Because of the non-anatomic mandibular denture teeth, a specific cusp/marginal ridge alignment of the opposing denture teeth is unnecessary. Therefore this type occlusion is useful for prognathic, retrognathic, and reverse articulation (crossbite) patients. It is not necessary to program the condylar inclination of the articulator with excursive records for a monoplane occlusion because no attempt is made to balance this occlusion. Generally the condylar inclination and incisal guidance are arranged to be parallel to the plane of occlusion.

Since opposing non-anatomic denture teeth are traditionally used for these patients, poor esthetics and compromised masticatory efficiency must be considered. Esthetics is compromised. However, studies have been inconclusive when comparing the masticatory efficiencies of patients with balanced and monoplane occlusions.

Because patients with a monoplane occlusion have no vertical overlap of the anterior denture teeth, when the patient protrudes, a mild disclusion (Christensen's Phenomena) of the most distal teeth often occurs. Clinicians must recognize and accept this condition and understand that this disclusion may not be as significant as that seen in a balanced occlusion patient. This will be discussed in greater detail later in this chapter.

Balanced Occlusion or Not

A question that has been discussed for decades is whether a balanced occlusion is required for most complete denture patients. A balanced occlusion is not required and, because of its complexity, not indicated for many patients. A balanced occlusion is required for two specific groups of patients. Those are, patients with a steep, vertical overlap of the anterior denture teeth (steep incisal guidance) and patients who require opposing anatomic or semi-anatomic denture teeth for esthetics or other reasons.

Why is a Balanced Occlusion Required in Patients Exhibiting a Significant Degree of Incisal Guidance?

As stated in Principle of Occlusion #4, significant posterior disclusion, which is caused by a moderate-to-steep vertical overlap of the anterior teeth, is contraindicated in complete denture patients.

Many patients with remaining natural anterior teeth exhibit significant disclusion of the posterior teeth (Christensen's phenomena) when they move from centric occlusion into excursive positions. This disclusion is caused by a combination of the incisal guidance (vertical overlap) of the anterior teeth and the movement of the head of the condyle down the articular eminence. Often only two or three anterior teeth are involved in this incisal guidance. If they are strong, natural teeth well anchored in bone, this is called an anterior disclusion and usually is considered a favorable type of natural occlusion. This occlusion reduces potentially destructive lateral forces from the posterior teeth.

Complete denture patients are different. Because of esthetic and/or functional requirements, some complete denture patients must have their anterior denture teeth arranged with a steep vertical overlap (incisal guidance). Unfortunately, because all contact occurs on the anterior denture teeth, the resultant forces are transferred to the anterior portion of the opposing ridges. These forces are usually excessive, cause trauma to the underlying hard and soft tissues, and may lead to excessive soft tissue abuse and eventual bone loss. To eliminate the effects of this posterior disclusion, it becomes necessary to attempt to distribute the occlusal forces over both anterior and posterior teeth, thereby gaining maximum anterior and bilateral posterior ridge support. This occlusion, by definition, is a balanced occlusion and is therefore indicated when there is a moderate-to-steep vertical overlap of the anterior teeth. Therefore, one primary indication for a balanced occlusion is for those patients with a moderate-to-steep vertical overlap of the anterior teeth and who make reasonably frequent contact of the anterior teeth leading to posterior disclusion.

Additionally, the steep vertical overlap of the anterior teeth often causes denture dislodgement throughout the day because of repeated parafunctional contact. A balanced occlusion is required for these patients to distribute the occlusal contact to at least some of the posterior teeth, thereby increasing denture stability.

Patients with a monoplane occlusion have no vertical overlap of the anterior teeth, and therefore have an incisal guidance of zero degrees. When these patients move into a protruded position, there is generally only a minimal separation of just the molars. Multiple anterior and posterior occlusal contacts are usually present that may extend to the second premolars. The extended area of these contacts, as opposed to the limited area of contacts with a steep incisal guidance patient, provides distribution of these forces over a broad enough area that excessive forces to any specific area of the ridges are usually eliminated. Also, with no vertical overlap of the anterior teeth, denture dislodgement because of parafunctional contacts is also usually eliminated. Denture instability caused by the occlusion is an unusual problem for these patients.

Therefore the clinician or the patient may desire a balanced occlusion because of the perceived functional or actual esthetic advantages of anatomic denture teeth. It is not required, however, except when desiring to spread functional or dislodging forces over a larger area or over a greater number of denture teeth.

From the previous comments it may be assumed by some that a balanced occlusion is necessary for all patients requiring a vertical overlap of the anterior teeth. There is an exception to this general assumption. Many patients with a significant vertical overlap also exhibit a significant degree of horizontal overlap of the anterior denture teeth. This often results in a mild-to-moderate incisal guidance that may not be a concern. Although there is a vertical overlap of the teeth, because of the significant horizontal overlap, many of these patients almost never have functional or parafunctional contact of the anterior teeth. Therefore almost no chance of trauma to the underlying anterior soft and hard tissues exists. Again, because of its simplicity, a monoplane occlusion is often acceptable for these patients.

A balanced occlusion is necessary for some patients. but because of the simplicity for both the clinician and laboratory technician and because patients' acceptance is high, a monoplane occlusion should be considered as the occlusion of choice for most patients.

Why is a Balanced Occlusion Required in Patients with Opposing Anatomic Denture Teeth?

A second primary indication for a balanced occlusion is for those patients requiring the use of opposing anatomic or semi-anatomic denture teeth. Principle #3 states that prematurities that prevent all anterior and posterior denture teeth inclines and surfaces from functioning as a unit must be eliminated. Therefore, with opposing anatomic or semi-anatomic denture teeth, the only way to eliminate excursive prematurities is through the creation of a balanced occlusion.

Lingualized Occlusion

Lingualized occlusion was developed in an attempt to simplify denture occlusion while maintaining the advantages and eliminating the disadvantages of both balanced and monoplane type occlusions. Among other disadvantages, a balanced denture occlusion is difficult to achieve because of the multiple opposing inclined surfaces that must be adjusted, the necessity of a good opposing residual ridge alignment, and the requirement for a repeatable centric relation position. A monoplane occlusion on both arches exhibits poor esthetics and the potential for a decreased efficiency when masticating food. A balanced or monoplane occlusion can be achieved while using the lingualized concept, which minimizes or eliminates most of the potential disadvantages listed earlier.

Opposing anatomic or semi-anatomic denture teeth are selected when creating a balanced lingualized occlusion, and anatomic teeth opposing non-anatomic teeth are selected for a nonbalanced lingualized occlusion. The maxillary teeth for both occlusions are arranged so that the lingual cusps are in contact with the mandibular teeth, and the tooth angled so that the buccal cusps lie slightly above the occlusal plane (Figure 9–6). This means that, in both centric occlusion and during excursive movements, the maxillary lingual cusps are the only cusps occluding with the opposing teeth and therefore are the functional cusps.

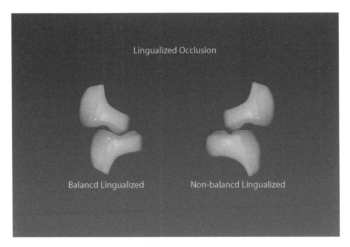

Figure 9–6 Examples of lingualized occlusion. A balanced lingualized tooth arrangement is seen on the left side. The arrangement of the opposing teeth for a nonbalanced lingualized occlusion is seen on the right side. Note that the buccal cusps are set above the occlusal plane to achieve no contact between the buccal cusp and the opposing teeth in the working movement. There are no cross-tooth prematurities to be concerned with in excursive movements.

There is a significant clinical advantage to having only the maxillary lingual cusps contact the opposing teeth in a balanced lingualized occlusion. While cross-arch contacts must be maintained, cross-tooth contacts are not present and not desired in the balanced lingualized occlusion. Because the maxillary buccal cusps never contact the mandibular teeth, prematurities seen in a traditional balanced occlusion are dramatically reduced. The advantages of a conventional balanced occlusion are still achieved while being greatly simplified with a lingualized occlusion.

To improve the esthetics and potential masticatory efficiency of a monoplane occlusion, a monoplane or nonbalanced lingualized type occlusion has also been developed. A monoplane lingualized occlusion is easily achieved and yet only slightly different from a conventional monoplane occlusion. Non-anatomic teeth arranged on a flat occlusal plane continue to be used on the mandibular arch, while anatomic denture teeth are selected for the maxillary arch. The non-anatomic teeth on the mandibular arch continue to provide the benefits of a monoplane occlusion, while the anatomic teeth used on the maxillary arch overcome the esthetics concerns of a conventional monoplane occlusion. Additionally, the selection of anatomic maxillary teeth may also address the potential loss of masticatory efficiency reported by some when using opposing monoplane teeth. This type of occlusion seems to eliminate the disadvantages of a conventional monoplane occlusion and has become popular and successful in the last few decades. It is also well received by patients.

Because both balanced and nonbalanced lingualized occlusions are easily achieved, and both reduce some of the disadvantages while increasing some of the advantages of conventional schemes, they are recommended for patients whenever possible.

Functional Inclines

Understanding the factors of occlusion is important in creating and maintaining a balanced occlusion. When completed, a balanced occlusion must exhibit bilateral anterior and posterior occlusal contacts in centric occlusion and excursive movements. In addition, the anterior and posterior teeth act as a unit in excursive movements because all prematurities have been eliminated from opposing inclined surfaces.

The term functional inclines (FI) indicates the inclines of the cusps of the anterior and posterior teeth that will contact when a patient moves into excursive movements. The inclines of the maxillary anterior teeth that face the palate and the inclines of the mandibular anterior teeth that face labially are the functional inclines. The posterior functional inclines are determined by the excursive movement. Generally, although other inclines may be involved, the following are the most frequent. Functional inclines for the posterior teeth:

1. In protrusive movements, the functional inclines face anteriorly for mandibular teeth and face posteriorly for maxillary teeth in protrusive movements (Figures 9–7 and 9–8).
2. In working movements, the functional inclines face buccally for the mandibular teeth and linquallu for maxillary teeth in working movements.
3. In nonworking movements, the functional inclines face lingually for the mandibular teeth and buccally for the maxillary teeth in nonworking movements.

Because of tooth anatomy and individual patient movement, other inclines on the teeth may be involved. Also all prematurities on any of the inclines must be eliminated for a balanced occlusion, while they are of minimal concern when using a monoplane occlusion. Understanding these inclines is important in the following discussion.

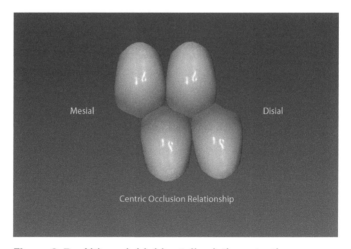

Figure 9–7 Although highly stylized, these teeth are arranged to illustrate the relative position of the tooth inclines when the teeth are arranged for centric occlusion. Horizontal overlap has been eliminated for better understanding.

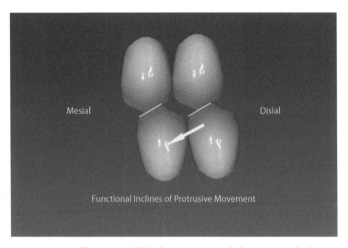

Mesial

Disial

Functional Inclines of Protrusive Movement

Figure 9–8 The mandible has assumed the protruded position, and the protrusive functional inclines of the opposing teeth are illustrated. The teeth have moved forward as controlled by the lateral pterygoid muscles and downward as controlled by the incisal guidance and the condylar inclination.

 Factors of Protrusive Occlusion

There are five factors of protrusive occlusion that must be considered when creating a balanced occlusion. Understanding the interrelationship between these factors will clarify how a balanced occlusion is achieved and how, once achieved, if one of the factors is altered at least one other factor must also be altered to regain the balance.

Although slightly altered by the author, the protrusive factors of occlusion have been identified as follows: degree of incisal guidance (IG), degree of condylar inclination (CI), inclination of the plane of occlusion (PO), angulations of the cusps of the posterior teeth in relation to the overall occlusal surface (CA), and the steepness of the compensating curve (CC). These factors are related in the following formulas, which simplify the understanding of the relationships of the factors. $CI \times IG = PO \times CA \times CC$

Although these factors affect all excursive movements of the posterior teeth, for simplicity, only the protrusive movement will be discussed and illustrated.

If the five protrusive factors of occlusion were completely under the control of the clinician, making necessary alterations would usually be relatively simple. However, the condylar inclination is beyond the control of the clinician, and the others can only be altered to a small degree. Therefore, when a problem develops, a combination of changes is necessary.

The author suggests the following formula to aid in the understanding of the 5 factors of protrusive occlusion. $IG \times CI = AFI$

This formula indicates that, for a balanced occlusion, to maintain posterior contacts and yet have no prematurities in the protrusive movement, the angulation of the functional inclines (AFI) of the maxillary and mandibular posterior teeth must match the influences of the incisal guidance and condylar inclination.

When a patient protrudes, the mandibular teeth move forward and downward. The distance of the protrusive movement is determined by the action of the lateral pterygoid muscles, while the angulation of the downward movement is determined by the steepness of the incisal guidance in the anterior and the steepness of the condylar inclination in the posterior. The incisal guidance and condylar inclination are sometimes called the "end controlling factors." Because the denture teeth are almost all anatomically closer to the incisal guidance than the condylar inclination, the incisal guidance (IG) has greater influence on the steepness of the required functional inclines of the teeth.

So how do clinicians make these functional inclines match the influences of the incisal guidance and condylar inclination, while still maintaining contact in excursive movement and not having prematurities? For complete denture patients the incisal guidance is determined by the esthetic and phonetic demands of the patient and is a slightly variable factor. The condylar inclination, however, is a fixed factor that is determined by the steepness of the articular eminence. The condylar inclination is usually programmed into the articulator by use of a protrusive record or lateral records made intraorally.

To illustrate these concepts, two imaginary patients will be described. The first patient has a 20 degree angulation of both the incisal guidance and condylar inclination. Therefore, to maintain contact of the posterior teeth in the protrusive movement, while not haveing prematurities, the functional inclines must be 20 degrees (Figure 9–9).

For the second patient, the incisal guidance is 15 degrees and the condylar inclination is 35 degrees. Remember that the incisal guidance has more of an influence on the angulation of the functional inclines than the condylar inclination. The required steepness of the functional inclines should reflect that. Even thought the teeth are close together in this illustration, note that a difference in the functional inclines still exists (Figure 9–10), These values have been chosen for illustration purposes but would be

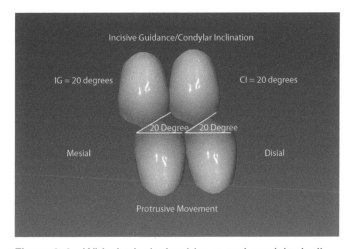

Figure 9–9 With the incisal guidance and condylar inclinations of this patient being 20°, it becomes necessary to have the protrusive functional inclines of all the posterior teeth be 20° A posterior tooth mold with 20° cusp angles, as supplied by a manufacturer, should be ideal for this patient. Contact of the opposing teeth in protrusive should be maintained and yet minimal adjustments to eliminate prematurities should be expected.

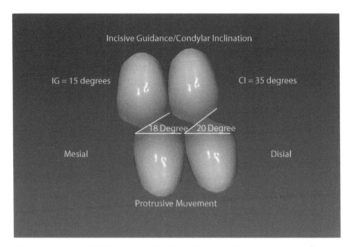

Figure 9–10 With the incisal guidance changed to 15^0 and the condylar inclination at 35^0, the functional inclines vary depending upon the relative position of the tooth to those controls. Because almost all teeth are closer to the incisal guidance, it has more of an influence than the condylar inclination. The cusp angle of the posterior teeth in this example is 22^0. Note that the second premolars have been slightly tipped to increase the effective cusp angle because the required functional incline has become larger than 20^0.

reasonably accurate. The closer these teeth are to the condylar inclination, the closer the inclines come to 35 degrees. In fact, the inclines of the second molars may be 25 degrees or more. Because the second molar is anatomically almost equidistance between the incisal and condylar inclinations, the inclination of its functional inclines is an average of the two (25 degrees). Table 1 demonstrates more examples (Table 9–1).

Table 9–1	FUNCTIONAL INCLINES - INCISAL GUIDANCE AND CONDYLAR INCLINATION			
Example	Incisal Guidance	First Premolar	Second Molar*	Condylar Inclination
A	20^0	20^0	20^0	20^0
B	30^0	30^0	30^0	30^0
C	30^0	28^0	25^0	20^0
D	0^0	8^0	17^0	35^0
E	20^0	22^0	27^0	35^0

Note that the incisal guidance has more influence over the functional inclines of the posterior teeth than the condylar guidance. However, the closer the tooth is to the condylar inclination, the closer the functional inclines match that guidance. Once again, these "values are provided for understanding the influences of the incisal and condylar guidances and are of no importance to know otherwise.

* Because the second molar is anatomically positioned about equidistant between the incisal and condylar inclination, the angulation of the functional inclines of the second molar is almost an average of the two guidances.

How does the clinician determine the cusp angle to be used when selecting the posterior teeth? If a nonbalanced lingualized occlusion is indicated, an anatomic maxillary tooth opposing a mandibular non-anatomic tooth would be the proper selection. However, the situation become more complicated when a balanced occlusion becomes necessary. In the example of the second patient previously described, it would seem that a tooth with a 20 degree cusp angle may be a good choice for the premolar areas. It would not, however, be a good choice for the molar area because there would be a loss of opposing tooth contact when the required functional inclines became greater than 20 degrees. Even though a tooth with a 30 degree cusp angle would not be a bad choice for the molar area, it would cause significant prematurities when moving into protrusive in the premolar area, and therefore would be a poor choice for that area. It may seem that a single set of posterior teeth with a single cusp angle as provided by the manufacturer (i.e. 20 degree), cannot match the changing functional incline requirements of the patient, and that teeth with differing cusp angles must be used. However, selecting teeth with differing cusp angles would be difficult for the clinician and cost prohibitive. This dilemma is resolved by altering the cusp angles of the denture teeth and creating "effective cusp angles" that can match the required angulation of the functional inclines.

Effective Cusp Angles (ECA)

As manufactured, posterior denture teeth exhibit differing cusp angles and cusp heights (Figures 9–1 and 9–2). Some have minimal or no cuspal angles and are called non-anatomic teeth, while the cuspal angles of semi-anatomic and anatomic teeth vary from approximately 10^0 to 45^0. For simplicity of illustration the cusp angles will be discussed from the buccal view here.

The cusp angle, as indicated by the manufacturer, is only accurate when the denture tooth is placed so that the long axis of the tooth is perpendicular to the plane of occlusion (Figure 9–11). If the long axis of the tooth is altered, the cusp angle of the

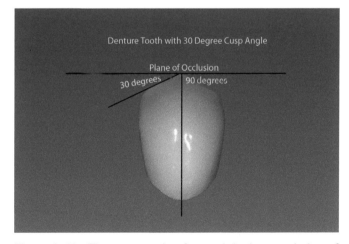

Figure 9–11   The cusp angle of a tooth is the angulation of the functional incline as measured from the long axis of the tooth. The cusp angulation of this tooth is 30^0.

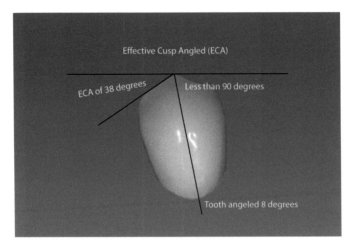

Figure 9–12   The effective cusp angle of a tooth is the angle of the functional incline as measured from a line parallel to the bench top. As a tooth is angled 8⁰, the effective cusp angle, and hence functional incline, change in a like manner. The effective cusp angle can also be altered by grinding the functional incline.

tooth relative to the occlusal plane is also changed. This altered cusp angle has been termed the effective cusp angle of the tooth (ECA) (Figure 9–12). With the two imaginary patients discussed earlier, it should now become clear that tilting the teeth to differing degrees becomes necessary to meet the differing required functional inclines of a patient. Thus a single mold of posterior tooth (i.e. 20 degrees) can allow contact in the protrusive movement of angles greater than 20 degrees. It should also become clear that, as the teeth are angled slightly more the further they are set posteriorly and as the plane of occlusion is slightly raised, a compensating curve is developed. Additionally, if the cusp angle of the tooth is altered by grinding, the tooth now has a different ECA. When the occlusion on a patient has been equilibrated to eliminate all excursive prematurities, the ECAs will be functional inclines.

 Example

In the case of another imaginary patient, the clinician has selected a balanced occlusion even though there is no esthetic or phonetic need for a vertical overlap of the anterior teeth. (Table 9–2, Example D)

Because there will be no vertical overlap of the anterior teeth, the clinician assumes that there is no need for selecting a posterior tooth with a steep cusp angle (i.e. 33 degrees) and therefore posterior teeth are selected with 20 degree cusp angles. The dental laboratory technician develops a balanced occlusion when arranging the denture teeth. The laboratory technician will have to equilibrate the cusps following processing to eliminate protrusive prematurities. This is because the cusp angles were steeper than

Table 9-2	FUNCTIONAL INCLINES - INCISAL GUIDANCE AND CONDYLAR INCLINATION			
Example	Incisal Guidance	First Premolar	Second Molar*	Condylar Inclination
D	0^0	8^0	17^0	35^0

* Because the second molar is anatomically positioned about equidistant between the incisal and condylar inclination, the angulation of the functional inclines of the second molar is almost an average of the two guidances.

the required angulation of the functional inclines, but at least posterior contact in the protrusive movement will be maintained.

At the trial insertion, the clinician determines that, for esthetic or phonetic reasons, a vertical overlap of the anterior teeth is necessary. The dental laboratory technician rearranges the denture teeth to achieve vertical overlap of the anterior teeth. (Table 9–3, Example E)

At that point, the technician notes that the incisal guidance is now 20 degrees and has resulted in a loss of posterior occlusal contacts when the articulator is moved into a protruded position. The technician no longer is concerned about protrusive prematurities, but now the 20 degree cusp angles are insufficient to maintain posterior protrusive contacts. To regain the posterior contacts, steeper cusp angles are needed. The technician knows that selecting and resetting new posterior teeth with steeper cusp angles is a choice. Replacing a 20^0 denture teeth with 30^0 might satisfy this requirement of maintaining contact in the molar area. From a cost and time standpoint, however, it is not the best choice. The technician knows that a better choice is to increase the ECA of the teeth by increasing the inclination of the plane of occlusion, the degree of the compensating curve, or a combination of both. For this patient the 20 degree teeth are rearranged using a steeper compensating curve, thereby making the ECA of the teeth more closely match the required angulation of the functional inclines, as provided by the incisal guidance and condylar inclination.

Table 9-3	FUNCTIONAL INCLINES - INCISAL GUIDANCE AND CONDYLAR INCLINATION			
Example	Incisal Guidance	First Premolar	Second Molar*	Condylar Inclination
E	20^0	22^0	27^0	35^0

* Because the second molar is anatomically positioned about equidistant between the incisal and condylar inclination, the angulation of the functional inclines of the second molar is almost an average of the two guidances.

Even though this is a good choice, the posterior height of the plane of occlusion and the degree of the compensation curve can only be moderately modified because of esthetic concerns. They can often be altered sufficiently, however, to satisfy functional demands of the tooth arrangement. However there are patients for whom, if a balanced occlusion is to be maintained, compromises in esthetics may be necessary. The desired extreme vertical overlap of the anterior teeth may not be possible.

Conclusion

The technician and the clinician must both have a complete understanding of occlusal concepts and the geometry of occlusion to satisfy the functional and esthetic needs of the patient. This understanding is necessary to make all anterior and posterior denture teeth inclines and surfaces function as a unit during excursive movements. Lingualized occlusions have more advantages and fewer disadvantages than conventional occlusal schemes. They can also be developed to create either a balanced or nonbalanced occlusion. Lingualized occlusions are usually more easily created by the technician and adjusted by the clinician, and are therefore indicated for most patients. Because of the simplicity and lack of problems or contraindications with a monoplane occlusion, a balanced occlusion is not required in most patients.

References

Bascom, P. W.: Masticatory efficiency of complete dentures. J Prosthet Dent. 1962;12:453-59.

Brewer, A. A.: Prosthodontic research in progress at the School of Aerospace Medicine. J Prosthet Dent. 1963;13:49-69.

Clough, H. E., Knodle, J. M., Leeper, S. H., Pudwell, M. L., Taylor, D. T.: A comparison of lingualized occlusion and monoplane occlusion in complete dentures. J Prosthet Dent, 1983;50: 176-79.

Graf, H., Brusixm. In Ramfjord, S. P., Ash, M. M., eds.: Occlusion. Dent Clin North Am. Philadelphia: W. B., Saunders Company, 1969;13:659-66.

Kydd, W. L.: Complete denture base deformation with vrie occlusal tooth form. J Prosthet Dent. 1956;6:714-18.

Lang, B. R.: Complete Denture Occlusion. In Engelmeier, R. L., ed. Complete Dentures. Dent Clin North Am. Philadelphia: W.B. Saunders, 1996;40:85-101.

Michael, C. G., Javid, N.S., Colaizzi, F. A., Gibbs, C. H.: Biting strength and chew forces in complete denture wearers. J Prosthet Dent. 1990;63:549-53.

Ortman, H. R.: Complete denture occlusion. In: Winkler, S., ed. Essentials of complete denture prosthodontics. 1st Ed. Philadelphia: W. B. Saunders Company, 1979;301-341.

Payne, S. H.: Study of occlusion in duplicate dentures. J Prosthet Dent. 1951;1:322-6.

Pound, E.: Using speech to simplify a personalized denture service. J Prosthet Dent. 1970;24:586-600.

Sheppard, I. M., Rakoff, S., Sheppard, S. M.: Bolus placement during mastication. J Prosthet Dent. 1968;20:506-10.

Wyatt, D. M., Macgregor, A.R., eds.: Designing complete dentures. Philadelphia: W.B., Saunders Company, 1976:385-387.

QUESTIONS

1. What is the difference between centric relation and centric occlusion?

2. What are the two major posterior occlusal schemes for complete denture patients?

3. What are the primary indications for a balanced occlusion?

4. What is a significant contraindication for selecting a balanced occlusion for a patient?

5. Both a steep vertical overlap of the anterior teeth and no vertical overlap result in some degree of separation of the posterior teeth when the patient makes a protrusive movement. Knowing that anterior disclusion of the posterior teeth is contraindicated in most patients, why is it often acceptable in a nonbalanced occlusion?

6. Why is an anterior disclusion of the posterior teeth a preferred occlusion of the natural teeth, but is contraindicated in complete dentures?

7. Why should lingualized occlusion be considered for patients?

8. What are the five factors of protrusive occlusion? Draw a formula that indicates their relationship.

9. What two factors control the angulation of the functional inclines of the posterior teeth, and which has the most influence on most of the teeth?

10. What are effective cusp angles?

ANSWERS

1. Centric relation is a positional relationship between the maxillary and mandibular arches. Centric occlusion is the occlusion of the denture teeth when the patient is in the centric relation position.

2. Balanced and nonbalanced.

3. a. Significant vertical overlap of the anterior teeth.

   b. If semi-anatomic or anatomic opposing posterior denture teeth are required because of esthetic concerns, the clinician believes they would improve the masticatory efficiency, the patient had existing dentures with anatomic or semi-anatomic denture teeth, or the necessity of a vertical overlap of the anterior teeth.

4. The patient's lack of achieving a repeatable centric relation position.

5. A steep vertical overlap of the anterior teeth results in unacceptable functional forces being directed to the anterior soft and hard tissues, while no vertical overlap of the teeth usually results in the contact of both the anterior and several of the posterior teeth. This distribution of contacts with no vertical overlap of the anterior teeth spreads the occlusal forces over an acceptably large area of the ridges and minimizes trauma to the underlying tissues.

6. The natural anterior teeth anchored in strong bone are able to bear strong excursive forces and eliminate or at least greatly reduce these destructive forces on the posterior teeth. Edentulous patients do not have natural teeth anchored in bone but they do have denture bases fitted to the residual ridges. Therefore any forces limited to the anterior teeth are immediately directed almost exclusively to the anterior ridges. Because these forces are not spread over a wide area of the edentulous ridges, soft tissue abuse and bone loss are common.

7. Both balanced and nonbalanced lingualized occlusions are easily achieved occlusal schemes. They reduce some of the disadvantages and increase some of the advantages of conventional schemes. Lingualized occlusion is recommended for patients whenever possible.

8. The factors are degree of incisal guidance (IG), degree of condylar inclination (CI), inclination of the plane of occlusion (PO), angulation of the cusps of the posterior teeth in relation to the overall occlusal surface (CA), and the steepness of the compensating curve (CC). These factors are related in the following formula, which simplifies their relationship.

$$CI \times IG = PO \times CA \times CC.$$

9. Incisal guidance and condylar inclination. Incisal guidance.

10. Effective cusp angles are the resultant cusp angles of denture teeth, once the long axis of the teeth are no longer perpendicular to the bench top, or once the cusp angle has been altered through occlusal adjustments.

CHAPTER

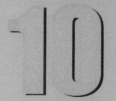

Maxillomandibular Records and Articulators

Dr. Kevin D. Plummer

161

The maxillomandibular records appointment occurs between the fabrication of the master casts and the arrangement of the denture teeth, and the trial insertion appointment. As might be imagined, this is an important appointment in which several goals must be accomplished. The maxillary record base and occlusion rim are used to transfer the correct orientation of the maxillary master cast relative to the condylar elements and axis-orbital plane of the articulator. This mimics the maxilla's relationship to the condyles and the patient's axis-orbital plane. The combination of both record bases and occlusion rims are used to transfer the correct horizontal and vertical position of the mandibular master cast relative to the maxillary master cast. This includes the proper centric relation position at the appropriate occlusal vertical dimension (OVD) for the patient (Figure 10–1). The occlusion rims are also used to record contour for the proper positioning of the anterior and posterior denture teeth. Before proceeding with the maxillomandibular records appointment, an articulator must be selected to use for the treatment procedures.

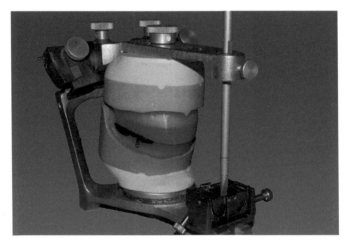

Figure 10–1   Record bases and occlusion rims properly oriented on the articulator.

Articulators for Complete Dentures

In the fabrication of dental prostheses, a mechanical device called an articulator is used to relate the opposing casts and simulate the movements that occur in the areas of the teeth. Although there are a myriad of articulators available with widely varying degrees of adjustability, most have similar physical characteristics. All have an upper and lower member to which maxillary and mandibular casts can be firmly attached and then removed as desired. All but the simplest articulators allow the maxillary cast to be attached to the articulator with an instrument called a facebow. A facebow relates the maxillary cast to the opening and closing axis of the articulator in the same relationship as the maxilla relates to the anatomical hinge axis of the patient. All articulators allow varying degrees of movement between the upper and lower members. Virtually all have some part that represents the condylar head in the patient (commonly called the condylar element or post on the articulator) and another part that represents the guiding surfaces or articular eminence (commonly called the condylar housing). The condylar elements and guidance surfaces should be thought of as cams that allow the articulator to replicate the movement observed intraorally. Most have an adjustable part that serves as a vertical stop in the front of the articulator (incisal pin) and helps maintain the vertical dimension as set on the articulator. There is usually some type of locking mechanism that will keep the upper member in the centric position in relation to the lower member of the articulator. These are the basic parts seen on most adjustable articulators (Figures 10–2A and 10–2B).

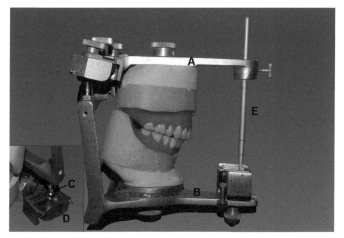

Figure 10–2A   Class III articulator. A: Upper Member B: Lower Member C: Condylar Element or Post D: Condylar Housing E: Incisal Pin

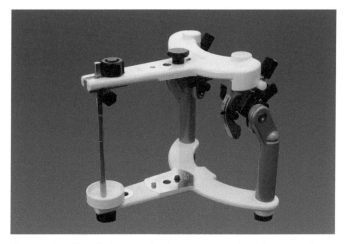

Figure 10–2B   Various articulators are suited for complete denture fabrication. The most common type are Class III articulators, which accept a facebow and can use protrusive or lateral records to set the condyles

No matter the number of adjustable parts or programmability, it is unlikely that any articulator will precisely duplicate the condylar movements in the temporomandibular joints. However, for complete denture patients and many dentate patients, exact accuracy is not necessary. The complexity of an articulator, its ability to be programmed, and the ability of the clinician to program the instrument will determine the accuracy of mimicking these anatomical movements. For an articulator to provide exacting accuracy, it must be precisely programmed. This programming is done by making recordings of patient mandibular movements and then forcing the articulator to duplicate these movements. These recordings are accomplished with various technologies, but all require precise fit and adjustability of the recording devices. To accurately record the patient movements, the device must be rigidly attached to the patient while the movements are being recorded. This is reasonably easy with the dentate patient because the device can usually be firmly attached directly to the natural teeth. However, for edentulous patients, the device must be attached to the record bases/occlusion rims, which are somewhat mobile because they are resting on movable tissues. Therefore, extreme accuracy in programming these articulators is difficult in complete denture patients. Fortunately this same accuracy is not required for edentulous patients, and complex articulators are not indicated for their treatment.

Even though an articulator may not reproduce movements in an identical pattern as that of the patient, it is still accurate enough to establish proper occlusal and esthetic placement of the artificial teeth. Because the completed dentures rest on movable tissues, the use of an articulator for the final occlusal adjustments is preferable to perfecting denture occlusions intraorally. This will be further discussed in the Chapter 14, Insertion.

Articulators are divisible into four classes. A class I articulator is a simple holding instrument capable of accepting a single static registration; vertical motion is possible. A class II articulator permits horizontal as well as vertical motion but does not orient the motion to the temporomandibular joints (Figure 10–3). A class III articulator simulates condylar pathways by using averages, or mechanical equivalents, for all or part of the motion; these instruments allow for orientation of the casts relative to the joints and may be arcon or nonarcon instruments (Figure 10–4 and 10–5). A class IV articulator will accept three dimensional dynamic registrations; these instruments allow for

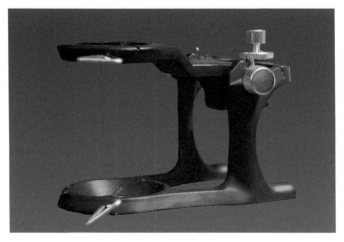

Figure 10–3 Class II articulators permit horizontal and vertical movement but do not orient the motion to the temporomandibular joints

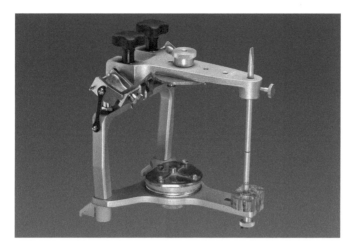

Figure 10–4 Class III articulators simulate condylar pathways with mechanical equivalents and allow for cast orientation relative to the temporomandibular joints. Arcon instruments have the condylar element on the lower member.

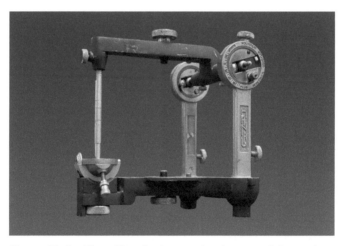

Figure 10–5 Class III articulators simulate condylar pathways with mechanical equivalents and allow for cast orientation relative to the temporomandibular joints. Non-Arcon instruments have the condylar element on the upper member.

orientation of the casts to the temporomandibular joints and simulation of mandibular movements.

The complexity of the occlusal scheme to be produced or replicated will dictate the complexity of the articulator to be used. Most dentures are fabricated on fairly simple articulators without complex settings. Articulators for denture fabrication usually fall into the Class III category and have the ability to use a facebow and accept some type of intraoral record for simple programming of the condylar elements.

Studies have shown that there is no need for a facebow orientation for most complete denture cases, provided that the occlusal vertical dimension is not changed

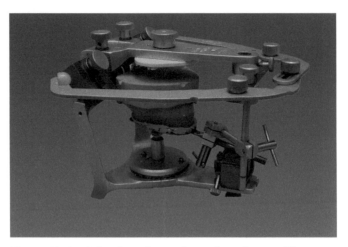

Figure 10–6   A facebow is used to orient the maxillary cast to the temporomandibular joints.

during the fabrication procedures. However, a facebow recording will place the dentures into a closer relationship with the anatomical closure axis of the patient and help minimize errors. Because using the facebow is a relatively easy procedure, it usually makes the articulating of the maxillary cast simpler and results in benefits making the denture fabrication process more accurate (Figure 10–6). The type of occlusal scheme (balanced versus nonbalanced) will also determine the need for interocclusal records to program the condylar inclination on the instrument.

The use of an articulator is essential for proper occlusal equilibration during the placement of the dentures. The use of a remount cast and remount index fabricated by the dental laboratory, will place the maxillary denture back on the articulator for the clinician prior to the placement appointment. A new centric relation record will orient the mandibular denture to the maxillary denture, and the occlusion can then be refined on the instrument (Figure 10–7). See Chapter 9, Occlusal Concepts, and Chapter 14, Insertion, for further information on denture occlusion.

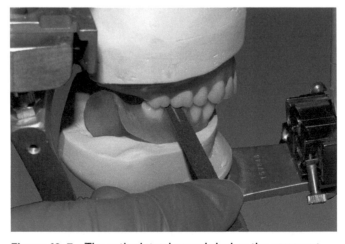

Figure 10–7   The articulator is used during the remount procedure to perform the final occlusal adjustments for the completed dentures

Maxillomandibular Records

The retention of the record bases is often a concern to the clinician and the patient at this time. This lack of adequate retention is usually caused by the requirements of the laboratory procedure during fabrication of the record bases. The laboratory technician must block out undesirable undercuts on the master cast prior to fabricating the record base in order to protect the cast during record base fabrication. This required blockout results in a space between the record base and tissues intraorally, and often causes a loss of retention of the record base. This lack of retention will be present until the dentures are processed and may be a major concern to the patient. The clinician must assure the patient that the record base is not the completed denture, and the retention will be present when the dentures are processed. Some clinicians prefer to have processed record bases fabricated on their master casts in order to minimize these problems. There is no blockout involved, and these are the actual denture bases that will be present in the completed dentures rather than an interim traditional record base. These record bases are processed just as if the denture was being completed. The occlusion rims are attached and eventually have the denture teeth arranged for trial insertion on these bases. A disadvantage of having processed record bases is the extra expense involved in needing a second processing step to attach the denture teeth to the base. The obvious advantages include the fact that the processed denture base can be evaluated for retention early in fabricating the dentures and additionally these bases will provide much better retention and stability during the making of maxillomandibular records and the trial insertion of the dentures.

Contouring the Occlusion Rims

The objective of this procedure is to shape the record bases and occlusion rim so that they will replace, in size and position, the teeth and supporting structures that have been lost. Correctly formed occlusion rims serve as excellent guides in the initial placement of artificial teeth (Figure 10–8).

Before the initial placement of the record base into the patient's mouth, the record base must be carefully inspected for sharp or rough surfaces or flanges. Once any irregularities are corrected, the record base should be comfortable for the patient. If the patient experiences discomfort, it may be necessary to use pressure disclosing paste to locate areas that may be causing the discomfort. Do not proceed if the patient is not comfortable. A slightly loose-fitting record base should be expected because most undercuts on the master cast were blocked out prior to record base fabrication. However, patients should be assured that these record bases are not the final denture, and that the completed denture will fit the ridges and soft tissues much better. The retention of slightly loose record bases may be improved by using a denture adhesive. However, extremely loose-fitting record bases should be evaluated for the cause. The final impression may have been unsatisfactory, and if that is determined to be the cause of the poor retention, now is the time to remake that impression.

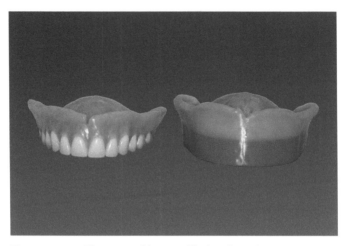

Figure 10–8   The record base will simulate the proper position of the teeth and establish the occlusal plane when contoured correctly.

 Labial/Buccal Contour

Wax is usually removed rather than added to the buccal and labial aspects of the maxillary occlusion rim to achieve adequate lip support from an esthetic and phonetic perspective. Because the laboratory technician probably had to block out labial undercuts prior to fabricating the maxillary record base, the upper lip may have the appearance of being over supported. Thinning or shortening the base may not fully correct the problem at this time. If it cannot be corrected, the patient must again be assured that this problem will not exist at denture insertion. The buccal surface of the rim almost always inclines labially from the border of the record base at about a 15 degree angle and is approximately 8–9mm labially from the center of the incisive papilla. A photograph of the patient when he or she had natural teeth could help in this determination. A comparison of the lip support with that from an existing denture, if one exists, is also helpful in making this determination.

In the posterior, wax should be added or removed to achieve a bilateral "buccal corridor" space for esthetic purposes. This space is created by sloping the maxillary occlusion rim inward in the posterior area. There should be pleasant amount of space on both sides of the occlusion rim, which reproduces the space seen between the buccal surfaces of the premolars and cheeks/lips in dentate patients. Obliterating this space is a common mistake when setting the width of the maxillary denture.

 Incisal Length and Esthetics

The anterior height of the maxillary plane of occlusion should be determined next. This is often called the incisal length of the occlusion rim. The incisal length will be the level at which the incisal edge of the maxillary central incisors will be positioned. Obviously esthetic and phonetic factors must be considered. Esthetically the length of the upper lip is an important guide because, generally speaking, the incisal edges of the central incisors should be slightly below the relaxed upper lip. It is common for the upper lip to drop slightly and become longer esthetically as wax is removed from the contours of maxillary occlusion rim. Therefore, only after achieving the proper labial/buccal contour of the maxillary occlusion rim, should the incisal length be considered.

Maxillary lip length must also be considered. The lip length can be evaluated by placing the tip of an index finger on the crest of the maxillary ridge in the anterior region and allowing the upper lip to rest down over the finger with the facial muscles relaxed. Observe the amount of the finger covered by the lip to get an approximation of the length of the lip. If the lip ends almost level with the crest of the ridge, the lip might be considered to be short. It the lip hangs down 4–5 mm below the crest of the ridge, it may be considered to be normal in length. If the lip hangs down 6 mm or more, it is generally considered to be long.

If the lip is short, a significant amount of the anterior teeth, and some of the denture base, may show in the completed denture even when the upper lip is relaxed. This may be a significant concern esthetically to the patient and should be discussed before any further treatment is completed. Surgery to minimize this problem is generally not indicated. If the upper lip appears normal in length, then the rim will often extend just below (1–2 mm) the resting length of the lip. Maxillary anterior teeth show on most patients when they smile. They do not, however, always show on patients when their muscles and lips are at rest. The amount of occlusion rim and eventually the denture teeth that show when the patient is at rest may vary, from not being visible at all to showing 4 mm or more, depending on the patient.

The phonetic contact of anterior teeth with the lips and tongue are essential for proper form and function in a complete denture. The contour and length of the occlusion rim should match these parameters. The proper position and support from the occlusion rim will affect the quality of speech sounds such as the "f" and "v" sounds, where the wet-dry line of the lower lip should gently contact the labial edges of the anterior occlusion rim. Sound such as "th" will also produce a gentle contact of the tongue with the lingual surfaces of the proposed position of the anterior teeth (Figure 10–9).

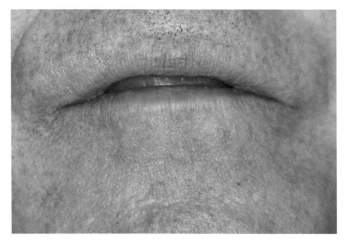

Figure 10–9 Proper contact of the wet/dry line of the lower lip with the labial edge of the maxillary occlusion rim during a "f"/"v" phonetic check.

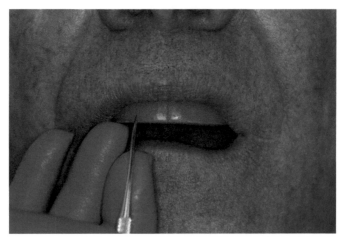

Figure 10–10   Midline is marked on the maxillary occlusion rim.

The midline of the anterior teeth should also be marked on the maxillary rim at this time. The philtrum of the lip is the most common guide for marking the midline (Figure 10–10). However, on some patients a different position may be more esthetic if the nose, philtrum of the lip, and chin are not in a line. Marking the midline on the rim will make this determination easier for the clinician. It will also serve to orient the maxillary rim correctly on the facebow fork, which will be discussed in a subsequent section.

 Forming the Plane of Occlusion

With the lip length determined, the plane of occlusion can now be formed (Figure 10–11). Three points will determine a plane, and at this point only the anterior length of

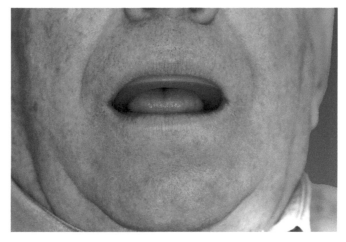

Figure 10–11   The anterior length is determined first and then the occlusal plane can be established.

the occlusion rim serves as one point. The posterior portion of the plane will be established using the anterior point along with other anatomical landmarks and esthetics. A Trubyte® Fox occlusal plane plate or tongue blade will help define the tentative plane of occlusion. However, esthetics is used to determine the final plane.

The Trubyte® Fox occlusal plane plate will be used to establish the anterior plane parallel to an interpupillary line, and the anterior-posterior plane parallel with Camper's plane (ala-tragus line). The occlusal plane of most natural posterior teeth is approximately parallel with these landmarks. This plane ideally would be parallel to the interpupillary line, equally split the distance between the opposing ridges, be at the level of the middle to upper third of the retromolar pad, be parallel to the remaining ridges, and be just below the corners of the mouth when the patient smiles (Figures 10–12 and 10–13). It

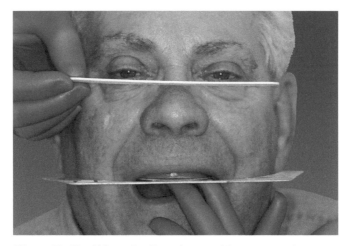

Figure 10–12   When the Fox plane guide rests on the occlusion rim, it should be parallel to the interpupillary line.

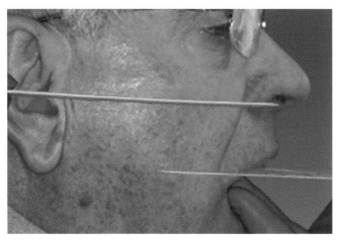

Figure 10–13   When the Fox plane guide rests on the occlusion rim, it should be parallel to the Ala-Tragus line (Camper's Plane).

will not often match all of the desired ideal critera on this list. Esthetics and function are certainly significant concerns for making the final determination. This initial estimate of the plane of occlusion is, therefore, tentative and may require adjustment during the setting of the teeth or at the trial insertion appointment.

Mounting the Maxillary Cast on the Articulator

The master casts must now be accurately positioned on an articulator so that proper occlusion will be developed during the tooth arrangement. The proper position of the maxillary cast relative to the condyles is an important concept for many prosthodontic procedures, and complete dentures are no exception. The orientation of the maxillary cast to the condylar elements of the articulator and axis-orbital plane must match the orientation of the maxillary arch to the hinge axis and axis-orbital plane of the actual patient. This is accomplished through use of the previously contoured maxillary record base/occlusion rim and a facebow. The correct orientation of the casts to the opening and closing hinge axis will minimize errors in occlusion that occur when there are discrepancies in the arc of closure. A facebow orientation will ensure that the proper relationship will minimize this type of error.

Facebows are generally classified as either kinematic or arbitrary. Kinematic facebows can precisely match the hinge axis position when used with the natural dentition. However, with the required used of movable record bases/occlusion rims with complete denture patients, that degree of accuracy is not normally achieved. They are not recommended for complete denture fabrication.

Arbitrary facebows rely on facial and anatomical landmarks to record the position of the maxilla relative to the hinge axis and axis-orbital plane (or base of the skull). They are accurate enough to place the articulator hinge axis within 6 mm of the true hinge axis more than 80% of the time. This creates an acceptably accurate arc of closure, which will minimize occlusal discrepancies in the dentures. Arbitrary facebows are similar enough to fall into the same approximate use pattern. Check with the facebow manufacturer for specific instructions for the particular facebow that will be used. Many arbitrary facebows use the external auditory meatus and an anatomical landmark based on the position of orbitale to make this three dimensional determination.

A fork is commonly attached to the anterior portion of the facebow with a series of adjustable fittings to allow three dimensional adjustments. The facebow is attached to the maxillary record base and occlusal rim during the clinical procedure, positioned on the patient, and the facebow recording is made. Four nonparallel notches are placed in the maxillary occlusion rim (two on each side), in the area usually occupied by the first premolar and the second molar. The notches will serve to orient the maxillary occlusion rim, which is then usually attached to the facebow fork using a vinyl polysiloxane (VPS) registration material (Figure 10–14). The adjustable fittings allow the fork attached to the maxillary occlusal rim and record base to be adjusted to align the facebow with the third point of reference to establish the axis-orbital plane (Figure 10–15).

Once the recording is made, the record base/occlusion rim and facebow are disinfected, the maxillary cast is placed in the record base, the facebow is positioned on the articulator, and the maxillary cast is attached to the articulator using mounting stone (Figure 10–16). The articulator manufacturer's instructions should be followed to accomplish this procedure. The master cast will need to be removed from this mount and

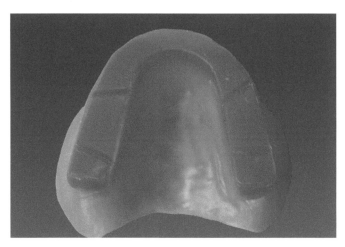

Figure 10–14   Four nonparallel notches 2 mm x 2 mm are placed on the maxillary occlusion rim in the area of the premolars and molars. Notches orient the rim to the face-bow fork.

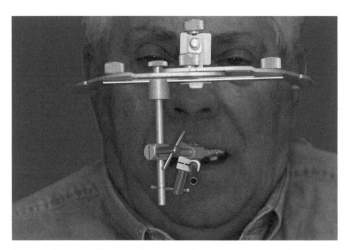

Figure 10–15   The maxillary occlusion rim is attached to the fork, which is then secured to the properly adjusted facebow using a series of adjustable toggles until the proper orientation is achieved.

returned during subsequent laboratory procedures. To facilitate this removal orientation grooves should be present in the master cast base and a lubricating agent should be applied to approximately fifty percent of the base surface before the mounting stone is used. If the decision is made to make the interocclusal recording prior to mounting the maxillary cast, the facebow can be set aside and the cast can be articulated at a later time. If the cast is to be articulated after using the maxillary rim to make the subsequent CR record, the occlusion rim and orientation grooves cannot be altered during the jaw relation procedure.

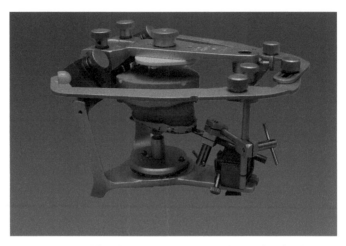

Figure 10–16   Maxillary cast and record base/occlusion rim supported by the facebow recording. The next step will be to attach the maxillary cast to the articulator using mounting stone.

Establishing the Occluding Vertical Dimension (OVD)

The centric relation (CR) position and occluding vertical dimension orientation of the mandibular cast on the articulator must match the centric relation position and occluding vertical dimension of that seen in the patient. The record bases/occlusion rims are used to transfer the correct horizontal and vertical position of the mandibular master cast relative to the maxillary master cast.

Once the maxillary plane of occlusion is established, the determination of the occlusal vertical dimension is made. When making this determination, the proper interocclusal distance must be maintained in order to minimize speech problems and potential soft tissue irritation. Failure to provide adequate interocclusal distance produces excessive interarch distance when the teeth are in occlusion. Most often the patient's face does not appear relaxed, and the lips cannot lightly touch when the patient is at rest. The patient might appear to be stretching the lower lip to get contact. This position does not allow the muscles that elevate the mandible to complete their contraction. Therefore these muscles will continue to exert force to overcome this obstacle. This often results in damage to the supporting tissues that includes soreness, possible ischemia, and eventual resorption. This excessive occlusal vertical dimension may also result in some facial distortion because the patient has difficulty closing the lips together properly. On the other hand, too much interocclusal distance can also cause problems. This overclosure or reduced occlusal vertical dimension at tooth contact can cause temporomandibular joint damage, facial distortion, loss of muscle tone, and possibly angular cheilitis. The patient often has the appearance of the "nose being too close to the chin."

The initial determination of the occlusal vertical dimension is often achieved by making multiple measurements of different facial parameters because there is no single method of accurately making this determination. One method begins by determining the proper resting vertical dimension (RVD) for a particular patient and subtracting approxi-

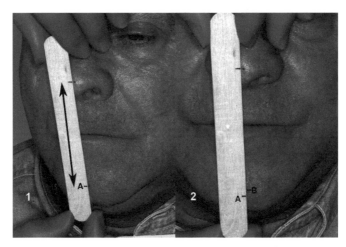

Figure 10–17 1. The resting vertical dimension (A) is established and marked on a tongue blade. The determination is made between two marks, one on the nose and another on the chin. 2. The rims are contoured to make even contact at 2–3 mm less than the resting vertical dimension. This 2–3 mm is the interocclusal distance and the resulting position (B) is the occlusal vertical dimension.

mately 2–3 mm (Figure 10–17). The resting position is theoretically a balance of muscles when the head is in a normal upright position. It can be determined by having the patient relax and letting the lips gently touch, or by having the patient maintain a prolonged "mmm" humming sound. This measurement should be attempted several times, letting the patient speak and relax between the measurements. Two to three millimeters is subtracted from the RVD and the resulting measurement is then the tentative occluding vertical dimension. Next the plane of occlusion of the record base and occlusion rim on the mandibular arch is altered so that it is at the middle of the retromolar pads in the posterior, and slightly below the corners of the mouth anteriorly. The maxillary and mandibular RBORs are inserted and the patient instructed to close into gentle contact. The occlusion rims are adjusted to allow for even contact at the tentative OVD. Opposing teeth should not touch during speech once the denture is completed, so no matter which method is used to determine the occlusal vertical dimension, there must be clearance between the opposing occlusion rims when the patient makes sibilant sounds. During sibilant sounds the teeth come as close together as they ever do during speech. Therefore, if the necessary interocclusal distance is present at this time it should be available once the dentures are inserted. This distance is often called the "closest speaking space," or interocclusal clearance. The anterior teeth may come extremely close together during this determination, but a range of 2–4 mm of interocclusal clearance in the premolar area is considered within the normal range. Esthetically, when the rims are in contact, the lips should gently touch and the chin should not look too close to the nose (Figure 10–18).

As the correct occluding vertical dimension is approached, it may become necessary to change the preliminary height of the maxillary plane of occlusion. If it appears as though the maxillary rim may be quite a bit longer than the mandibular rim, the initial length of the maxillary rim should be modified. In most instances, the maxillary and mandibular rims will not be grossly different in height at the correct occluding vertical

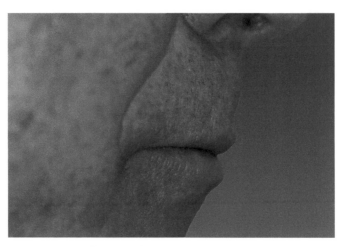

Figure 10–18 Esthetically, when the rims are in contact, the lips should touch and the chin should not appear to be too close to the nose

dimension, with the maxillary rim usually slightly larger than the mandibular. Always keep esthetics, phonetics, and function in mind when making these changes. If the facebow recording and horizontal records are both being made before the maxillary cast is mounted on the articulator, all adjustments of the maxillary rim must be made prior to the facebow recording. Changes to the rims after making the facebow recordings will change the fit of the rims into the facebow fork.

 Determining the Centric Relation Position

The correct horizontal relationship for fabricating complete dentures is always the centric relation position. Many techniques for establishing centric relation for dentate patients are not applicable for edentulous patients because of the unique nature of the record bases on the residual ridges of the edentulous patient. Edentulous patients do not need to be deprogrammed prior to making the CR recording.

The clinician must be able to manipulate the patient's mandible to the centric relation position, as it is: 1) the starting reference point for complete denture fabrication, 2) repeatable and it can be verified, and 3) is a functional position for denture occlusion. Complete dentures should always be fabricated so their initial and complete final occlusal position is coincident with the centric relation arc of closure. At the proper occluding vertical dimension, this position then becomes the centric occlusion position for the patient.

Because the centric relation position is somewhat dependant on head posture, the head should be held fairly upright. The position of the dentist's hands is an important factor in making accurate centric relation records and maintaining record bases in their correct position. The nondominant hand is inverted and placed in the mouth so that the soft tissue of the thumb and index fingers lies on the opposing buccal surfaces of the maxillary and mandibular occlusion rims, between the occlusal surfaces in the first molar

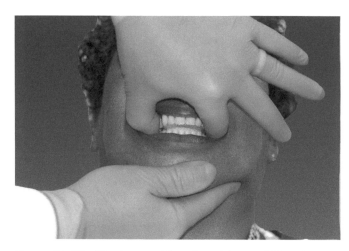

Figure 10–19   The inverted hand position stabilizes both the maxillary and mandibular record bases during the CR record-making procedure. Note the thumb on the symphysis of the mandible to guide the patient but not displace the mandibular record base.

region. As the patient closes, the tissue of the fingers is allowed to move buccally so that the force of the closure maintains both bases in position with a minimum of displacement of the supporting tissue. The other hand is used to help guide the patient to centric relation position. Care should be exercised to avoid displacing the mandibular record base in the posterior direction (Figure 10–19).

Because it is sometimes difficult to get the patient into the CR position, it is a good idea to practice this position with the patient prior to attempting to make the recording. Remember, you are attempting to capture the most superior/anterior relaxed position from which the patient can make rotational and repeatable recordings. This is the centric relation position and is the only verifiable position the patient can assume. Most patients cannot assume a relaxed centric relation position from a vertical dimension that is grossly open from the desired final occlusal vertical dimension. Therefore, the patient should be close to the correct OVD prior to attempting to achieve the CR position. It is advisable to instruct the patient to "let your jaw relax, close slowly and easily on your back teeth, and stop as soon as you feel the first contact". Some patients will automatically assume the CR position. Some, however, simply cannot relax and close into this position. These patients may be very difficult and take all the skills of the clinician to achieve and verify the position. Practice with the patient until both the clinician and the patient are familiar with the desired position and procedure. In some instances, other methods must be used to position the jaw in centric relation. Some of these include:

1. Having the patient completely relax the mandible while the clinician gently shakes the mandible up and down. When the patient gets in a completely relaxed state, the mandible should hinge up and down in a repeatable arc. This is the centric relation position. Gently continue to shake and lift the mandible until the correct OVD is reached.
2. Placing the tip of the tongue in the top and back of the mouth.

3. Telling the patient to "Stick out the upper teeth." This misnomer sometimes will help the patient make the correct mandibular movement.
4. Tipping the chair and patient back to allow gravity to help position the mandible.
5. Using a mirror so that the patient can see the CR mandible position.

When the patient is closing in centric relation, inform him or her that the closure is correct so that he or she becomes aware of the position by feel. Most patients will learn the desired technique by means of these instructions.

The maxillary master cast has now been properly placed on the articulator using a face-bow recording. The mandibular occlusion rim has been adjusted so that there is unrestricted contact with the maxillary occlusion rim at the correct occluding vertical dimension, and it is in centric relation. This horizontal relationship will now be captured with some type of recording material. However, because we must make the recording at the correct OVD, space must now be created to allow room for the record material. If this space is not created, the OVD will be unacceptably increased during the record-making procedure. This space is created by vertically reducing approximately 2 mm of wax from the occlusal surface of the mandibular occlusion rim in the premolar and molar areas bilaterally (Figure 10–20). It is very important that, when the patient closes into contact on the anterior occlusion rims, minimal pressure is applied to the rims by the patient. It is also necessary to ensure that the anterior contact does not displace the record base and occlusion rims during this procedure.

The opposing record bases/occlusion rims will be related to each other by making an interocclusal recording. Modeling compound, wax or VPS is often used for this recording. Some type of orientation grooves are necessary to be able to relate the opposing occlusion rims once the interocclusal recording is made. The orientation grooves used to make the facebow recording on the maxillary arch should still be present. VPS material will not stick to the mandibular rim, so mechanical retention or adhesive is necessary to keep the registration material in place on the mandibular rim. Undercut

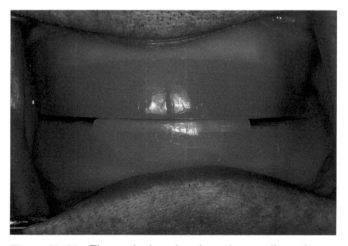

Figure 10–20 The occlusion rims have been adjusted to the occlusal vertical dimension and wax has been removed to allow for placement of the record material for recording the vertical and horizontal mandibular position.

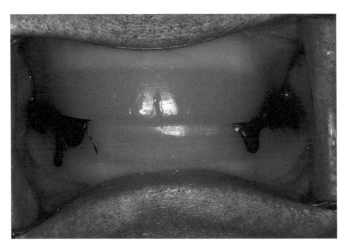

Figure 10–21   A modeling compound record has been made intraorally.

grooves or adhesives are both acceptable methods for retention. The retention is not necessary if modeling compound or wax is used to make the recording because it will stick to the mandibular occlusion rim. Whichever material is used, the maxillary occlusion rim is covered with a thin film separating medium, often Vaseline, the patient is closed into the material at the correct OVD and in the CR position, and the material is allowed to polymerize or cool until rigid. Due to the short set time of VPS recording materials, the clinician should manipulate the patient into the proper CR position with both rims in the mouth and approach the correct OVD. Just before contact of the anterior of the rims, an assistant should place the recording material between the rims. The patient should then be guided and closed to the final position. If modeling compound or wax is used, it will be placed on the mandibular rim extraorally, properly heated, tempered, and then placed in the patient's mouth to make the record (Figure 10–21).

Retrieve and reassemble the rims and check to see if there is contact of the opposing record bases in the posterior areas. If the record bases are touching, they may have been displaced from their correct position on the ridge, and a new interocclusal record must be made after relieving these contact areas. The recording of the indices should be sharp and well defined (Figure 10–22). The record bases and occlusion rims should be stable when reassembled.

Excess recording material is trimmed from the occlusion rim, and the occlusion rims are placed back in the patient's mouth. If the record appears to be correct, proceed with articulating the mandibular cast. If there is any question about the mandible being in the correct CR position, the record should be remade.

Articulating the Mandibular Cast

The maxillary cast is either already positioned on the articulator using the facebow record or is positioned at this time following the articulator manufacturer's instructions. Once the maxillary cast is properly positioned, the occlusion rims are placed on their

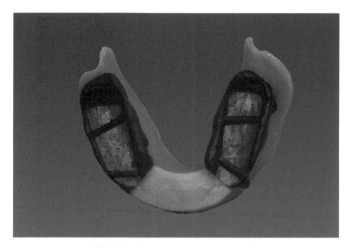

Figure 10–22 Well-defined notches have been recorded, and there is even, smooth contact over the entire record surface.

respective casts, and the records are seated together. Observe the casts for possible contact in the posterior areas. If they make contact, the cast must be trimmed until there is no cast-to-cast contact. Secure the mandibular cast to the maxillary cast to prevent movement during the articulation procedure. The articulator must be checked to verify that the position of the incisal pin is correct and that the upper member of the articulator is locked in the CR position. The settings of the articulator should match the manufacturer's instruction for the instrument being used. Secure the mandibular cast to the lower member of the articulator using mounting stone (Figure 10–23) (Figure 10–1). Orientation grooves and proper lubrication should be used for the mandibular cast as described for the maxillary cast earlier.

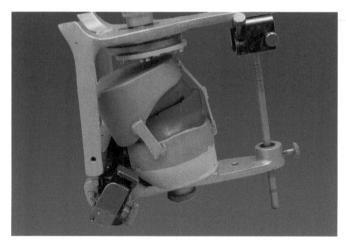

Figure 10–23 Mandibular cast and record base/occlusion rim secured into centric relation record and related to the maxillary cast. The mandibular cast is ready to attach to the articulator with mounting stone.

Some clinicians make a verification of the CR record after the mandibular cast has been articulated. This is simply a repeat of the initial recording made intraorally. The second recording should match the original cast mounting. To verify the first recording the upper and lower members of the articulator should be in the same relationship when the second record is introduced between the occlusion rims. The pin is raised off the incisal support and the centric holding latch is released. The occlusion rims are returned to the casts and firmly seated into the new record. There must be no movement of the condylar heads away from their initial positions. If the second record does not verify the first recording. then a determination must be made about which recording is accurate. The clinician should note the discrepancy between the two recordings and make a third recording. If this third recording matches the first recording, then the initial recording is verified. If it does not match the first recording, but matches the discrepancy seen with the second recording, then the mandibular cast should be removed from the articulator and re-articulated. It may be necessary to verify this third recording. Verification records may not be applicable to all types of articulators and are not a guarantee that the record is correct.

Completing the Maxillomandibular Records Appointment

To complete this visit, it will be necessary to select the correct denture teeth that will be used in the arrangement of the teeth. This will be covered in the Chapter 11, Tooth Selection.

References

Fayz, F., Eslami, A.: Determination of Occclusal Vertical Dimension: A Literature Review. J Prosthet Dent 59:321-323, 1988.

Hickey, J.: Centric Relation—A Must for Complete Dentures. Dent Clin N Am, 587-600, Nov 1964.

Niswonger, M.: The Rest Position of the Mandible and Centric Relation. J Am Dent Assoc: 1572-1582, 1934.

Pleasure, M.: Correct Vertical Dimension and Freeway Space. J Am Dent Assoc 43: 160-163, 1951

Rahn, A. O., and Heartwell, C. M., editors: Textbook of Complete Dentures. 5th Ed. New York: Lippincott, 1993.

Swerdlow, H.: Vertical Dimension Literature Review. J Prosthet Dent 15:241-247, 1965.

The Glossary of Prosthodontic Terms. J Prosthet Dent 94:10-92, 2005.

Wagner, A. G.: Comparison of four methods to determine rest position of the mandible. J Prosthet Dent 25:506, 1971

Weinberg, L.: An evaluation of basic articulators and their concepts, Part I. Basic concepts. J Prosthet Dent 13: 622, 1963.

Weinberg, L.: An evaluation of basic articulators and their concepts, Part II. Arbitrary, positional, semiadjustable articulators. J Prosthet Dent 13: 645, 1963.

Weinberg, L.: An evaluation of basic articulators and their concepts, Part III, Fully Adjustable Articulators. J Prosthet Dent 13:873-888, 1963.

Yurkstas, A., and Kapur, K.: Factors Influencing Centric Relation Records in Edentulous Mouths. J Prosthet Dent 14:1054-1065, 1964.

QUESTIONS

1. What is the objective of contouring the occlusion rims?

2. Which measurements can serve as a guide for the initial anterior contours of the maxillary occlusion rim?

3. How can phonetics help determine the proper occlusion rim contour?

4. The orientation of the maxillary cast to the condylar elements of the articulator and axis-orbital plane must match the orientation of the maxillary arch to the hinge axis and axis-orbital plane of the actual patient. How is this accomplished?

5. Which anatomical landmarks are typically used by arbitrary facebows to achieve proper orientation?

6. What is the normal range for interocclusal distance?

7. Why is the centric relation position so important for complete denture fabrication?

8. What does a facebow record accomplish when articulating a maxillary cast?

9. Why is recording extreme accuracy of mandibular movements not possible with fully edentulous patients?

10. What affects the accuracy of an articulator with regard to mimicking anatomical movements of the patient?

ANSWERS

1. To shape the record bases and occlusion rim so that they will replace, in size and position, the teeth and supporting structures that have been lost. Correctly formed occlusion rims serve as excellent guides in the initial placement of artificial teeth.

2. The buccal surface of the rim almost always inclines labially from the border of the record base at about a 15 degree angle and is approximately 8–9 mm labially from the center of the incisive papilla.

3. The proper position and support from the occlusion rim will affect the quality of speech sounds such as the "f" and "v" sounds, where the wet-dry line of the lower lip should gently contact the labial edges of the anterior occlusion rim. Sounds such as "th" will also produce a gentle contact of the tongue with the lingual surfaces of the proposed position of the anterior teeth.

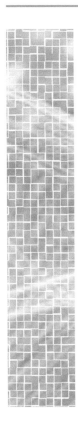

4. This is accomplished through use of the previously contoured maxillary record base/occlusion rim and a facebow recording.

5. Many arbitrary facebows use the external auditory meatus and an anatomical landmark based on the position of orbitale to make this three dimensional determination.

6. A range of 2–4 mm of interocclusal distance is considered to be within the normal range.

7. This position is: 1) the starting reference point for complete denture fabrication, 2) repeatable and can be verified, and 3) a functional position for denture occlusion. Complete dentures should always be fabricated so their initial and complete final occlusal position is coincident with the centric relation arc of closure. At the proper occluding vertical dimension, this position then becomes the centric occlusion position for the patient.

8. A facebow relates the maxillary cast to the opening and closing axis of the articulator in the same way that the maxilla relates to the anatomical hinge axis of the patient.

9. The record bases that are attached to the recording devices are somewhat mobile because they are resting on movable tissues.

10. The complexity of an articulator, its ability to be programmed, and the ability of the clinician to program the instrument will determine the accuracy of mimicking anatomical movements.

CHAPTER

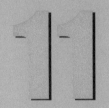

Tooth Selection

Dr. Philip S. Baker

The growing demand for esthetic dentistry clearly demonstrates increased public awareness of the benefits of a pleasing smile and, as shown in recent studies, this interest is not limited to younger patients. In contrast to previous generations, today's middle-aged and older adult is much more likely to be concerned with maintaining a healthy and youthful dental image. Because of this emphasis on the esthetic aspects of treatment, selection of appropriate denture teeth plays an extremely important role in patient satisfaction.

The selection of denture teeth for complete dentures seems to be an area in which many dentists feel uncomfortable. The academic background of these clinicians may play a significant role in their hesitance to deal with esthetic details. Concern with facts, figures, and logic often took precedence over artistic development in their education. In frustration, they may delegate this task to auxiliary personnel, including laboratory technicians. By doing so, these dentists lose an opportunity to develop the esthetic skills that are vital to many other aspects of dental treatment and deprive themselves of a tremendous source of satisfaction and accomplishment. In any case, the ultimate responsibility for denture tooth selection remains with the clinician.

As with any skill, excellence in denture esthetics can be developed with patience and persistence. In the selection of denture teeth to meet the esthetic desires of a patient, the clinician must: 1) correctly interpret the esthetic desires of the patient, 2) recognize the practicality of those desires and discuss this information with the patient in treatment planning and again throughout treatment, and 3) coordinate the patient's realistic desires with the dentist's personal esthetic and functional philosophies in construction of the definitive prostheses.

Information necessary for the selection of appropriate denture teeth may actually begin with introduction of the dentist and patient. Valuable direct and indirect information is gathered through careful observation as the patient describes their problems and desires. The clinician should observe the patient's posture, personality, oral and facial characteristics, dress, speech, habits, and mannerisms. The clinician should evaluate the patient both emotionally and physically. Compare the patient's assessment of their condition and desires with these clinical observations. Unrealistic expectations should be dealt with well before treatment begins, and the patient continually reminded of any limitations as care progresses. Negative factors, such the requirement for a severe Class II anterior occlusion (Figure 11–1), that are pointed out to the patient after the dentures are completed, are often perceived as an excuse for error.

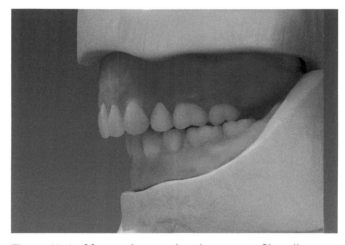

Figure 11–1 Mounted casts showing severe Class II anterior malocclusion.

Anterior Mold Selection

Existing Information

If the patient was relatively satisfied with his or her previous appearance, diagnostic casts of the patient's natural dentition, which may be in the possession of the patient or available from a previous care provider, may be ideal sources of information. The size and form of the natural teeth can often be matched. However the clinician must be careful not to agree to perpetuate any existing condition that may prove harmful if incorporated into new dentures.

Photographs can be an invaluable aid in tooth selection. Request that the patient bring in any personal photographs clearly showing their natural permanent teeth. Approximate tooth size, existing diastmas, anterior tooth alignment, and shade may be obvious in old photographs. However, many patients will bring in photographs that are decades old, and they must be reminded that the physical changes that have occurred over those decades make it impossible to match the esthetics of the natural dentition or dentures as seen in very old pictures. It is very important to safely store and return all personal photographs to the patient as soon as possible to preclude loss or damage.

A simple mathematical proportion may be developed using three known values in reference to the photograph and the patient: the interpupillary distance and width of the central incisor from the photograph, and the interpupillary distance on the patient. Solving for X gives the original width of the patient's central incisor.

$$\frac{\text{photo interpupillary distance}}{\text{patient's actual interpupillary distance}} = \frac{\text{photo central incisor width}}{X}$$

Any old dentures can serve as a guide for both the patient's likes and dislikes. If the patient is satisfied with the size and shape of the teeth, these are usually the best choice for new dentures. However, to repeat, the clinician must not agree to perpetuate any existing condition that may prove harmful to the patient. An irreversible hydrocolloid impression of the existing denture can be made extraorally, and a stone cast poured for later reference. These casts may become very important to the laboratory technician during tooth arrangement.

The patient's significant others are also an important source of information for tooth selection. In addition, observing the teeth of close relatives can be helpful. Any esthetic concerns brought up by this important group should be recognized and noted for future consideration.

The frontal outline form and size of the face, and lateral view of the patient's profile have been considered gross guides in tooth selection. There is, however, no scientific evidence to indicate that these are valid guides in the tooth selection process.

Although the size and shape of the residual ridges cannot actually determine a specific mold selection, they are important guides to overall size. Large maxillary ridges will usually require teeth with a "width of six anteriors on a curve" (canine to canine) of at least 53 mm. Small ridges will usually be less than 50 mm. (Figure 11–2)

Record Bases and Occlusion Rims

Record bases and occlusion rims play a basic role in complete denture prosthodontics as the means of transferring information from the clinic to the laboratory. For patients

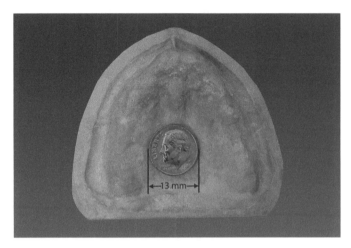

Figure 11–2 Example of an extremely small edentulous maxilla, with a coin placed to illustrate scale.

unable to supply records of their natural teeth, record bases and occlusion rims can also be used in denture tooth selection. To be useful in the selection of denture teeth, the occlusion rims must be correctly contoured to provide adequate lip support and meet esthetic and phonetic demands. Additionally the plane of occlusion must be formed and the vertical dimension of occlusion established.

The midline, high smile line and the "relaxed" corners of the mouth are scribed into the wax intraorally. The high smile line indicates the normal minimum incisogingival height of the maxillary anterior teeth to avoid an unsightly display of gingival base material (the so-called "gummy" smile). The distance between the corners of the mouth measured along the incisal region of the facial curvature of the occlusion rim represents an appropriate width for the six anterior teeth.

For patients with obvious contraction or distortion of the corners of the mouth, the interalar width technique may prove more reliable. It is based upon the observation that the centerline of the natural canine teeth is roughly in vertical alignment with the outer edge of the ala of the nose. Clinicians need to add 7 mm to the interalar measurement to produce the width of the six maxillary anterior teeth, from distal of canine to distal of canine. Generally, for African-American patients, one size smaller category mold than indicated by this value should be used, because of anatomical differences.

Commercial Guides

Many forms of commercial guides are available to the dentist to aid in selection of denture teeth, including physical mold guides (Figure 11–3). Although normally designed for a specific manufacturer's system, the information obtained can often be used with any other system.

One device is the Trubyte® Tooth Indicator (Figure 11–4), which can be used for estimating the size as well as outline and profile forms of maxillary anterior denture teeth. Tooth width and length are based upon an average 16:1 ratio of the bizygomatic width and height of the face in relation to the width and length dimensions of the

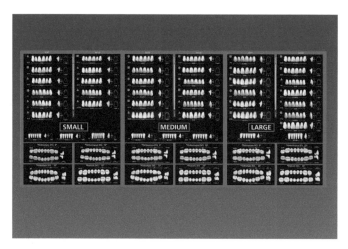

Figure 11–3   An example of a physical mold guide. Note that, although the denture teeth used in mold guides appear to be the normal denture teeth as sold by the particular company, the denture teeth in the mold guide may be of poor quality and should not be used in actual dentures. (Photo courtesy Ivoclar Vivadent, Inc.)

natural maxillary central incisor. The indicator's face plate has two registration bars, one on the left side and one at the bottom, which are moved along slots and locked into position against the skin of the zygomatic region and underside of the chin, with the mandible at rest. Maxillary central incisor width and length are read directly from the corresponding scale, as indicated by the position of the bar surface in contact with the patient's face.

Outline form is shown by comparing the facial form in relation to the vertical lines of the indicator, and is classified in the manufacturer's directions as square, square tapering, tapering, or ovoid (Figure 11–5). In the square form, the sides of the face roughly parallel the vertical lines. For the square tapering form, the upper face outline will parallel the lines and the lower will taper inward. The tapering form will exhibit a diagonal from the forehead to the angle of the mandible. The ovoid face shows an overall curved outline. This information is recommended for selecting denture teeth by some denture tooth manufacturers. However, there is no scientific data to validate this recommendation. This does not mean that it is not useful information and should not be used.

The Trubyte® Tooth Indicator may also be used to determine the patient's profile form for matching to the denture teeth. With the device held in place, the operator observes the relative straightness or curvature of the profile (Figure 11–6). Three reference points are used: the forehead, the base of the nose, and the point of the chin. If these points lie in a straight line, the profile is considered straight. If the forehead and point of the chin lie posterior to the base of the nose, the profile is curved. Again, while useful, there appears to be no scientific findings that validate the use of this information.

Another guide for maxillary anterior tooth selection is the Ivoclar Vivadent BlueLine™ FormSelector™ (Figure 11–7), which features a caliper, the Facial Meter, for correlation of the patient's interalar dimension with tooth mould width. This system also incorporates cards with actual-sized photographs of the six maxillary anterior teeth.

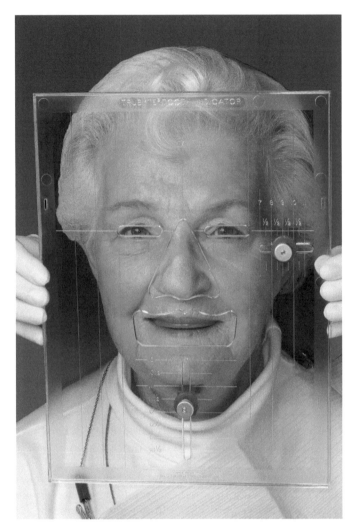

Figure 11–4   The Trubyte® Tooth Indicator. (Photo courtesy
DENTSPLY® International, Inc.)

These cards are helpful in selecting tooth form (soft or bold) and tooth length (short to long).

Additional Guides

While no study to date has confirmed predilections for tooth form, size, or shade, the factors of sex, age, and personality may be considered to develop a pleasing and harmonious restoration. Delicate, small, and curved or tapering forms are considered more feminine, while bold, large, and square forms tend toward the masculine. With age, the teeth become less rounded at the incisal edges and interproximal contacts, exhibiting an overall loss of curvature. Aging also produces a decreasing display of the maxillary anterior teeth and a greater display of the mandibular. The curve of the smile line also tends to flatten over time.

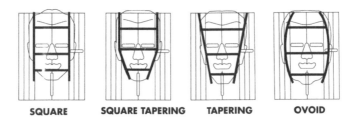

SQUARE   SQUARE TAPERING   TAPERING   OVOID

Figure 11-5   Use of the Trubyte® Tooth Indicator to determine facial outline form. (Drawing courtesy DENTSPLY® International, Inc.)

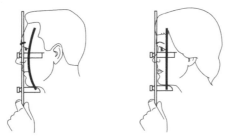

Figure 11-6   Determining facial profile with the Trubyte® Tooth Indicator. (Drawing courtesy DENTSPLY® International, Inc.)

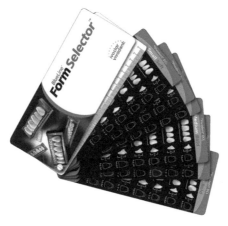

Figure 11-7   The Ivoclar Vivadent BlueLine™ Form Selector™. (Photo courtesy Ivoclar Vivadent, Inc.)

Posterior Mold Selection

The selection of the mold of the posterior teeth that will be used for the dentures is the responsibility of the dentist. Almost all denture tooth manufactures have a guide to recommend the posterior teeth based on the size of the anterior teeth. Therefore, an

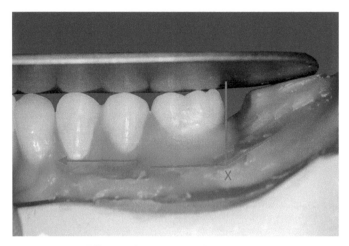

Figure 11–8 Effects of setting teeth over the steep slope leading from the residual ridge to the retromolar pad. X indicates the beginning of the slope from the residual ridge leading to the retromolar pad. Note the arrow indicating the potential movement of the mandibular denture during function if a second molar were placed on the slope leading to the retromolar pad.

initial mold selection is indicated following the selection of the anterior teeth. Remember that manufacturer's recommendations are based on averages and opinions, and may not be acceptable for a particular patient. The final posterior mold selection may not be possible until the anterior teeth have been arranged and the remaining posterior space has been evaluated.

The overall mesiodistal length of the posterior teeth is governed by the length of the edentulous mandibular ridge. Posterior denture teeth are not set on the slope leading from the residual ridge to the retromolar pad because of its tendency to act as an inclined plane when the patient chews food. The mandibular denture sliding down this slope may lead to severe irritation to the lingual aspect of the anterior ridge (Figure 11–8).

Prior to setting the posterior teeth recommended by the mold guide, a measurement is made from the distal surface of one of the mandibular canines to the beginning of the slope of the ridge leading up to the retromolar pad. This measurement, in millimeters, will be used to evaluate the recommended mold, and to select and alternative if necessary. If no slope is apparent, measure to the beginning of the retromolar pad. The mold selection designated by the guide may be correct, but because of inadequate space, a premolar or molar may be omitted from the tooth arrangement.

The selection of the occlusal scheme of the mandibular teeth is covered in Chapter 9, Occlusal Concepts.

 Shade Selection

Shade selection for denture teeth is usually made with a shade guide, which consists of a number of tooth-shaped tabs with varied degrees of hue, value, and chroma, and

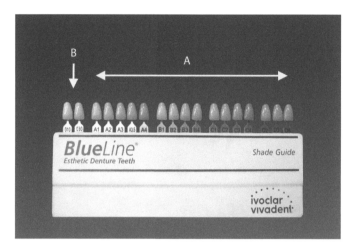

Figure 11–9 The BlueLine™ Shade Guide. A = Vita Classic A – D shades. B = Bleach shades. Note the exceptionally white shades (010 and 030) intended to match natural teeth that may have been bleached. (Photo courtesy Ivoclar Vivadent, Inc.)

sometimes characterization (Figure 11–9). The tabs represent the range of shades available for denture teeth. Although manufacturers have recently attempted to develop shade cross-matching with other company's products, the shade guide specifically designed by the maker of a selected product line is recommended for the most predictable and consistent results. Both anterior and posterior shade selections are done simultaneously and are the same shade in most manufacturers' systems.

The selection of shade is very difficult for some patients because it is not a scientific procedure. The following aids are helpful:

1. The shade of teeth on any previous dentures is often the shade of choice for patients.
2. Although teeth tend to darken over time, there is no specific shade of artificial teeth that can be used for a given age group.
3. The selection of tooth shade may be based upon the facial complexion. The least conspicuous shade is often the best choice.
4. Make use of any pre-extraction shade determination.
5. Recently extracted teeth may be useful, but caution is advised. Extracted teeth tend to lighten in shade with drying or storage in disinfectant solutions.
6. Listen to the patient's desires.

Many patients have the misconception that their natural teeth were "pure white," so the clinician must be careful when beginning the shade selection. Showing the patient the entire shade guide is not recommended—at least until an initial shade range is selected. This is because many patients will immediately focus on the lightest shade available regardless of skin complexion and other considerations.

Compare possible shades by holding several likely tabs adjacent to the patient's face. The operator may squint his eyes to reduce light intensity. The tab that disappears from vision first is in better harmony with the facial coloring than the other shades.

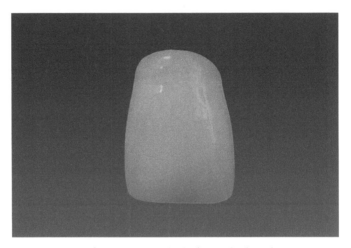

Figure 11–10   Shade tab with dark cervical region.

Do not allow the shade at the cervical of the tabs to distract the eye in this process. That area of the denture teeth will lie beneath the base material of the denture, and does not represent a final factor in tooth shade selection (Figure 11–10). Once a preliminary shade has been determined, the actual shade guide tooth should be observed in three locations: 1) outside the mouth and beside the cheek, 2) under the upper lip with just the incisal edge exposed and 3) under the upper lip with the mouth open and two-thirds to three-fourths of the tooth exposed.

Selection of the shade for the denture teeth should be made, within reason, with the consent of the patient and the patient's significant other. It is very frustrating to have newly completed dentures deemed unacceptable simply because the significant other does not approve of the shade or mold of the teeth. It is always wise to select a range of two or three shades that seem natural for the patient and then let the patient and the significant other make the final decision.

Many patients desire very light shades, and it is the dentist's responsibility to point out that such a choice may appear unnatural. However, some elderly patients do have very lightly shaded natural teeth, especially with the advent of bleaching. The greatest error in tooth selection is choosing teeth that are too light in shade and too small in size.

It is very important that the clinician enter the mold and shade selection in the patient's chart for future reference. If a repair or denture replacement becomes necessary, it may prove very difficult or impossible to exactly match the previously selected tooth mold and shade. Even a very minor change in shade or mold selection can lead to failure in the eye of the patient.

References

Groba, R. E.: Dollars and sense of dentures in your practice. Dental Economics November 2006;96:84-6.

Mavroskoufis, F., Ritchie, G. M.: Nasal width and incisive papilla as guides for the selection and arrangement of maxillary anterior teeth. J Prosthet Dent 1981;45:592-7.

Scrandrett, F. R., Kerber, P. E., Umrigar, Z R.: A clinical evaluation of techniques to determine the combined width of the maxillary anterior teeth and the maxillary central incisor. J Prosthet Dent 1982;48:15-22.

Young, H. A.: Selecting the anterior tooth mold. J Prosthet Dent 1954;748-60.

QUESTIONS

1. The collection of information for use in denture tooth selection begins:
   a) during contouring and marking of the occlusion rims.
   b) at the esthetic try-in appointment.
   c) with the introduction of the dentist and patient.
   d) after the casts have been mounted on the articulator.

2. Sources of information for anterior tooth mold selection include:
   a) patient photographs.
   b) diagnostic casts of the patient's natural dentition.
   c) existing dentures.
   d) record bases and occlusion rims.
   e) all of the above.

3. The high smile line scribed into the wax of the maxillary occlusion rim usually indicates the minimum incisogingival height of the maxillary anterior teeth to avoid a "gummy" smile.
   a) true
   b) false

4. The factors of age, sex, and personality can be useful in developing an esthetically pleasing denture. This has been proven in several scientific studies.
   a) both statements are true.
   b) both statements are false.
   c) the first statement is true, and the second is false.
   d) the first statement is false, and the second is true.

5. The selection of molds for denture teeth is the responsibility of the:
   a) dental assistant.
   b) patient.
   c) dentist.
   d) laboratory technician.

6. The overall mesiodistal width of the mandibular posterior teeth is governed by the amount of space available from the distal end of the canine tooth to the beginning of the slope to the retromolar pad.
   a) true
   b) false

7. Recently extracted teeth may be unreliable sources of shade information due to the effects of drying or storage in disinfectant solutions.
   a) true
   b) false

8. The most important source of shade information is the:
   a) tooth manufacturer.
   b) dentist.
   c) patient.
   d) photograph.

9. The shade that stands out most strongly when the operator squints the eyes is the best choice for harmony with the patient's complexion.
   a) true
   b) false

10. The most common errors in denture tooth selection are too light in shade and too small in size.
    a) true
    b) false

ANSWERS

1. c

2. e

3. a

4. c

5. c

6. a

7. a

8. c

9. b

10. a

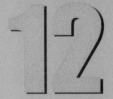

Tooth Arrangement

Dr. Carol A. Lefebvre
Dr. John R. Ivanhoe

The anterior and posterior denture teeth must be arranged to meet the esthetic, functional, and phonetic needs of the patient. Esthetic and functional guidelines were used when contouring the occlusion rims at the maxillomandibular records appointment, and the desired anterior and posterior facial and buccal contours as well as the plane of occlusion were established. The midline was also marked. These previously contoured occlusion rims serve as the guide for the preliminary arrangement of the denture teeth.

Generally the teeth are arranged in the following order: (1) maxillary anterior teeth—following the maxillary occlusion rim, (2) mandibular anterior teeth—using the occlusion rims and maxillary teeth as guides, (3) mandibular posterior teeth—using the anterior teeth, retromolar pads, and residual ridges as guides and (4) maxillary posterior teeth—using the mandibular posterior teeth as guides.

General Considerations for the Arrangement of the Anterior Teeth

1. The midline of the teeth should coincide with the facial midline (Figure 12–1).
2. For most patients, the position of the incisal edge of the maxillary anterior teeth provides esthetics and phonetics, while the position of the cervical portion, or necks, of the teeth and the fullness of the maxillary denture base determines lip support (fullness of the lips) (Figure 12–2).
3. The labial surfaces of the maxillary anterior teeth should generally be placed slightly labial to the surface of the labial flange. When viewed from the tissue side of the denture, a small but consistent amount of tooth should be present beyond the denture flange (Figure 12–3).
4. A vertical overlap of the anterior teeth is not indicated unless specifically determined by the clinician.

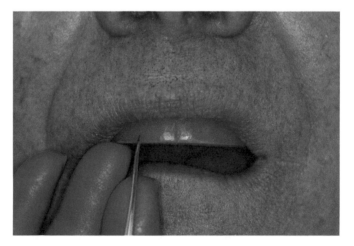

Figure 12–1   When arranging the central incisors, the dental laboratory technician will match the midline as marked by the clinician. The midline will often match the middle of the philtrum of the patient.

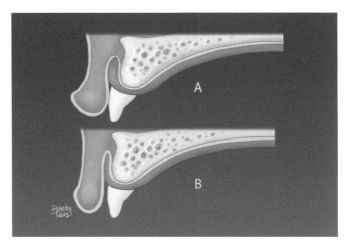

Figure 12–2   The position of the incisal edge of a maxillary anterior tooth generally provides for phonetics and esthetics, whereas the cervical portion, or necks, of the teeth and the fullness of the denture base determine lip support. Note that the position of the necks of the teeth and the increased fullness of the denture base provides more lip support in diagram A than it does in diagram B.

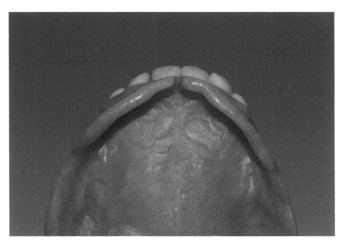

Figure 12–3   Note that, generally, a small but consistent amount of tooth should extend beyond the denture flange when viewed from the tissue side of the denture.

Maxillary Anterior Tooth Arrangement

Although asymmetry can be esthetically pleasing, and an irregular alignment of the anterior teeth may be quite esthetic, (Figure 12–4) most patients desire the incisal edges of all teeth to be on the same plane, no rotation of the individual teeth, no diastmas, and a

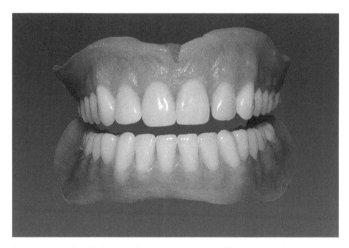

Figure 12–4 This tooth arrangement illustrates the esthetic effects of completing an irregular arrangement of the anterior teeth. Note that, by rotating the canines properly, the distal halves of the teeth are not visible. This dramatically improves the esthetics of the tooth arrangement.

very light tooth shade. Patients also generally desire no more than a moderate horizontal overlap of the opposing anterior teeth.

The exception is patients with existing dentures, who desire the arrangement of the teeth of the new denture to mimic those of the existing denture. Occasionally patients receiving immediate complete dentures also desire that the arrangement of the denture teeth match the arrangement of the natural teeth. For these patients, it is advisable to ask if they desire that the new tooth arrangement mimic the existing one. If so, an irreversible hydrocolloid impression of the existing denture should be made, a cast poured, and the cast forwarded to the dental laboratory technician to be used as a guide in the tooth arrangement. If the denture is to match existing natural teeth then a pre-extraction cast of the natural teeth should be included.

For the average complete denture patient, the maxillary central incisors should be positioned so that the midline is in harmony with the midline of the face, and so that the long axes are parallel with the long axis of the face. The labial position should match the labial surface of the occlusion rim, as was contoured during the maxillomandibular records appointment. A correctly marked midline will generally match the middle of the philtrum, (Figure 12–1) will usually coincide with the middle of the incisive papilla, and may or may not match the position of the labial frenula.

The alignment of the maxillary lateral incisors can be slightly altered to create a natural-appearing denture. Changes include altering the: (1) inclination of the long axis, usually distally (2) relationship to the incisal edges of the central incisors, (3) tooth width, (4) levels of the gingival margins, (5) tooth shade, and (6) shapes of incisal edges, angles, and proximal surfaces. However, as previously mentioned, most patients do not desire a characterized arrangement of the teeth, but prefer a symmetrical arrangement.

The maxillary canines are generally positioned so that the incisal cusp tip is at the same level as the central incisors. The long axis of the maxillary canine should be vertical or inclined distally, with the cervical portion appearing prominent because of its labial position in relation to the lateral incisor. For esthetic purposes, the canine should be rotated so that the distal half of the facial surface of the tooth is barely visible when viewed from the anterior (Figure 12–4).

Mandibular Anterior Tooth Arrangement

When arranging the mandibular anterior teeth, it is generally desirable to have some horizontal and/or vertical separation of the opposing anterior teeth while in centric occlusion. This arrangement will minimize premature contact of the anterior teeth, eliminating potentially excessive forces on the weaker anterior residual ridges. It should be noted that the maxillary anterior residual ridge is composed primarily of cancellous bone, which will rapidly resorb in some patients when subjected to excessive forces. The incisal edges of the mandibular teeth should not be placed forward of a plane perpendicular to the center of the labial vestibule, and under no circumstances should they be positioned over the anterior land area of the cast (Figure 12–5). Positioning the teeth in such a manner will generally result in significant denture instability during function due to the cantilever effect caused by positioning the mandibular teeth anterior to the residual ridge. Mandibular canines should usually be positioned in the same relative manner as the maxillary canines.

The mandibular central incisors are not initially arranged with the maxillary anterior teeth vertically overlapping the mandibular, unless specifically determined by the clinician. Vertical overlap is generally indicated for esthetic, phonetic, or functional

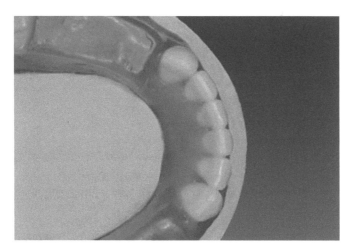

Figure 12–5   Because of potential undesirable cantilever forces, the incisal edges of the mandibular anterior teeth should not be arranged beyond the center of the vestibule. These teeth are in excellent position. To minimize a significant horizontal overlap of the opposing anterior teeth, the incisal edges may occasionally be positioned over the land area. However, position of the teeth in this manner is a compromise.

reasons. Vertical overlap of the anterior teeth is not allowed when arranging the teeth for a nonbalanced type of occlusion. Therefore, when vertical overlap of the teeth is required, the dental laboratory technician must anticipate the arrangement of the posterior teeth in a balanced occlusion.

The degree of horizontal and vertical overlap of the anterior teeth determines the incisal guidance of the arrangement. The teeth should not be arranged with such a steep incisal guidance that the posterior teeth disclude in excursive movements. Christensen's phenomena, the space that occurs between opposing occlusal surfaces during excursive movements, is not acceptable for complete denture patients. Generally, an incisal guidance more than 20 degrees greater than the anterior-posterior angulation of the plane of occlusion is contraindicated. It is difficult, if not impossible, to create a balanced occlusion with an excessively steep incisal guidance. The dental laboratory technician should attempt to minimize the steepness of the resultant incisal guidance whenever possible. This can be accomplished by either decreasing the vertical overlap or increasing the horizontal overlap as much as is permissible (Figure 12–6). Decreasing the steepness of the incisal guidance minimizes the separation of the posterior teeth during excursive movements and hence the requirement for excessively steep cusp heights, compensating curves, and/or effective cusp angles when arranging the posterior teeth.

The opposing anterior teeth should contact lightly in the protrusive and working movements. Anterior teeth that do not contact in the protrusive movement cannot incise thin foods such as lettuce, which may be a significant problem for many patients.

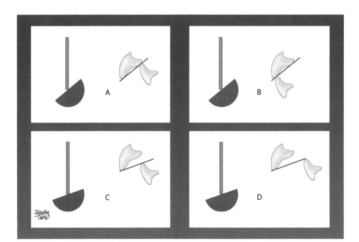

Figure 12–6   The incisal guidance of the articular is the result of the horizontal and vertical overlap of the anterior denture teeth and may be altered, within limits, by the dental laboratory technician while arranging the denture teeth. The incisal guidance of the denture teeth and incisal table is approximately 45 degrees in diagram A. In diagram B the vertical overlap of the teeth has been reduced, but the incisal guidance has not changed because the horizontal overlap was also decreased. The incisal guidance in diagram C has been reduced because the vertical overlap of the teeth has been decreased while the horizontal overlap has remained constant. The incisal guidance in diagram D has also been reduced by increasing the horizontal overlap while maintaining the vertical overlap.

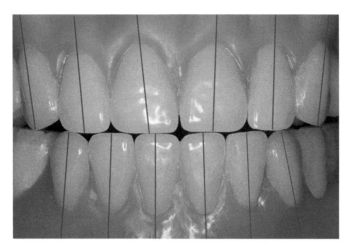

Figure 12–7   The long axis, incisal edges, and facial alignment of these teeth have been arranged to provide excellent esthetics. These teeth have a horizontal overlap when in centric occlusion. However, this illustration demonstrates the "kissing contacts" desired when the teeth are moved into the protruded relationship.

The dental laboratory technician should ensure that the individual tooth orientations combine to make the complete arrangement harmonize with the shape and relative positions of the residual ridges (Figure 12–7).

General Considerations for Posterior Tooth Arrangement

1. As mentioned previously, vertical overlap of the anterior teeth is occasionally indicated due to the esthetic, phonetic, or functional demands of the patient. However, because the need for an overlap is often not obvious during the maxillomandibular records appointment, initially a nonbalanced type occlusion is generally created for patients. If, at the trial insertion appointment the need for vertical overlap becomes obvious, it is necessary to make protrusive or lateral interocclusal records to set the condylar inclination of the articulator. Additionally, the clinician must determine the desired vertical overlap, select anatomic mandibular denture teeth, and return the arrangement to the dental laboratory technician. The denture teeth must be rearranged into a balanced occlusion and the trial insertion appointment repeated.

2. To minimize mandibular denture dislodgement during function, denture teeth should not be placed beyond the point at which the residual ridge begins to slope up toward the retromolar pad. If insufficient anteroposterior space exists to place all four posterior teeth, the first premolar or second molar is generally eliminated, depending upon the space available. A second molar will not be placed in this arrangement

(Figure 12–8). For improved masticatory function, it is generally better to eliminate the first premolar rather than the second molar, when possible (Figure 12–9).

3. When completing a nonbalanced occlusion, the mandibular posterior teeth are arranged on a flat occlusal plane with the long axes of the posterior teeth arranged perpendicular to the plane of occlusion (Figure 12–10). For balanced occlusion, the posterior teeth are arranged to a

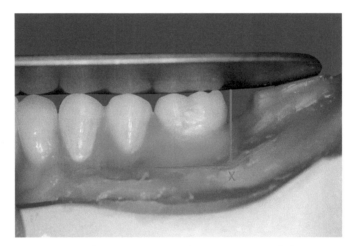

Figure 12–8 To minimize mandibular denture dislodgement during function, denture teeth should not be placed beyond the point at which the residual ridge starts to slope up toward the retromolar pad. A second molar will not be placed in this arrangement. Although not seen, X indicates the beginning of the slope up to the retromolar pad.

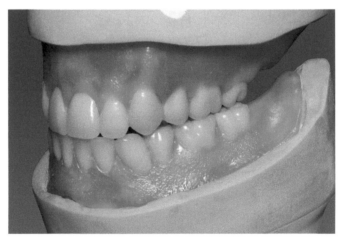

Figure 12–9 To improve chewing potential, the first premolars have been eliminated from this arrangement, due to the lack of space for all four posterior teeth.

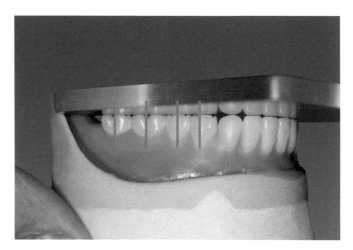

Figure 12–10   Note that the mandibular posterior teeth are arranged on a flat occlusal plane with the long axes of the posterior teeth arranged perpendicular to the plane of occlusion for a nonbalanced occlusion.

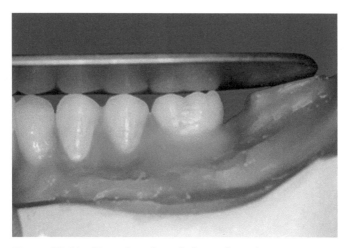

Figure 12–11   Note that, for a balanced tooth arrangement, a curved template is used. This creates an anterior-posterior and medial-lateral curvature of the occlusal surfaces. In complete dentures, this is called a compensating curve and is necessary to create the excursive contacts required for a balanced occlusion.

compensating curve (Figure 12–11). See Chapter 9, Occlusal Concepts, for further explanation.

4. The central grooves and centers of the marginal ridges of the teeth should lie in one continuous line, which may be straight or have a slight curvature with the concavity being directed lingually or palatally (Figure 12–12).

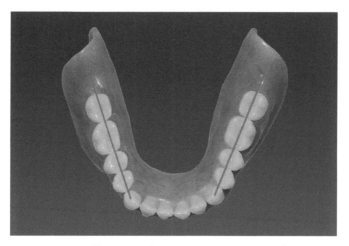

Figure 12–12   The central grooves and centers of the marginal ridges of the teeth in this arrangement lie in one continuous line, which may be straight or have a slight curvature with the concavity being directed lingually or palatally.

 ## Mandibular Posterior Tooth Arrangement

The antero-posterior placement of the mandibular posterior teeth is relatively easy to determine. The distal surfaces of the canines are the most anterior position for placement of the first premolars. The distal limit to placement of mandibular molars is the beginning of the incline of the retromolar pad (Figure 12–8). By not arranging mandibular teeth on the incline, the patient will not function in this area, and thus denture dislodgement during chewing is minimized. If no incline exists to serve as a guide, the denture teeth should not be placed over the retromolar pad. The maxillary teeth should not be placed on the slope leading down to the hamular notches.

The medial-lateral placement of the mandibular posterior teeth is well established. The premolars should be arranged so that the buccal surface of the first premolar aligns with the buccal surface of the canine. In achieving this relationship, the central groove of the first premolar should align with either the contact point between the canine and lateral incisor or the tip of the canine (Figure 12–13). Posteriorly the mandibular molars, particularly the second molar, should be positioned almost directly over the remaining residual ridges (Figure 12–14), To help create this alignment, a line can be drawn along the crest of the mandibular residual ridges. Because this line cannot be seen once the record base is seated, it is necessary to mark the land areas of the cast, indicating where a continuation of this line would cross the land area (Figure 12–15). A guideline can now be visualized connecting the anterior (canine) to posterior (crest of ridge) guides. The correct alignment of the premolars and molars is indicated when the central grooves are centered on this line and all central grooves align with each other (Figure 12–12).

The vertical placement of the mandibular posterior teeth is also well described. In the anterior, the teeth are set to the height of the canines. Posteriorly, the plane of

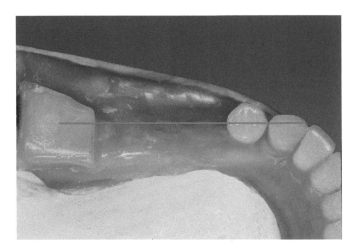

Figure 12–13 To maintain the proper alignment of the buccal surfaces of the mandibular canines and first premolars, the central groove of the first premolar should be aligned along a line extending from the tip of the canine and the mesial contact point of the canine and lateral incisor.

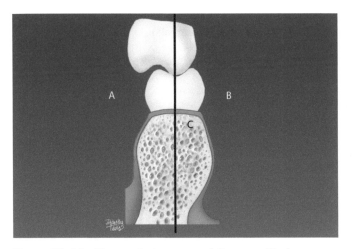

Figure 12–14 The central groove of the mandibular second molar is positioned almost directly over the remaining residual ridge.

occlusion is generally placed at the level of the middle to upper one-third of the retromolar pad and ideally is located midway between the maxillary and mandibular residual ridges and parallel to both ridges (Figure 12–16). When alteration of the vertical height of the occlusal plane become necessary, generally because of a lack of interocclusal clearance, the plane should be lowered whenever possible. Lowering the plane will decrease the height of the denture teeth above the mandibular residual ridges, decrease cantilever forces, and increase the stability of the mandibular denture.

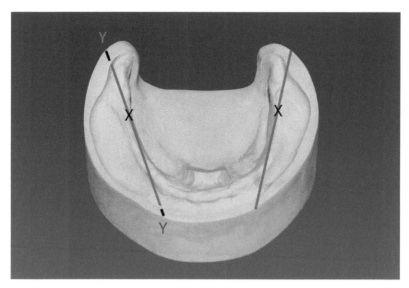

Figure 12-15 The green lines indicate the center of the residual ridges on this master cast. It is important that as many posterior teeth as possible be positioned directly over the residual ridges for proper function and denture stability. The ideal position of the distal-most denture tooth (usually second molar) is indicated (X). This tooth should ideally be place directly over the residual ridge and just anterior to the slope leading to the retromolar pad. The most posterior tooth is generally the most important tooth to center over the residual ridge. This is because anteriorly the premolars must align somewhat with the canine and therefore are often placed slightly buccal to the ridge crest. Note that, on the right side, marks have been drawn on the land areas of the cast (Y) indicating the extension of the green line. When the record bases and occlusion rims are placed on the cast, a straight edge can be placed between these marks, and a line can be drawn into the occlusion rim indicating the center of the ridges. This line indicates the proper buccal-lingual alignment of the posterior teeth.

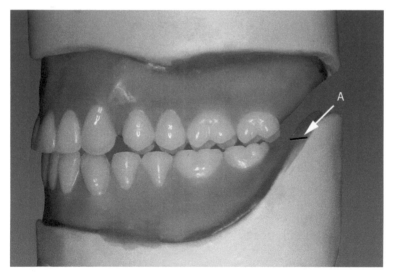

Figure 12-16 Ideally the posterior plane of occlusion is located at the level of the middle to upper one-third of the retromolar pad (A), midway between the opposing residual ridges, and parallel to both ridges.

Maxillary Posterior Teeth

When arranging the teeth for the trial insertion appointment, the posterior teeth are initially arranged primarily to obtain good centric occlusion contacts. There is less concern for potential excursive prematurities at this time because the potential for excursive prematurities for a nonbalanced occlusion are minimal. If a balanced occlusion is being created, the condylar inclinations of the articulator have not yet been set and therefore excursive contacts and prematurities cannot be properly evaluated at this time.

For a lingualized occlusion, either balanced on nonbalanced, the maxillary posterior teeth are arranged so that the buccal cusps of the opposing teeth are approximately 0.5 mm above the antagonist teeth when the articulator is moved into the working position (Figure 12–17). Cross-tooth contact of opposing working side posterior teeth is not indicated (Figure 12–18). This arrangement minimizes the difficulty in arranging the denture teeth and in correcting excursive prematurities at insertion.

For a conventional balanced occlusion, the buccal and lingual cusps of the opposing teeth are arranged into a "tight" intermeshing design (Figure 19). When correctly arranged there is: (1) minimal spacing between the opposing occlusal surfaces in centric occlusion, (2) anterior and bilateral cross-arch contact in all excursive movements, and cross-tooth contact on the working side (Figure 12–18).

Additionally, an arrangement that results in the buccal surfaces of both the maxillary and mandibular teeth being aligned vertically is contraindicated because of the potential for cheek biting. Therefore, the maxillary posterior teeth, especially second molars, must be arranged to provide adequate buccal overlap to minimize cheek biting (Figure 12–20). To provide this alignment, ideally the lingual cusps of the maxillary teeth are centered on the central grooves and marginal ridges of the mandibular teeth (Figure 12–21), which allows the buccal surfaces of the maxillary teeth to be more

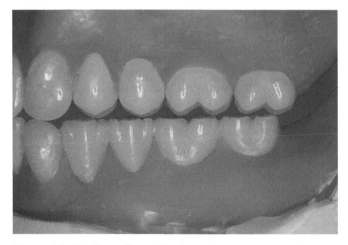

Figure 12–17 For a lingualized tooth arrangement, the buccal cusps of the maxillary teeth should be at least 0.5 mm above the mandibular buccal cusps when the teeth are in the working movement. This is an example of a nonbalanced lingualized arrangement.

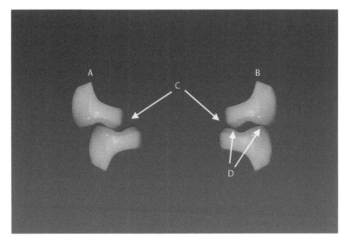

Figure 12–18 Cross-tooth contacts (D) are not seen with lingualized occlusion arrangements (A) however, these contacts are necessary for a conventional balanced occlusion (B). C indicates cross-arch contacts.

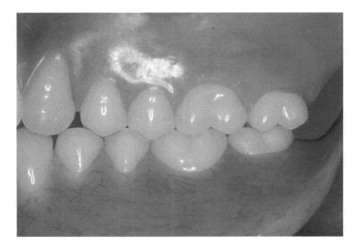

Figure 12–19 A "tight" alignment of the posterior teeth is necessary to achieve a conventional balanced occlusion. The requirements for cross-tooth contacts in excursive movements and a "tight" alignment of the teeth complicate the tooth arrangement and eventual occlusal correction procedures for balanced occlusion.

buccally positioned than the buccal surfaces of the mandibular teeth (Figure 12–20). However, in attempting to maintain the opposing teeth over their respective residual ridges this ideal alignment may not be possible. Therefore, it may be necessary to slightly move one or more teeth, particularly the second molars, in a non-ideal tooth position to prevent this vertical alignment. However, when arranging the mandibular teeth, the central grooves of the teeth should continue to align and fall within a triangle as drawn from the cusp tip of the canine and continuing to the buccal and lingual of the retromolar pad. (Figure 12–22).

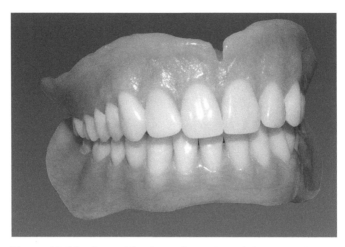

Figure 12–20 Buccal horizontal overlap of the posterior teeth, especially for the second molars, is required to minimize potential cheek biting. The arrangement may consist of conventional overlap with the maxillary teeth more buccally positioned than the mandibular teeth, as in this illustration, or it may be in the form of a reverse articulation (crossbite) alignment, as seen in Figure 23.

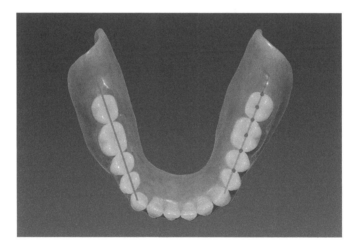

Figure 12–21 To achieve the conventional buccal overlap of the posterior teeth, the lingual cusps of the maxillary teeth are positioned to contact the central groves and middle of the marginal ridges of the mandibular teeth. The ideal positioning of teeth is illustrated by the red dots in this illustration.

Long-term studies indicate that, when the natural teeth have been extracted, the mandibular ridge resorbs downward and outward while the maxillary ridge resorbs upward and inward. Because of these resorptive patterns, it may be necessary to create a reverse articulation (crossbite) for the posterior teeth. The reverse articulation (crossbite) may exist on all the posterior teeth (Figure 12–23) and is termed a full or complete

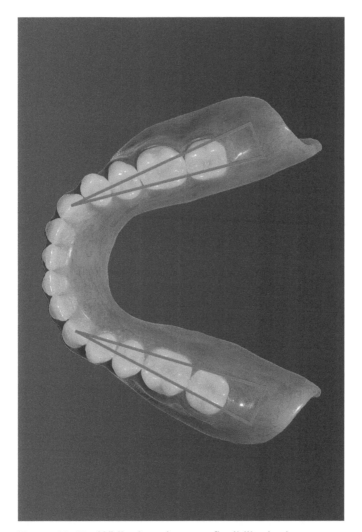

Figure 12–22 While there is some flexibility in the exact positioning of the mandibular teeth in relation to the residual ridge, the central grooves of the mandibular teeth should be arranged within a triangle, as drawn from the cusp tip of the canine and continuing to the buccal and lingual of the retromolar pad.

reverse articulation (crossbite). The maxillary buccal cusps become the functional cusps in this type of occlusion. However, a reverse articulation (crossbite) alignment of the teeth may occur only in the second molar area, while a normal alignment exists in the first premolar area (Figure 12–24). This may be called a partial reverse articulation (crossbite), and it results in the second premolars and first molars being arranged as transition teeth. Then central grooves of the teeth should continue to be aligned. This arrangement is acceptable and in fact, esthetic in many patients. When arranging teeth in a reverse articulation (crossbite) situation, the teeth may require occlusal adjustment to allow proper alignment.

When completed, both a balanced and nonbalanced occlusion will have bilateral contacts of all posterior teeth while in centric occlusion to minimize forces on the anterior residual ridges. Many clinicians do not desire anterior contacts while in centric

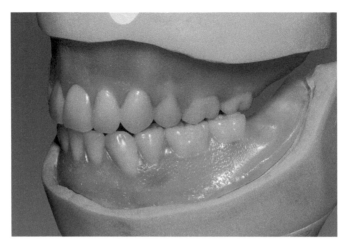

Figure 12–23 Complete reverse articulation (crossbite) of the posterior teeth. Note that all maxillary teeth are positioned more palatally than the mandibular teeth, resulting in the buccal cusps serving as the functional cusps in this type arrangement. This arrangement may be required because of the resorptive patterns of the opposing ridges.

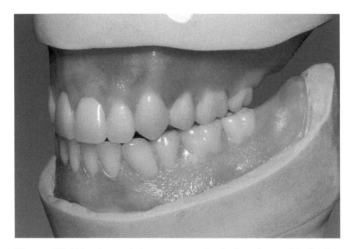

Figure 12–24 A partial reverse articulation (crossbite) of the posterior teeth. Note that the first premolar is in a normal alignment, the buccal surfaces of the first molars are in a vertical alignment (not ideal but necessary from an esthetic perspective), and the second molars are in a reverse articulation (crossbite) alignment.

occlusion. In excursive movements, a nonbalanced occlusion should exhibit bilateral simultaneous contact of the posterior teeth for one or more millimeters around the centric occlusion position. Christensen's phenomena may exist beyond this area. Generally a balanced occlusion will exhibit more excursive posterior contacts distributed over a wider range of movements than a nonbalanced occlusion. A balanced occlusion will have both bilateral contacts of the posterior teeth and simultaneous anterior contacts in all excursive movements. Protrusive contacts should exist from centric occlusion until

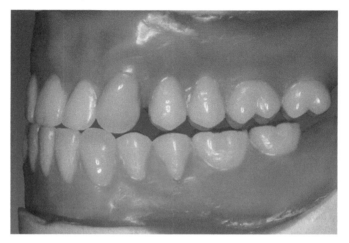

Figure 12–25 For a balanced occlusion to have good "timing," one or more posterior contacts, bilaterally, must be maintained through the entire excursive movement. In this example, the casts have been moved into a protruded relationship until the incisal edges of the opposing central incisors are in contact. Note that multiple contacts are present posteriorly. Contacts must also be present on the opposite side of the arch.

the central incisors are in the incisal edge-to-incisal edge position (Figure 12–25). Working and nonworking contacts should exist until the working side canines are cusp tip-to-cusp tip (Figure 12–26). When contacts correctly exist through this range, the tooth arrangement is said to have "good timing." This arrangement will require some occlusal adjustments to eliminate prematurities on some teeth, which cannot be completed until the condylar guidances have been correctly set on the articulator.

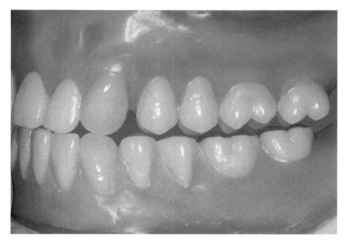

Figure 12–26 The dentures depicted in Figure 25 have been moved into a working position. Note that multiple contacts exist, and the canines are edge-to-edge. Nonworking contacts on the opposite side of the arch must also be present.

References

Fenton, A. H.: Selecting and arranging prosthetic teeth and occlusion for the edentulous patient. In Zarb, GA., Bolander CL., eds. Prosthodontic Treatment for Edentulous Patients. 12th ed. St. Louis: Mosby Inc; 2004. pp. 308-328.

Parr, G. R.: Arranging the artificial teeth for the trial denture. In Rahn, A. O., Heartwell, C. M., editors. Textbook of complete dentures. 5th ed. Philadelphia: Lea & Febiger; 1993. pp. 351–356.

Rahn, A. O.: Developing complete denture impressions. In Rahn, A. O., Heartwell, C. M., editors. Textbook of complete dentures. 5th ed. Philadelphia: Lea & Febiger; 1993. pp. 323–350.

Sowter, J. B.: Custom impression trays. In Barton, R. E., ed. Removable Prosthodontic Techniques. Revised edition. Chapel Hill: University of North Carolina Press; 1986. pp. 58-79.

Tallgren, A.: The continuing reduction of the residual alveolar ridges in complete denture wearer: a mixed-longtidunal study covering 25 years. J Prosthet Dent 1972;27:120-32.

The Glossary of Prosthodontic Terms. J Prosthet Dent 2005;94(1):23, 69.

QUESTIONS

1. For most patients, when considering the arrangement of the maxillary anterior teeth, what determines esthetics? What determines the fullness of the lips (lip support)?

2. Most patients desire symmetrical arrangement of the anterior teeth with minimal variations that might provide a more natural look. Which two groups of patients might be an exception to this statement?

3. Alterations of the maxillary lateral incisors can be made to help create a more natural-appearing denture. What changes might be considered?

4. The alignment of the canines is important from an esthetic standpoint. How should canines be arranged in comparison to the central and lateral incisors?

5. Why is it important to minimize the vertical overlap of the anterior teeth when arranging these teeth for a balanced occlusion?

6. In what direction do the crests of the residual ridges resorb following extractions, and what might these resorptive patterns result in?

7. What anatomical feature limits the most posterior position of a mandibular molar?

8. Ideally, how should the plane of occlusion relate to the retromolar pad, the interocclusal space between the ridges, and the ridge crests themselves?

9. If an adjustment is necessary to the vertical position of the plane of occlusion, which arch should be favored and why?

10. How should the buccal surfaces of the opposing, primarily second molars be aligned and why?

ANSWERS

1. For most patients, the position of the incisal edge of the maxillary anterior teeth determines esthetics, while the cervical portion, or necks, of the teeth and the fullness of the maxillary denture base determine lip support (fullness of the lips).

2. The exceptions are those patients with existing dentures, who would like the arrangement of the teeth of the new denture to mimic those of the existing denture. Occasionally patients receiving immediate complete dentures also desire that the arrangement of the denture teeth match the arrangement of the natural teeth.

3. Changes include: (1) inclination of the long axis, (2) relationship to the incisal edges of the central incisor, (3) tooth width, (4) levels of the gingival margins, (5) tooth shade, and (6) shapes of incisal edges, angles, and proximal surfaces.

4. The long axis of the maxillary canine should be vertical or distally inclined with the cervical portion (neck) prominently oriented because of its labial position in relation to the lateral incisor. For esthetic purposes, the canine should be rotated so that the distal half of the facial surface of the tooth is not visible when viewed for the anterior.

5. Decreasing the steepness of the incisal guidance minimizes the separation of the posterior teeth during excursive movements, and hence the requirement for excessively steep cusp heights, compensating curves, and/or effective cusp angles. This reduction simplifies the arrangement of the teeth and eliminates prematurities in both the laboratory and clinic remount phases of treatment.

6. Long-term studies indicate that, when the natural teeth are lost, the mandibular residual ridge resorbs downward and outward, while the maxillary residual ridge resorbs upward and inward. Because of these resorptive patterns, it is often necessary to create a reverse articulation (crossbite) for the posterior teeth.

7. The most distal mandibular molar should be set no further posteriorly than the beginning of the incline leading to the retromolar pad.

8. The plane of occlusion should ideally split the distance between the maxillary and mandibular ridges, be parallel to both ridges, and be at the level of the middle to upper one-third of the retromolar pad.

9. If interarch space or esthetics are significant problems, the position of the plane of occlusion may be adjusted either superiorly or inferiorly to a small degree. When making adjustments to the height of the occlusal plane, the mandibular arch should be favored whenever possible because of the decreased stability of the mandibular denture.

10. A buccal horizontal overlap of the posterior teeth, especially second molars, is required when arranging the opposing teeth. An arrangement that results in the buccal surfaces of both the maxillary and mandibular teeth being aligned vertically is contraindicated because of the possibility of creating a cheek-biting situation.

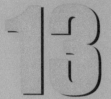

Trial Insertion Appointment

Dr. Kevin D. Plummer

The esthetic and functional tial insertion is the clinician's final opportunity to ensure that the dentures will meet the esthetic, phonetic, and functional demands of the patient and his or her significant other. Additionally it is the final opportunity to ensure that the opposing casts are in the correct horizontal and vertical relationship on the articulator before the dentures are processed. Using the criteria for denture tooth arrangement found in Chapter 12 (Tooth Arrangement), all mechanical requirements of anterior and posterior tooth position should be verified on the articulator. The clinician must critically and objectively evaluate the degree to which the dentures meet the desired goals of each previous step. If there is any concern about some aspect of the denture, it must be addressed now.

If all of the previous procedures have been accomplished well, and the patient is reasonable in his or her expectations, this can be a short and rewarding appointment. If shortcuts were taken, and the patient is exacting or has unrealistic expectations, this can be a long and frustrating appointment. In either case, it is much easier to make final adjustments at this point while the dentures and teeth are still in wax. Once a denture is processed, changes can be expensive or even impossible to accomplish without starting over.

The trial insertion appointment will make assessments of the esthetic position of the denture teeth, facial support, phonetics, occluding vertical dimension (OVD), occlusal scheme, and the centric occlusal position. This procedure will also give the patient an opportunity to see the esthetic results from the previous deliberations during the maxillomandibular records appointment and the tooth selection process. This is also an excellent opportunity for the patient's significant other to see the proposed new prostheses. It is often the significant other's response to the new dentures that will have the most influence on the patient's acceptance of their new appearance.

The trial insertion appointment should begin with adjustment of the record bases to ensure comfort and proper fit. If retention is a problem, it is advisable to use an adhesive to keep the record bases stable during the trial insertion procedure. The stability and retention is necessary for proper inspection and will also give the patient confidence about his or her new dentures. After fitting the record bases, a systematic evaluation of the procedures completed during the maxillomandibular records appointment is conducted, beginning with the evaluation of the OVD and centric occlusion position. Most clinicians make a quick assessment of the esthetics, but the tendency to concentrate on that area should be avoided until the vertical and horizontal relationships of the mounted casts have been evaluated.

Evaluation of Occluding Vertical Dimension

The same parameters used to determine the rest vertical dimension (RVD) and the OVD at the maxillomandibular records appointment should be used once again to check for the proper interocclusal clearance, phonetics, and vertical position of the occlusal plane. The OVD is evaluated first using sibilant sounds, as was done when making the maxillomandibular records. The presence or lack of an acceptable degree of interocclusal clearance is used to evaluate the OVD. This interocclusal clearance is seen as a very slight separation of the anterior teeth during sibilant sounds and a little more space in the posterior areas (Figure 13–1). There should be no contact of the

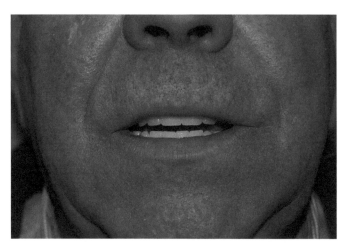

Figure 13–1   Evaluating the interocclusal distance

opposing teeth during speech. If contacts exist, the tentative OVD may have been too great, resulting in the OVD being too close to the RVD. This is often called excessive OVD. The correct amount of interocclusal distance must be regained by decreasing the OVD. If the desired decrease is more than 2 mm, a new interocclusal record must be made in the CR position at the new OVD. To provide room for the recording material when making the new records, the posterior teeth must be removed from either the maxillary or mandibular arch. If the anterior teeth prevent the proper OVD position from being obtained, they must also be removed from the same occlusion rim from which the posterior teeth were removed. The OVD is reestablished and a new maxillo-mandibular recording is made in CR. The mandibular cast is removed from the articulator and re-articulated using the new recording. Many clinicians will verify this new mounting by making another maxillomandibular record and ensuring that it matches the cast relationships. The maxillary cast is not removed because it was mounted using the facebow and that relationship must not be lost.

An excessive amount of space between the teeth may indicate that the tentative OVD might have been "overclosed" or insufficient. If the desired change is more than 2 mm, then a new interocclusal record made in the CR position is needed. Because of the excessive interocclusal distance, there is usually ample space between the opposing teeth for a new record. Therefore, no posterior teeth need be removed prior to making a new maxillomandibular recording. Again the mandibular cast should be re-articulated on the articulator, and this mounting should be verified.

If the vertical relationship is deemed incorrect, but within 2 mm of being correct, the correction can be made on the articulator. This minimal change is possible on the articulator because the facebow mounting established an arc of closure on the instrument similar to that of the patient. Studies have shown a negligible error would be present from making this minor change. If the necessary change is greater than 2 mm, or if no facebow was used when mounting the maxillary cast, then the clinician should make a new centric relation record at the proper OVD. This demonstrates the importance of using a facebow when mounting the maxillary cast on the articulator. By capturing this relationship, the clinician can make interocclusal records that will verify on the articulator at a slightly increased or decreased OVD, and also can make simple changes to the

OVD on the articulator without making new interocclusal records. It also simplifies the mounting the maxillary cast.

The patient's skeletal relationships may also play a part in evaluating the OVD. For example, a Class II patient may have what seems to be excessive vertical and horizontal clearance due to the normal relationships of the residual ridges in that skeletal position. Class III patients may exhibit almost no interocclusal distance during speech. This relationship must be taken into account when evaluating the function of the prostheses.

Evaluation of Centric Relation Record

An attempt was made during the maxillomandibular records appointment to articulate the mandibular cast on the articulator in the centric relation position as it relates to the maxillary cast (Figure 13–2). Two methods are commonly employed by clinicians to evaluate and verify that the opposing casts are in the correct relationship on the articulator at the esthetic trial insertion. The first is to simply visually inspect the closure of the dentures on the articulator and intraorally. They are evaluated for complete closure and evidence of multiple occlusal contacts with no slide present.

If the visual inspection is questionable or if the clinician prefers, a new centric relation record is made to verify the horizontal position. The new centric relation record is made at a slightly increased OVD to prevent contact of the denture teeth and possible errors from record base movement. As explained earlier, the facebow recording of the maxillary cast makes this procedure possible. Place approximately 1.5 mm of passive wax on the occlusal surfaces of the mandibular teeth and soften by immersing in water at 130°F (Figure 13–3). Place the denture intraorally and guide the patient to close into the wax when the jaws are in centric relation. Closure must be short of tooth-to-tooth contact due to the chance that contact may displace the denture base (Figures 13–4 and 13–5). The wax record is not acceptable if the teeth penetrate the record to make contact. Carefully repeat the closure to verify that the patient can close into the record without

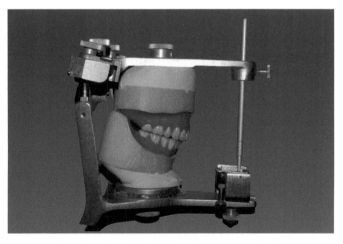

Figure 13–2   Initial horizontal and vertical position of the dentures at the wax trial insertion stage

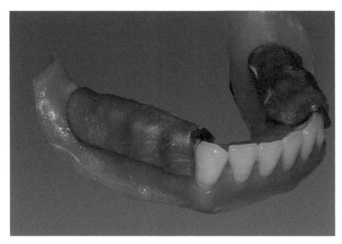

Figure 13–3   Aluwax™ placed on the posterior teeth prior to making the verification record

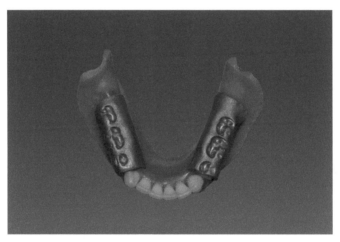

Figure 13–4   Recording at a slightly increased occluding vertical dimension for verification of the centric relation position – occlusal view

deviation from the centric arc of closure. The new recording verifies the initial recording if the opposing denture teeth close completely into the record with no slide. On the articulator, the unlatched condylar element should remain in its correct position within the condylar housing with no visible movement when the dentures on their casts are seated into the record (Figure 13–6). If the record verifies the original horizontal position, the clinician can continue with the remaining steps in the trial insertion visit. If the record fails to match the current horizontal position, another record should be made—just in case the first verification record was made in an incorrect position. If the second record matches the first verification record, the clinician should consider re-articulating the case and rearrange the teeth to function correctly at the new horizontal position. If the cast is re-articulated, another verification record should be made to check the new horizontal position.

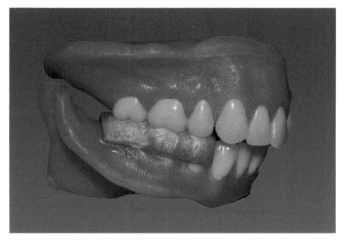

Figure 13–5 Recording at a slightly increased occluding vertical dimension for verification of the centric relation position – lateral view

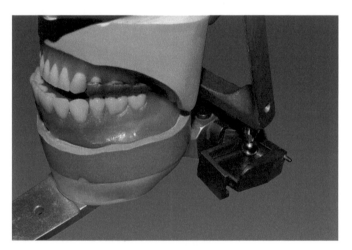

Figure 13–6 Condyle post remains in contact with the back wall of the condylar housing when the dentures are fully seated in the record.

 Eccentric Records

Complex occlusal schemes that require precise mechanical equivalents of the true mandibular movement on the articulator will require eccentric records to set the condylar guidance. Protrusive position records, or lateral position records, are commonly used for this purpose. Refer to the articulator manual for the preferred method for the machine being used. Lateral, or protrusive, records allow the slope of the articular eminence to be recorded, so adjustments of that parameter can be accomplished on the articulator. The record captures the relative angle of the articular eminence as the condyle travels down the slope. This will make the final adjustment of eccentric positions in a balanced denture occlusion much more accurate.

Intraoral protrusive records are made by recording the opposing dentures while the patient is in a protrusive position (usually with the anterior teeth end-to-end). It is important to stabilize the dentures during this record because the anterior contact may cause the record bases to become unstable. The protrusive record is used to adjust both condylar elements. Intraoral lateral records are made with the patient in a lateral position (usually the canines will be end-to-end). The left lateral record records the movement down the slope of the right articular eminence and is used to adjust the right side of the articulator. The right lateral record records the movement down the slope of the left articular eminence and is used to adjust the left side of the articulator. The casts are seated into the record and the condylar housing, or guide, is adjusted into contact with the condylar element, which has moved forward and down. These records are made more easily when teeth are present, and therefore are usually made at the trial insertion appointment. This allows for adjustments to be made before processing and also will provide for proper articulator settings for the insertion or placement appointment.

Facial Support, Esthetics, and Phonetics Evaluation

Facial support, esthetic placement of the denture teeth, and phonetics must be carefully evaluated. Much of the support of the lips surrounding the mouth comes from the proper position and angulations of the teeth and the supporting structures. In a denture, this translates to the artificial teeth and the wax supporting those teeth, and replacing missing tissues. The proper position and support will affect the quality of speech sounds such as the "f" and "v" sounds where the wet-dry line of the lower lip should gently contact the incisal edges of the anterior maxillary teeth (Figure 13–7). Sound such as "th" will also produce a gentle contact of the tongue with the lingual surfaces of the

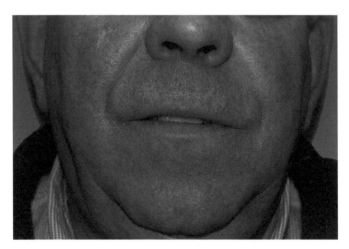

Figure 13–7 The "f" and "v" sound produces a gentle contact of the wet-dry line off the lower lip with the incisal edges of the maxillary teeth.

anterior teeth. The placement of the maxillary anterior teeth should follow basic esthetic guidelines for tooth length and position (See Chapter 12, Tooth Arrangement). The mandibular anterior teeth should be basically the same height as the resting lower lip and follow the same curvature as that lip. The evaluation should include rest and functional positions.

The midline, shade, and other esthetic factors, such as individual tooth position preferences, diastemas, and personalized esthetic concerns should be evaluated and corrected if necessary before having the patient review the wax trial insertion. The patient should evaluate the prostheses using a full-sized mirror at a conversational distance. Avoid letting the patient use a small hand-held mirror until after the total esthetic results have been evaluated. After a general appraisal, the patient can be more critical with a smaller mirror if necessary. After the clinician and patient are satisfied, the patient's significant other should be allowed to inspect the prostheses and make their concerns known. Listen carefully to patient's concerns at this point of the evaluation. If the clinician fails to satisfy the patient's or the significant other's small esthetic demands, it may result in a general dissatisfaction of the prostheses that may be hard to isolate at subsequent follow up appointments.

Final Evaluations

If a custom gingival denture base shade is to be used, it must be selected at this time (Figure 13–8). Additionally this is the final chance to ensure that the posterior palatal seal has been prepared into the maxillary master cast. Some clinicians have the patient sign a consent form that indicates their satisfaction with the esthetic results at this time. Many times this consent form will help when patients have questions concerning the esthetic results of the final processed dentures. Only after the clinician, patient, and significant other are satisfied with all of the above-mentioned criteria should the dentures be submitted to the laboratory for denture processing (Figures 13–9-12).

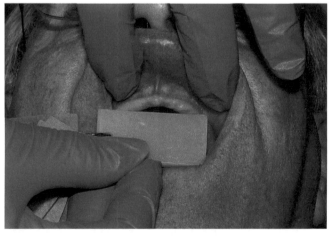

Figure 13–8   A gingival shade tab is used to pick a custom resin shade.

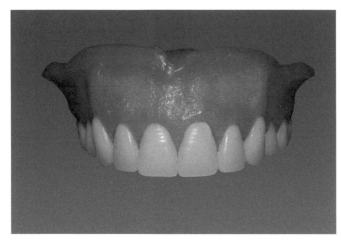

Figure 13–9   Final wax-up ready for processing

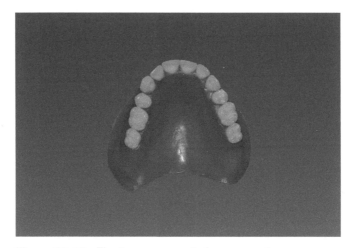

Figure 13–10   Final wax-up ready for processing

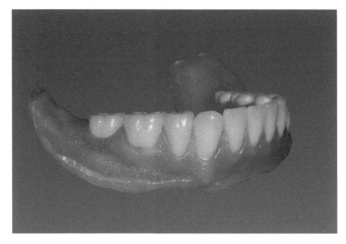

Figure 13–11   Final wax-up ready for processing

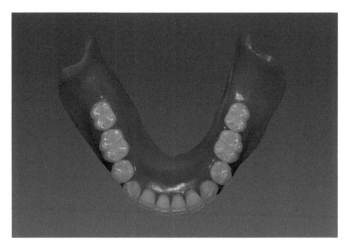

Figure 13–12   Final wax-up ready for processing

References

Swoope, C. C.: The try-in—a time for communication. Dent Clin North Am 1970 Jul; 14(3): 479-491.

Travaglini, E. A.: Verification appointment in complete denture therapy. J Prosthet Dent 1980 Nov; 44(5):478-483.

QUESTIONS

1. What assessments should be made during the esthetic and functional try-in appointment?

2. If the interocclusal distance is inadequate and the teeth touch at the rest vertical dimension, how is space obtained to make a new centric maxillo-mandibular record at the proper occluding vertical dimension?

3. If changes need to be made in the vertical position of the teeth, but the change is less than 2 mm, those changes can be made by altering the occluding vertical dimension on the articulator. True or False?

4. What type of eccentric records can be used to program semi-adjustable articulators to make the final occlusal adjustments in lateral positions more accurate?

ANSWERS

1. The trial insertion appointment will make assessments of the esthetic position of the denture teeth, facial support, phonetics, occluding vertical dimension (OVD), occlusal scheme, and the centric occlusal position. This procedure will also give the patient an opportunity to see the esthetic results from the previous deliberations during the maxillomandibular records appointment and the tooth selection process.

2. To provide room for the recording material when making the new records, the posterior teeth must be removed from either the maxillary or mandibular arch. If the anterior teeth prevent the proper OVD position from being obtained, they must also be removed from the same occlusion rim from which the posterior teeth were removed.

3. True, if a facebow recording was used to position the maxillary cast on the articulator.

4. Protrusive or lateral excursive records

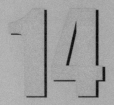

CHAPTER 14

Insertion

Dr. Kevin D. Plummer

The insertion of the completed dentures should follow a systematic sequence of procedures, including evaluating the denture base, attaching the mandibular remount cast to the articulator using an interocclusal record, correcting occlusal prematurities, conducting a final check of the prostheses, and issuing patient instructions. For some patients, this visit may be time consuming, but it is absolutely necessary that adequate time be scheduled to thoroughly complete each procedure and answer any and all patient questions and concerns.

Both dentist and patient anticipate with pleasure the appointment for the insertion of the dentures. However, patients receiving their first complete dentures are familiar with neither the physiologic requirements of dentures nor with the use and care of the dentures. One of the most important steps in the insertion appointment is to educate the patient on what to expect from dentures. During insertion procedures is an opportune time to discuss instructions and address concerns of the patient about the use and care of the new prostheses. Providing a written letter of instruction at a previous appointment will make this discussion clearer to the patient (Figure 14–1).

INSTRUCTIONS TO DENTURE PATIENTS

A. WHAT TO EXPECT FROM YOUR NEW DENTURES

1. You must learn to manipulate your new dentures. Most patients require at least three weeks to learn to use new dentures, and some patients require more time.
2. Dentures are not as efficient as natural teeth so you should not expect to chew as well with dentures as with your natural teeth. Dentures are better than no teeth at all. Start with small bites of easy to manage foods. Do not try to bite with your front teeth. Use the area of the canine teeth to bite foods, but it is even better to cut the food into small pieces before attempting to chew.
3. Speaking will feel awkward for a while. Diligent practice usually enables a patient with new dentures to speak clearly within a few days.

B. ADJUSTMENTS

1. You must return to your dentist for follow-up treatment after the dentures have been inserted. In nearly every instance, it is necessary to make some minor adjustments to the denture.
2. Most patients must make some adjustments in their attitude and habits in order to wear dentures successfully.
3. If you develop soreness, do not become alarmed. Call your dentist for an appointment. Do not expect soreness to go away by itself.
4. If you are unable to reach your dentist during weekends or holidays, remove your dentures to prevent excess tissue damage.

C. CLEANING

1. Your dentures and supporting ridges must be cleaned carefully after each meal. "Denture breath" is a result of dirty dentures.
2. Clean your *gums* with a soft brush and toothpaste.
3. Clean your *dentures* with liquid dish detergent, and gently brush with a soft denture brush. Many toothpastes are too abrasive to use on the polished denture surface.

(Continued)

4. Soak your dentures at night in a denture cleaner or a water/mouthwash solution.
5. Always keep your dentures wet when not wearing them to prevent warping.

D. YOUR ORAL HEALTH

1. Nature did not intend for people to wear dentures. You must, therefore, be very careful of the supporting tissue.
2. In addition to keeping the dentures meticulously clean, you must rest the tissues at least eight hours a day. Most patients find it convenient to leave their dentures out at night.
3. The tissues that support your dentures are constantly changing. This will result in denture looseness. However, looseness can result from many causes. With time, your dentures will need either refitting or replacement. In any event, you should call your dentist for an appointment when you notice exccessive looseness.
4. Annual examinations of the supporting tissue for abnormalities and to assess the function and fit of the denture are important for your overall dental health.

Figure 14–1   Example of a printed instruction sheet for a denture patient

Evaluating the Denture Base

Before the insertion appointment, the clinician should inspect the denture bases to determine that the polished surfaces are smooth and devoid of scratches, that no imperfections on the tissue surface remain, and that the borders are round with no sharp angles—especially in the frenum areas.

Next, each denture base should be individually evaluated for accuracy of adaptation to the tissues and for areas of excessive tissue/denture base pressure. Excessive pressure will result in irritation to the tissue and pain to the patient, and must be eliminated. It is most likely to occur in those areas in which the rigid denture base must slide into an undercut or contact tissues that are almost noncompressible (Figure 14–2). To identify pressure areas, the intaglio surface (tissue side of the denture) should be painted with a thin film of pressure disclosing paste using uniform brush strokes (Figure 14–3). The denture is then inserted and removed. When removed, the pressure-disclosing paste and brush strokes will be undisturbed in areas of no tissue/denture base contact, exhibit minimal uniform contact in those areas with the desired tissue/denture base contact, or be wiped off in those areas of excessive pressure (Figure 14–4 and 14–5). Prior to relieving the resin in the areas of excessive contact areas, this procedure should be repeated to verify that the markings are correct. It may be advisable to have the patient insert and remove the denture, as the method and path of insertion may vary with two individuals.

Once positively established, excessive pressure caused by the resin being placed and removed from undercut areas are addressed and carefully removed by relieving them with an acrylic bur (Figure 14–6). This procedure is repeated until positive tissue/denture base contact exists and excessive pressure has been relieved. Excessive pressure in the area of an undercut can occur on the denture flange and, when relieving the area, it must be remembered that tissue/denture base contact is absolutely necessary to retain the border seal of the denture and the resulting retention. Excessive removal of denture

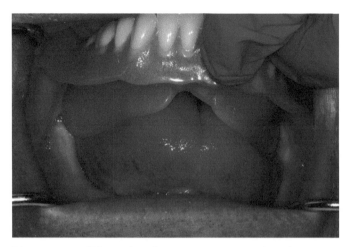

Figure 14–2   Bilateral undercuts prevent seating the mandibular denture. This area must be adjusted in order to have the denture seat properly.

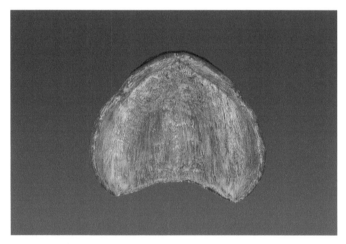

Figure 14–3   The initial application of pressure disclosing paste should leave brush marks visible.

base resin will result in a loss of retention. Areas of exostosis or areas of bone covered with tissue that is not displaceable, such as the midpalatal suture, often appear as pressure areas even when the denture is seated with little pressure. When these areas appear in the pressure-disclosing paste, they are relieved by grinding. Multiple insertions are usually necessary, as relieving one pressure area may reveal another. The most common pressure areas are on the buccal slopes of the tuberosities on the maxilla. These occur due to typical processing shrinkage of the acrylic resin and may prevent the denture from making uniform contact with the palate and the palatal seal area. Use only finger pressure when evaluating these pressure areas. Do not let the patient bite on the dentures to place pressure. Uncorrected premature occlusal contact may cause the pressure disclos-

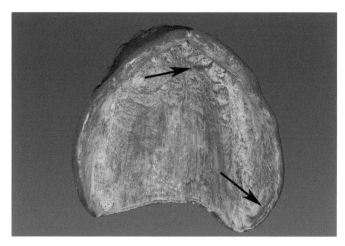

Figure 14–4   Arrows indicate areas of pressure or wipe-off from an undercut.

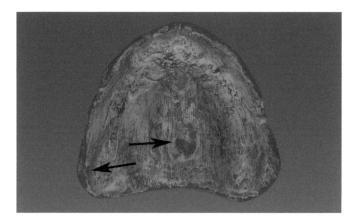

Figure 14–5   Arrows indicate areas of excessive pressure.

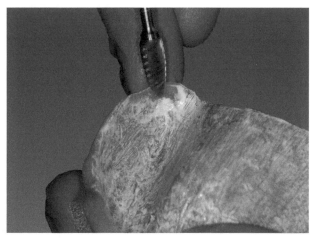

Figure 14–6   An acrylic bur is used to adjust the pressure areas identified by the pressure disclosing paste.

ing paste to be displaced, mimicking pressure areas. A final check of pressure areas may be made with biting pressure after the occlusion has been adjusted.

Evaluating Borders

The third step in the insertion appointment is to evaluate the borders and the contour of the polished surfaces in the mouth. This will determine whether the border extensions and contour are compatible with the available spaces in the vestibules, the borders are properly relieved to accommodate the frenum attachments and the reflection of the tissues in the hamular notch area and the dentures are stable during speech and swallowing.

Apply disclosing wax to the borders of the maxillary denture in the same manner as the impression compound or heavy bodied vinyl polysiloxane siloxane material that was applied during the border refining procedures (Figure 14–7). Instruct the patient to open the jaws as in yawning, push the lower jaw forward, and move the lower jaw from right to left. Disclosing wax is very displaceable, and slight overextensions that might have been developed during border molding can be determined (Figure 14–8). Relieve any existing overextensions (length or thickness) by grinding and then polish the relieved area. Apply disclosing wax to the remaining borders of the maxillary denture and instruct the patient to smile, speak, laugh, and swallow. Relieve any overextended areas by grinding, and then polish the relieved surface. Apply disclosing wax to the mandibular denture borders in the same manner. Carefully evaluate the area of the insertion of the masseter muscle to make sure adequate space exists on the mandibular denture for the muscle movement during chewing (Figures 14–9 and 14–10). The altered exterior surface of the denture base is smoothed most often with a slurry of pumice and water. It is polished with polishing compound and a soft cloth wheel. Finishing and polishing points may be used for small areas. Whichever method is used, all finishing and polishing is completed at a slow speed to prevent heating the acrylic resin, which may cause warping.

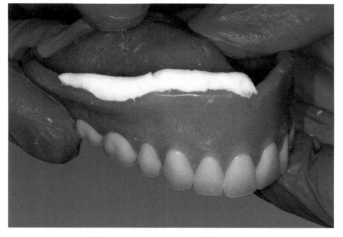

Figure 14–7 Disclosing wax applied to a border for evaluation.

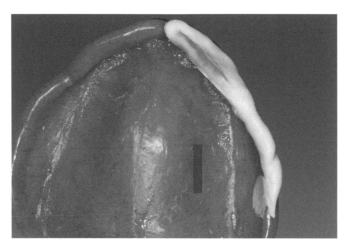

Figure 14–8   The exposed acrylic resin should be slightly reduced in height where it shows through the wax.

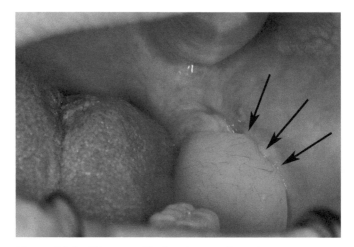

Figure 14–9   The mandibular denture base is overextended in the area of the masseter muscle.

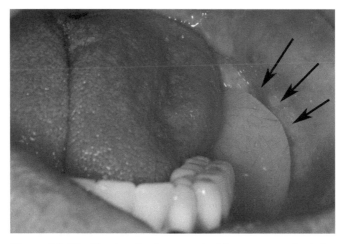

Figure 14–10   The border is corrected for proper adaptation.

Correcting Occlusion

The fourth step in the insertion procedures is the occlusal correction. Occlusal harmony in complete dentures is necessary if the dentures are to be comfortable, function efficiently, and to preserve the supporting structures. It is difficult to see occlusal discrepancies intraorally with complete dentures. The resiliency of the supporting soft tissues and the ability of the tissues to displace in varying degrees tend to disguise premature occlusal contacts. The tissues permit the dentures to shift; as a result, after the first interceptive occlusal contact, the remaining teeth appear to make satisfactory contact. Patients are seldom aware of faulty occlusion in complete dentures; yet they always seem to notice an improvement after the fault has been corrected. The eye cannot be relied upon to observe occlusal discrepancies, and the patient cannot be depended upon to diagnose occlusal faults. It is the responsibility of the dentist to find and correct these occlusal discrepancies and ensure that the dentures are free of occlusal disharmony.

It must be assumed that there are occlusal faults in all complete dentures until proved otherwise. Occlusal faults can be determined by obtaining an interocclusal record from the patient and remounting the dentures on an articulator. These faults can be corrected with careful selective grinding procedures. Remounting the dentures on the articulator and selective grinding procedures should be carried out at the time of placement of the dentures. Postponing this important step will lead to a deformation of the underlying soft tissues, discomfort, and destruction of the supporting bone. Later, the occlusal errors may be concealed, making them impossible to locate and correct because of distorted and swollen tissues.

Occlusal disharmony in the completed dentures may result from processing changes that occur within the acrylic resin during the packing and decasting of the denture, undetected errors in registering jaw relations, errors in mounting casts on the articulator, differences in tissue adaptation between the processed denture bases and the record bases that were used in recording maxillomandibular relations, and changes in the supporting structures since the impressions were first made. This is particularly true if the patient is using other dentures.

There are many intraoral methods for correcting occlusal disharmony. However, the intraoral methods are not accurate enough to ensure proper occlusal contacts of opposing dentures. The resiliency of the supporting tissues allows the dentures to shift; therefore, markings are frequently false and misleading. The denture bases can move from the basal seat, causing the teeth in the opposite side of the arch or the opposite end of the arch to contact prematurely and produce an incorrect marking. Placing articulating paper on one side of the arch may induce the patient to close toward or away from that side. Arch-shaped articulating paper should be placed to minimize this problem, if an intraoral adjustment is attempted.

Adhesive green wax can be placed on the occlusal surfaces of the mandibular denture. Points of penetration that occur upon closing with the jaws in centric relation may be marked with a pencil and relieved where indicated. This method may also locate points of interference during functional movements. Again, the disadvantage of this method is that shifting of the dentures over resilient supporting tissues may give false markings.

Patient Remount and Selective Grinding

The patient remount method is to rearticulate the dentures on an articulator by means of interocclusal records made in the patient's mouth. This is by far the most accurate occlusal adjustment procedure. It has the following advantages:

1. It reduces patient participation.
2. It permits the dentist to see the procedures better.
3. It provides a stable working foundation; bases are not shifting on resilient tissues.
4. The absence of saliva makes possible more accurate markings with the articulating paper or tape.
5. Corrections can be made away from the patient, thus preventing occasional objections when patients see their new dentures being altered.

To carry out a patient remount procedure, orient the mandibular denture to the maxillary denture by means of an interocclusal record with the jaws in centric relation. Place approximately 1.5 mm of passive-type wax on the occlusal surfaces of the mandibular teeth and soften by immersing in water at 130°F. Place the denture intraorally and guide the patient to close into the wax when the jaws are in centric relation. Closure must be short of tooth-to-tooth contact due to the chance that contact may displace the denture base. The wax record is not acceptable if the teeth penetrate to make contact. Carefully repeat the closure to verify the patient can close into the record without deviation from the centric arc of closure (Figure 14–11). Other materials can be used for this record but passive-type wax is the material of choice due to its excellent working time, short term high accuracy and ease of use.

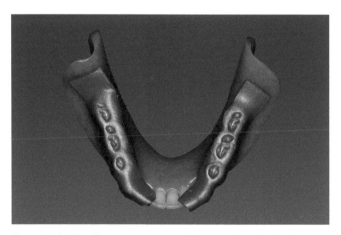

Figure 14–11 A remount record in centric relation is made with Aluwax™ as close to the proper occlusal vertical dimension as possible.

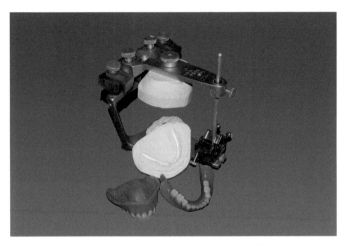

Figure 14–12 The articulator, mounted maxillary remount cast, the mandibular remount cast, and the dentures are generally all returned from the dental laboratory. Remount casts are made by blocking out undercuts on the processed dentures and making stone casts. The dentures can be removed and replaced on these casts.

The maxillary remount cast was fabricated and placed on the articulator by using a remount index made in the dental laboratory immediately after the dentures were processed, in order to preserve the facebow record. The dental laboratory generally returns the articulator with the properly positioned maxillary remount cast and a mandibular remount cast (Figure 14–12). After properly orienting the mandibular denture to the maxillary denture by means of the interocclusal record, seat the mandibular remount cast in the denture and attach it to the mandibular member of the articulator with mounting stone (Figures 14–13 and 14–14).

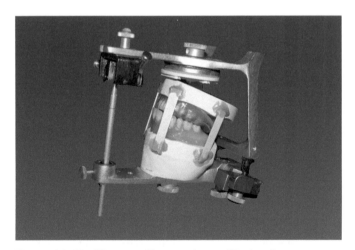

Figure 14–13 The maxillary and mandibular dentures properly related to each other and secured in their respective remount casts. The casts are secured together for the mounting procedure.

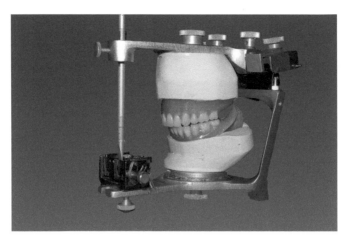

Figure 14–14   Completed remount procedure. Dentures reoriented to the articulator in the centric relation position.

To verify what has been recorded is the patient's centric occlusion position, make another wax interocclusal record in the same manner as the first. Replace the dentures on the articulator and, with the condylar elements unlatched, place the teeth in the indentations in the wax record. The condylar elements should rest against the stops. Repeat the procedure until two consecutive records are accepted.

When cusp form posterior teeth are used, and balanced occlusion is desired, it is best to have an even distribution of tooth contacts bilaterally. This involves a cusp-to-fossa marginal ridge relation of maximum intercuspation when the jaws are in the terminal hinge position (See Chapter 9, Occlusal Concepts). When the teeth move to and from centric to eccentric positions, the maxillary cusps track in three approximate directions (Figure 14–15). An articulator that travels in a straight path does not travel the same path as the condyles in the fossae. It has been generally accepted that the error is so negligible that the resiliency of the supporting tissues accommodates for the error. There is no scientific proof that this assumption is correct, and this may not be true in all situations.

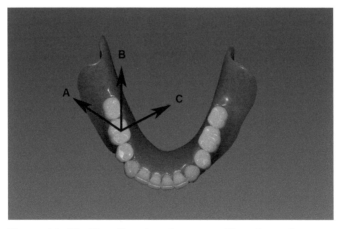

Figure 14–15   The direction that a maxillary lingual cusp will track during mandibular movement. A: Nonworking movement B: Protrusive movement C: Working movement

Undoubtedly this error is tolerated by the majority of patients. When the jaws are moving to and from centric and eccentric positions, within the functional range of the teeth in gliding occlusion, the teeth can be altered to maintain harmonious contact on the articulator. This harmonious contact from fossae to cusp tips will not be exactly repeated in the mouth, but is accepted as the most accurate adjustment possible.

When the teeth are altered by selective grinding to make simultaneous cusp tip-to cusp tip contact on both sides of the arch, and the jaws are in a right or left lateral position, balanced occlusion in a static eccentric position exists. Some of these static contacts may be repeated in the mouth. When the mandible is in a straight protruded relation with the maxillae and the posterior teeth are altered to make cusp contacts at the same time the anterior teeth make incisal edge-to-incisal-edge contact, balanced occlusion in protrusion exists. One may expect this static occlusal and incisal edge relation to exist in the mouth when the mandible is protruded to the same forward position.

When teeth are arranged and the anteroposterior horizontal relations of the jaws are even (considered normally related), the buccal cusps of the mandibular posterior teeth and the lingual cusps of the maxillary posterior teeth maintain the occluding vertical dimension by contacting in the fossae and on the marginal ridges of their antagonists. When the horizontal position of the mandible is in a more forward position than the maxillae or in a situation where the mandible is larger in a lateral direction than the maxillae, the posterior teeth are frequently arranged in a reverse relation (crossbite, or reverse articulation). The buccal cusp tips of the maxillary posterior teeth and the lingual cusp tips of the mandibular posterior teeth maintain the occluding vertical dimension. After the occlusal surfaces of the teeth have been altered by grinding to achieve balanced occlusions with the jaws in centric relation, the cusps that maintain the occluding vertical dimension are not altered in subsequent adjustments.

Selective Grinding of Anatomic Teeth in a Balanced Occlusion

In the first step of selective grinding, cusp form teeth are altered by reshaping to obtain balanced occlusion when the jaws are in centric relation. Occlusal balance in a lateral direction is obtained by having all of the posterior teeth and the canines in contact on the working side and posterior contact only on the non-working side. In protrusive balance, the anterior teeth should make incisal edge contact at the same time that the tips of the buccal and lingual cusps of the posterior teeth contact.

Adjust the horizontal and lateral condylar inclinations of the articulator to the settings dictated by a protrusive interocclusal maxillomandibular relation record (See Chapter 10, Maxillomandibular Records and Articulators). The incisal pin should be raised off the table and secured.

With the condylar elements against the centric relation stops, close the articulator until the posterior teeth are in contact. The anterior teeth should not be in contact. Examine the lingual cusps of the maxillary posterior teeth and the buccal cusps of the mandibular posterior teeth. Record the area or areas of premature contact with articulating paper. The contacts may be in varying amounts and may involve more than one cusp or tooth. These varying situations make critical evaluation necessary prior to grinding procedures in the centric position.

Before grinding or adjusting the centric contacts, the excursive position contacts should also be evaluated. With the right condylar element in the centric position, place the lingual cusps of the maxillary posterior teeth in the nonworking relation with the buccal cusps of the mandibular posterior teeth. This procedure also places the buccal and lingual cusps of the maxillary and mandibular posterior teeth and the canines in their working position on the opposite side. The teeth are placed in these positions and not shifted from the centric to the eccentric position with the teeth in contact. When the teeth on the nonworking side are not in the correct relation, the error appears on the nonworking or working side. If the nonworking contact is excessive, the working side teeth will not be in contact. If the working side contact is excessive, the excess prevents contact on the nonworking side. If the teeth on the working side are too long, there will be no contact on the nonworking side. If a single tooth is high on the working side, there will be contact neither on the nonworking side nor on the working side. Record any premature contacts with articulating paper and repeat the procedure with the left side as the working side and record the premature contacts. If the cusp is high in the centric and in the eccentric position, reduce the premature cusp.

If the cusp is high in the centric and not in the eccentric position, deepen the fossae or the marginal ridges. After all interceptive contacts have been removed in the centric and full eccentric position, do not reduce the maxillary lingual cusp or the mandibular buccal cusp and do not deepen the fossa or marginal ridge of any tooth. This will maintain the centric and eccentric holding cusp relationships.

To refine the teeth to retain contact when the articulator is being moved to and from centric and eccentric position, additional adjustments are needed. On the working side, reduce the inner inclines of the buccal cusps of the maxillary teeth and the lingual cusps of the mandibular teeth (BULL rule). On the nonworking side, reduce the inner inclines of the mandibular buccal cusps. If it is necessary to eliminate a centric cusp to correct balancing prematurities, eliminate the mandibular buccal cusp. This maintains the centric occlusal contact on the maxillary lingual cusp, which will better direct the forces of mastication against the mandibular denture. The mandibular denture is generally less stable than the maxillary and will retain length to the lingual cusp, which is often necessary to establish protrusive balance. To achieve balance in protrusive excursion, reduce the distal inclines of the maxillary cusps and the mesial inclines of the mandibular cusps. After completing the selective grinding procedures to establish and maintain the desired occlusion refine the occlusal anatomy.

Selective Grinding of Lingualized Balanced Occlusion

Correcting occlusal disharmonies in a balanced lingualized occlusion is similar to a fully balanced occlusion with the exception that only the lingual cusps of the maxillary teeth or their antagonist surfaces are adjusted. The same basic approach is used to evaluate where the disharmony exists and then correct it by reducing the mandibular fossae or marginal ridges in centric relation position. After the centric relation position is refined, the eccentric movements are adjusted on the slopes of the mandibular cusps as indicated in the fully balanced occlusal adjustment section. Since only the lingual cusps of the maxillary teeth are in contact this balanced set up is much less complicated to adjust.

Selective Grinding of Nonanatomic Teeth

When noncusp form posterior teeth or a nonbalanced lingualized occlusal scheme are used, and selective grinding procedures are instituted, the occlusal surfaces of the maxillary posterior teeth are altered to make harmonious contact on the right side and on the left side when the jaws are in centric relation.

Secure the condylar elements on the articulator against the condylar housings and place articulating tape over the occlusal surfaces and incisal edges of all of the mandibular teeth. Tap the teeth together to record the contacting areas. Using an acrylic bur, grind the occlusal surfaces of the teeth until simultaneous even contacting areas on the right and left are developed. The anterior teeth should be slightly out of contact in the centric relation position, but can make a "kissing" contact during lateral excursive movements. Smooth gliding movements from the centric position to eccentric positions should be developed by careful adjustment of opposing surfaces during excursive movements of the articulator. Exercise care to maintain the occlusal surfaces of the mandibular arch on a plane.

Stripping Method for The Occlusal Equilibration of Nonanatomic Teeth

The simplest technique to refine the occlusion for cuspless, nonanatomic teeth or a nonbalanced lingualized occlusal scheme is the carborundum stripping technique, which was originally published by Dr. Gronas in 1970. It, like all procedures in dentistry, if followed correctly, will yield excellent results. The primary purpose of nonanatomic posterior teeth, when set on a flat plane, is to eliminate cuspal inferences. Therefore, it is necessary during the selective grinding procedure in this technique to maintain the previously established flat occlusal scheme. A rotary instrument usually produces irregularities in the flat occlusal surfaces. Waterproof carborundum abrasive paper is the most ideal material to use with this method. A fine 320-grit paper is used for acrylic resin teeth. Strips of the abrasive paper should be cut in varying widths to allow for the reduction of individual teeth or to reduce entire quadrants. It should be remembered that the flatness of the occlusal surfaces of the mandibular teeth must be maintained throughout the entire grinding procedure.

Locate the premature contacts with articulating ribbon or paper (Figure 14–16). If there is a grossly tipped tooth that is above the occlusal plane, reduce the tooth with a stone or bur until a flat occlusal plane is obtained. Place a carborundum strip of the appropriate width with the abrasive side against the teeth that are to be reduced (maxillary), and gently close the articulator in centric relation. Apply tight pressure to the upper member of the articulator, and pull the strip briskly between the teeth (Figure 14–17). Always pull the strip in the same plane as the flat occlusal surfaces of the teeth in order to avoid rounding of the bucco-occlusal angle of the teeth. Evaluate the occluding vertical dimension carefully throughout the procedure, as the rapid reduction of the occlusal surfaces could allow over closure past the original vertical dimension. Reduction of the contacts with the strips is continued by stripping an equal number of times until uniform bilateral contacts on the posterior teeth are obtained (Figure 14–18). Finish the reduction with finer grits of sandpaper strips in order to produce a smoother flat surface.

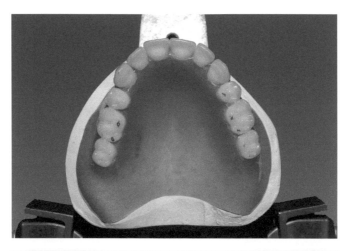
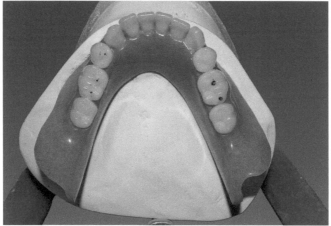

Figure 14–16 Initial centric occlusion marks on a nonbalanced, lingualized occlusion.

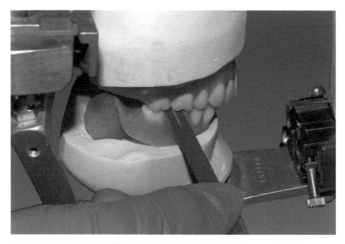

Figure 14–17 Using a carborundum strip to refine the centric occlusal stops on a nonbalanced, lingualized occlusion.

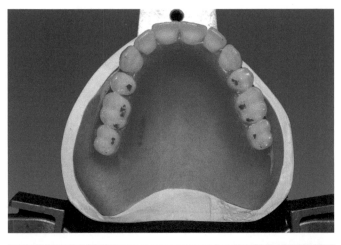

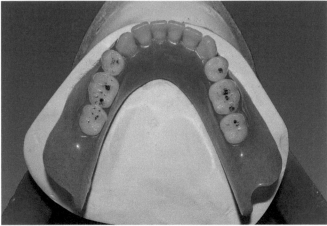

Figure 14–18   The final revised centric occlusal contacts on a nonbalanced, lingualized occlusion.

Check each eccentric position (working, nonworking, protrusive) and remove any premature contacts with a carborundum strip or an acrylic bur while maintaining a flat occlusal plane. The anterior teeth should be slightly out of contact in the centric relation position, but can make a "kissing" contact during lateral excursive movements. Smooth gliding movements from the centric position to eccentric positions should be developed by careful adjustment of opposing surfaces during excursive movements of the articulator.

 Final Checks of The Prostheses

Once all adjustments have been made to the denture intaglio surfaces and the occlusion has been finalized, the dentures should be evaluated for proper contour and thickness. Improper contour can affect the final fit of the prostheses and make muscles work against stabilization instead of enhancing it. Contours of most external surfaces should be slightly concave from the necks of the teeth to the denture borders. Occasionally surfaces are left bulky for lip or cheek support, but that is an exception to the norm. The palate should be 2–3 mm thick for proper strength and be thinned to blend with the posterior palate after the posterior palatal seal is finalized. All surfaces should be smooth and highly polished (Figures 14–19-25).

After completing all final checks, it is time to let the patient try out the new dentures. This is the clinician's opportunity to help the patient understand the limitations of the prosthetic devices they are wearing, give tips on making the new dentures work properly, provide care instructions for both the mouth and the prostheses, and reassure the patient that he or she will be successful with diligence about the learning process for using dentures (Figures 14–26 and 14–27).

A written letter of instruction should be given the patient to help them recall the conversation and instructions they have received. A definitive recall appointment should

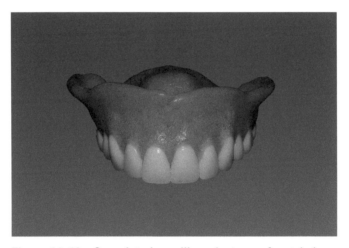

Figure 14–19   Completed maxillary denture – frontal view

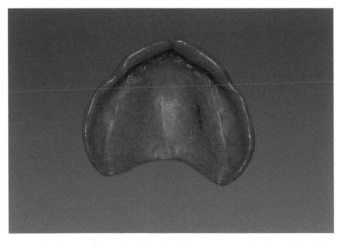

Figure 14–20   Completed maxillary denture – intaglio view

be arranged in case the patient has problems that need additional attention. A good rule of thumb is to see the patient the next day, after one week, and possibly about one month after insertion. It is important to stress the importance of annual recalls to make sure no damaging wear patterns develop that could cause injury to underlying supporting structures. The need for periodic examinations of the soft tissue intraorally as patients get older should also be emphasized.

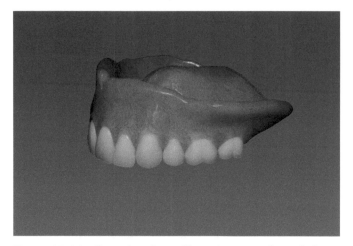

Figure 14–21   Completed maxillary denture – lateral view

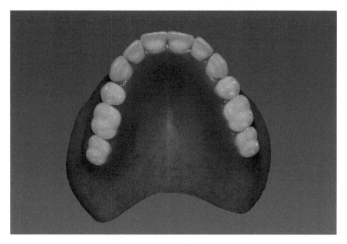

Figure 14–22   Completed maxillary denture – occlusal view

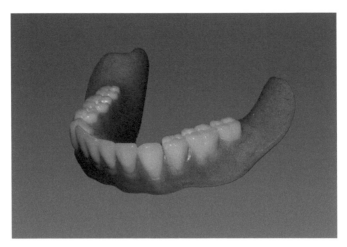

Figure 14–23   Completed mandibular denture – lateral view

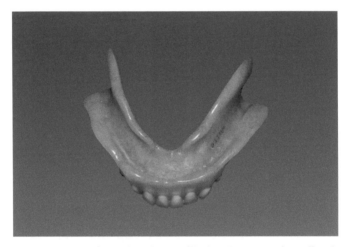

Figure 14–24   Completed mandibular denture – intaglio view

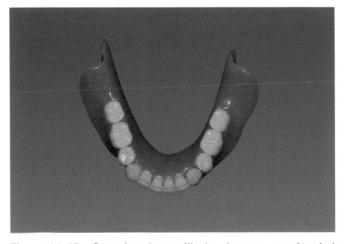

Figure 14–25   Completed mandibular denture – occlusal view

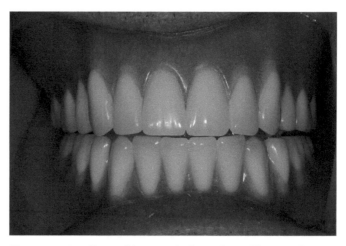

Figure 14–26   Frontal intraoral view of maxillary and mandibular complete dentures (nonbalanced, lingualized occlusion).

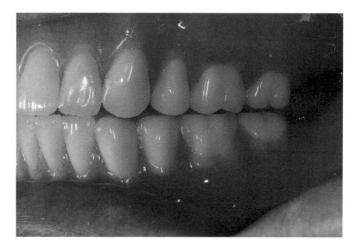

Figure 14–27   Lateral intraoral view of maxillary and mandibular complete dentures (Nonbalanced, lingualized occlusion).

References

Firtell, D. N., Arnett, W. S., and Holmes, J. B.: Pressure indicators for removable prosthodontics. J. Prosth. Dent., 54:226, 1985.

Firtell, D. N., Finzen, F. C., and Holmes, J. B.: The effect of clinical remount procedures on the comfort and success of complete dentures, J. Prosth. Dent., 57:53, 1987.

Gronas, D. G.: A carborundum stripping technique for the occlusal adjustment of cuspless teeth. J, Prosth, Dent,, 23:218, 1970.

Jankelson, B.: Adjustment of dentures at time of insertion to compensate for tissue change. J.A.D.A., 64:521, 1962.

Leary, J. M., Diaz-Arnold, A. M., and Aquilino, S. A.: The complete denture remount procedure. Quint. Int., 19:623, 1988.

Logan, G., and Nimmo, A.: The use of disclosing wax to evaluate denture extensions. J. Prosth. Dent., 51:281, 1984,

Rahn, A. O., and Heartwell, C. M., editors: Textbook of Complete Dentures. 5th Ed. Philadelphia: Lippincott, 1993.

Sussman, B. A.: Insertion of a full upper and lower denture, J. Ontario Dent. Assoc., 34:16, 1957.

Young, H. A.: Denture insertion, J.A.D.A., 64:505, 1962.

QUESTIONS

1. What should be done to evaluate the fit of the intaglio surface of a denture for proper fit?

2. Should the patient bite on the dentures to help mark possible pressure areas on the intaglio surface?

3. Is an intraoral occlusal adjustment of complete dentures the most accurate method to evaluate and correct occlusal disharmony in complete dentures?

4. What procedure makes it possible to make a new interocclusal record at the insertion appointment at a slightly open OVD without loss of accuracy?

ANSWERS

1. Each denture base should be individually evaluated for accuracy of adaptation to the tissues and for areas of excessive tissue/denture base pressure. Excessive pressure will result in irritation to the tissue and pain to the patient, and must be eliminated. It is most likely to occur in those areas in which the rigid denture base must slide into an undercut or contact tissues that are almost noncompressible. To identify pressure areas, the intaglio surface (tissue side of the denture) should be painted with a thin film of pressure-disclosing paste using uniform brush strokes. The denture is then inserted and removed. When removed, the pressure-disclosing paste and brush strokes will be undisturbed in areas of no tissue/denture base contact, exhibit minimal uniform contact in those areas with the desired tissue/denture base contact, or be wiped off in those areas of excessive pressure.

2. Use only finger pressure when evaluating these pressure areas. Do not let the patient bite on the dentures to place pressure. Uncorrected premature occlusal contact may cause the pressure-disclosing paste to be displaced, mimicking pressure areas.

3. It is difficult to see occlusal discrepancies intraorally with complete dentures. The resiliency of the supporting soft tissues and the the ability of the tissues

to be displaced in varying degrees tend to disguise premature occlusal contacts. The tissues permit the dentures to shift; as a result, after the first interceptive occlusal contact, the remaining teeth appear to make satisfactory contacts. Occlusal faults can be determined by obtaining an interocclusal record from the patient and remounting the dentures on an articulator.

4. The facebow positioning of the maxillary cast simulates the correct arc of closure position.

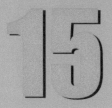
Post Insertion

Dr. Kevin D. Plummer

Correcting the many possible problems associated with the use of dentures requires persistence on the part of patients and skill and experience on the part of dentists. Dentists also need thorough knowledge of anatomy, physiology, pathology, and psychology. They must be capable of differentiating between normal and abnormal tissue responses. They must distinguish between a physical disorder that is aggravated by the psychic and emotional processes of a patient and one that is solely physical. When dentists have knowledge of the basic sciences and the skill and experience to investigate these denture-related problems, they will readily see that, in the majority of instances, the problems are real and not psychosomatic.

Compatibility

Even though it is not living tissue, a denture is compatible when it is accepted by the oral environment. The acrylic resin of the denture should be inert. The artificial teeth should be placed in positions that do not produce trauma when they are in function and that are in balance with the various muscle groups of the face. The forces of occlusion should be directed toward the most acceptable support. The artificial teeth should be arranged so that, when they make contact, they are in harmony with mandibular positions and movements. When the mandible is at the vertical dimension of rest, sufficient interocclusal distance must exist to allow for full contraction of the elevator muscles of the mandible before the occlusal surfaces of the posterior teeth make maximum contact. The artificial teeth should be arranged to give support to the lips and cheeks, and they should be compatible with their actions and those actions of the tongue. The denture bases should cover the basal seat areas to achieve a "snowshoe" effect of maximum support. The soft tissues that are supported by bone should be recorded in their undisplaced form to ensure even contact with the tissue side of the denture bases and to minimize the pressure to the underlying bone.

Problems with Mastication

The artificial nature of dentures means that they cannot function as efficiently as natural teeth function. Patients will not be able to perform certain functions, such as chewing extremely hard or chewy and sticky foods. Incising with the front teeth is usually difficult with dentures because they have little support directly under the incisor area. The patient will need to learn these limitations and be helped through a training period to become more comfortable with the limitations of their artificial teeth. Knowing that the canine area will be more efficient for incising, that smaller portions will be easier to handle, and that some foods may be "off limits" will help the patient have more realistic expectations.

Soft Tissue Considerations

Stress-Bearing Mucosa

Traumatic lesions of the stress-bearing mucosa of the palate and the crest and slopes of the residual ridges are usually the result of imperfections in or on the surface of the tissue side of the denture base. Pressure areas on the tissue side of the denture can develop from imperfections developed during the impression procedures or as a result of damage to the master cast. Disharmony in occlusion in either the centric or the eccentric jaw positions can also produce traumatic lesions in these areas (Figure 15–1). Lesions occurring in the mucosa that covers the palate and the crest of the residual ridges are usually small, well circumscribed, and indurated. The presence of excessive keratin often causes the area to appear white.

Lesions that are hyperemic and painful to pressure during function are usually a result of pressure directed toward an area of exostosis, a sharp spur of bone, or a foreign body. These areas may not produce a noticeable soreness at the insertion appointment because the abuse of the tissue occurs over time and is associated with the function of the dentures.

Occasionally, severe irritation and a detaching of the overlying mucosa occur. This may be encountered over the mylohyoid ridge, the cuspid eminences, the alveolar tubercles, and areas of exostosis. This is usually produced by the denture flange during the insertion and removal of the denture or from excessive friction when the denture moves during function.

Hyperemic, painful, and detached areas of epithelium that develop on the slope of the residual ridges are usually the result of disharmony of occlusion when the teeth are

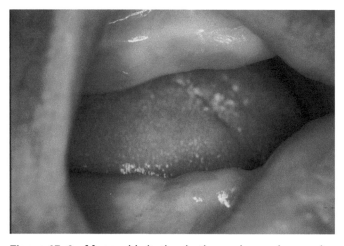

Figure 15–1   Mucosal irritation in the canine and premolar area, where a large excursive prematurity existed in lateral functional movements

making unbalanced contact in eccentric jaw positions (Figure 15–2). A horizontal torque or shearing force causes these lesions.

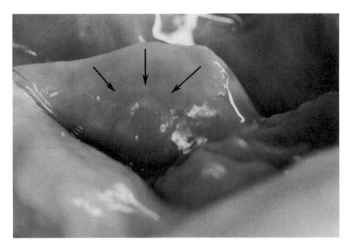

Figure 15–2   A large ulceration on the lingual slope of the anterior mandibular ridge caused by excessive movement of the denture base in an anterior direction during function

Basal-Seat Mucosa

Two problems associated with the basal-seat mucosa are hypertrophy and inflammation. Inflammatory reactions of the mucosa covering the basal seat are usually the result of the patient not removing the dentures to allow the tissues to rest. The constant pressure of the dentures retards the normal blood supply, which oxygenates the tissues and removes the waste products. This is a generalized inflammation and is usually not restricted to one area, but covers all of the mucosa.

A generalized soreness of the crest and slopes of the residual ridges accompanied by pain in the muscles attached to the mandible may be the result of insufficient interocclusal distance. The constant pressure from the denture bases, because the teeth are always in contact produces hyperemia in the mucosa. The muscles of mastication may also become sore because they cannot reach a relaxed position, and are always slightly overstretched.

Hypertrophy, an abnormal increase in the size of the oral mucosa, is unusual in the stress-bearing mucosa. However, in the midpalatal suture area, hypertrophy of the mucosa can occur. Small nodules, which are defined as 'papilloma-like hypertrophy," develop throughout the area (Figure 15–3). A poor-fitting prothesis with poor retention usually leads to this type of tissue reaction.

Transitional Submucosa

Hypertrophy can also occur in the areas of transitional submucosa, such as border extensions. The lesions occurring in the border extension areas are usually laceration-type

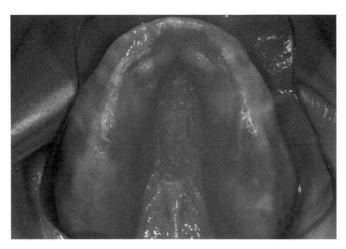

Figure 15–3   Papillary hyperplasia in the center of the palate caused by a loose and poorly fitting maxillary denture

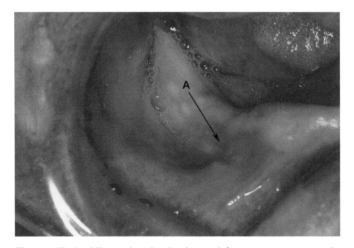

Figure 15–4   Ulceration in the buccal frenum area caused by an overextension of the denture base (A).

fissures. The fissures vary in length and depth, are painful, and often become ulcerated. These lesions result primarily from overextension of the border, but can result from sharp or unpolished borders (Figure 15–4). The lesions can occur in any border area; however, they are most frequently encountered in the frenum attachments, the retrornylohyoid space, the retromolar pad, the masseter groove, the hamular notch, the floor of the mouth, and the soft palate (Figures 15–5-7).

Lining Mucosa

Abrasions appearing on the mucosa of the cheeks and lips are frequently the result of cheek biting, rough margins on the teeth, or unpolished denture bases. Cheek biting may be associated with a lack of horizontal overlap of the posterior teeth or the transition from a normal to crossbite or reverse-articulation occlusal scheme (Figure 15–8). Occasionally tongue biting can occur if the horizontal overlap is improper on the lingual cusp areas (Figure 15–9).

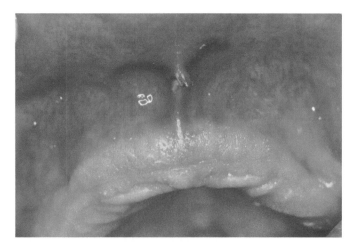

Figure 15–5 Ulceration and irritation caused by improper design of the notch and flange in the area of the maxillary labial frenum

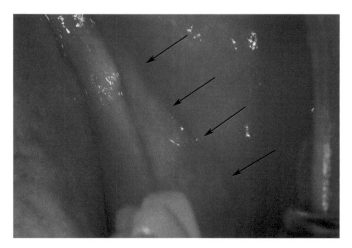

Figure 15–6 Irritation caused by a slightly overextended border or a sharp edge on a properly extended border

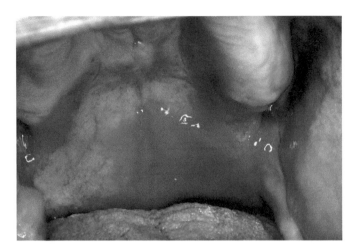

Figure 15–7   Ulceration of the hamular notch caused by overextension of the posterior border or too much pressure from the palatal seal of the maxillary denture. This can be extremely painful, and patients may believe the soreness is located in the throat or mandibular retromylohyiod area.

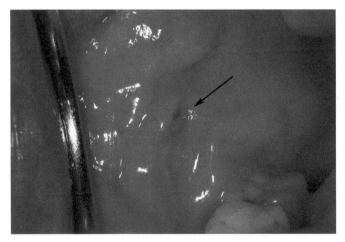

Figure 15–8   Abrasion caused by cheek biting due to lack of horizontal overlap of the posterior teeth

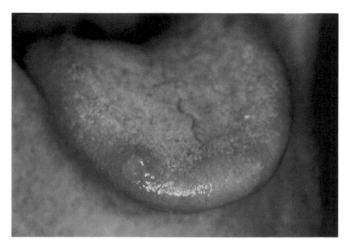

Figure 15–9   Tongue injury due to improper horizontal overlap of the lingual cusp area of the artificial teeth

Treatment Procedures

Examine each denture for stability and retention with the mouth at rest and also with the mouth in function. To check functional stability and retention, instruct the patient to speak, laugh, yawn, wipe the lips with the tip of the tongue, and swallow. The patient can also gently chew on a cotton roll or small piece of gauze to simulate chewing on tough food. If these procedures cause pain or dislodgement of the denture, the borders should be checked with disclosing wax to determine if they are properly adjusted. Poor retention may be due to borders that were shortened too much during initial placement or subsequent adjustments. Adding disclosing wax may temporarily alleviate this problem and may indicate that a permanent repair to add flange length is needed. There may also be pressure areas on the tissue surface of the denture that prevent the denture base from fully seating against tissue and reducing the interfacial surface tension, which results in a loose denture. Pressure disclosing paste should be used to identify and correct those areas. Indelible marking sticks may also be used to transfer information from muscle activity or pressure to the denture base, to facilitate adjustments. Marking a suspected problem area and inserting the denture will transfer the mark to the denture base resin for evaluation.

To check for undesirable undercuts, apply pressure disclosing paste to the tissue side of the denture. Instruct the patient to insert and remove the denture. An undercut appears when the paste is removed from the denture, as if it were dragged from the surface. When it has been definitely established that an undercut exists and that the denture is abusing the mucosa, alter the tissue side of the denture base by grinding with an acrylic bur. It is better to grind too little than too much because tissue contact with the denture must be maintained. Always smooth and polish all ground areas. To check for pressure from occlusal prematurities, pressure disclosing paste is applied to the entire tissue side of the denture. Instruct the patient to insert both dentures and tap the teeth together with the jaws in centric relation. Instruct the patient to exercise care when inserting the maxillary denture and not to apply finger pressure to the denture. When the teeth have been tapped in place, an area of displaced paste on the tissue side of the denture is a sign of pressure. It is best to repeat the procedure to verify the marking. The pressure area may result from premature tooth contact or an imperfection of the denture base. The cause must be determined before institution of corrective measures. To determine if the pressure area is produced by faulty occlusion, institute patient remount procedures or mark the occlusal contacts intraorally using articulating paper. When occlusion causes the pressure, adjust the occlusion. When the denture base causes the pressure (Figure 15–10), relieve the denture base by grinding with an acrylic bur; then smooth and polish. It is possible that both denture base and occlusion may need correction.

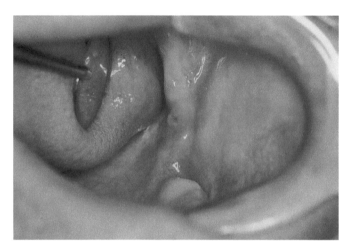

Figure 15–10   Injury caused by the maxillary and mandibular denture bases pinching soft tissue between each other, if the bases do not have proper clearance during function

When a generalized inflammatory condition exists or hyperkeratosis is present in the stress-bearing mucosa, evaluate a lack of interocclusal distance. Another common problem associated with the lack of interocclusal distance is an audible "clicking" of the teeth during speech and chewing. If the interocclusal distance is not adequate, alter the teeth to provide adequate space. If the teeth cannot be altered enough to provide the proper interocclusal distance, the teeth may need to be removed from the resin denture base and rearranged. This procedure requires a new interocclusal record at the corrected occlusal vertical dimension. The denture will have to be reprocessed after arranging the teeth in the proper relationship. If the reduction of the occlusal vertical dimension creates interferences that cannot be adjusted between the anterior teeth, they may need to be removed and rearranged also.

 ## Problems with Maxillary Denture

Dislodgment during functions is a result of overfilled buccal vestibule; overextension in the hamular notch area; inadequate notches for frenum attachments; excessively thick

denture base over the distobuccal alveolar tubercle area— leaving insufficient space for the forward and medial movement of the anterior border of the coronoid process; placing the maxillary anterior teeth too far in an anterior direction; placing the maxillary posterior teeth too far in a buccal direction; or placing the posterior palatal seal too deep—causing excessive displacement of soft palate tissues. Lack of occlusal harmony can also cause dislodgement of the denture during function. When the teeth do not make harmonious contact, the lever action tilts the denture base, and there is a loss of the seal between the tissues and the denture base. The result is loss of stability and retention.

Dislodgment when the jaws are at rest is a result of underfilled buccal vestibule, inadequate border seal, excessive saliva, or xerostomia. When the maxillary denture slowly loses retention, the consistency of the saliva, excessive saliva, or the lack of saliva is usually involved. When the drop or loosening of the denture is sudden, the cause is usually mechanical.

Problems with Mandibular Denture

Dislodgment during function is the result of overextension in the masseter groove area; extending in a lateral direction beyond the external oblique line; overextension of the lingual flanges; placing the occlusal plane too high; causing dislodgment when the tongue tries to handle the bolus of food; underextension of the lingual flanges, causing the border to become the playground for the tongue; improper contour of the polished surface; or overextension in the retromolar pad area, causing contact between the denture base that covers the alveolar tubercle and the denture base that covers the retromolar pad when the mandible is protruded. This contact dislodges the mandibular denture in the anterior section.

Other Common Problems

Commissural cheilitis, inflammation of the angles of the mouth, is frequently attributed to excessive interocclusal distance (reduced occluding vertical dimension). However, placing the maxillary posterior teeth too far in a lateral direction eliminates the buccal corridor. When the crowns of the teeth are against the cheeks, the saliva collects at the necks of the teeth and makes its escape in the area of the canines. Commissural cheilitis can also develop when the occlusal plane of the lower teeth is too high. This prevents the regular action of the cheek from eliminating the saliva from the lower buccal vestibule, so the saliva will exit through the corners of the mouth.

Gagging and Vomiting

Patients who develop a gagging or vomiting problem with dentures are frequently difficult to treat, and the difficulty is primarily one of determining the cause. Some patients have a hypersensitive gagging reflex evident prior to and during the denture construction. The insertion or removal of complete dentures may elicit gagging. However, occasionally a patient develops a gagging problem *after* denture insertion.

A complete denture patient may develop a gagging or vomiting problem as a result of loose dentures; poor occlusion; incorrect extension or contour of the dentures—particularly in the posterior area of the palate and the retromylohyoid space; underextended denture borders; placing the maxillary teeth too far in a palatal direction and the mandibular teeth too far in a lingual direction so that the dorsum of the tongue is forced into the pharynx during the act of swallowing; an increased vertical dimension of occlusion; and psychogenic factors. Patients may refuse to swallow for fear that the dentures will dislodge and strangle them. As a result of not swallowing, the saliva accumulates and triggers the gagging reflex. A common problem often overlooked is that the posterior border of the denture is too thick. It should be thinned to blend into the palate and not create an uncomfortable bump in the posterior.

Burning Tongue and Palate

The burning sensation that some patients experience in the anterior third of the palate may result from pressure on the nasopalatine area. Relief of the denture over the incisive papilla is usually effective.

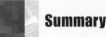

Summary

Problems associated with real, identifiable causes can be eliminated by careful observation and physical correction of the cause. Occasionally a patient will return numerous times with vague problems, which are difficult to diagnose and correct. These patients may really be having a difficult time adjusting to the psychological realities of denture wearing and need time to overcome the fears they have associated with the prostheses they now wear. Patience and understanding along with further education will sometimes help these patients make this transition. The use of a powdered adhesive may make the dentures more stable and help the patient gain confidence in the use of the dentures. Also, be sure to investigate the esthetic result of the dentures with these patients; they may actually have esthetic concerns (their own or those of a significant other) that they feel uncomfortable discussing, and may be using other problems as an excuse to make the dentures appear unsuitable.

References

Bell, D. H., Jr.: Problems in complete denture treatment. J. Prosth. Dent, 19:550, 1968.

Berg, H., Carisson, G. E., and Helkimo, M.: Changes in shape of posterior parts of upper jaws after extraction of teeth and prosthetic treatment. J. Prosth. Dent., 34:262.1975.

Collett, H. A.: Oral conditions associated with dentures. J. Prosth. Dent., 8:591,1956.

Conny, U., and Tedesco, L.: The gagging problem in prosthodontic treatment. Part 1—Description and causes. J. Prosth. Dent., 49:601, 1983.

Conny, U., and Tedesco, L.: The gagging problem in prosthodontic treatment, Part 11—Patient management. J. Prosth. Dent., 49:757, 1983.

Harris, W. T., and Mack, J. F.: Conditioning dentures for problem patients. J. Prosth. Dent., 34:141, 1975.

Kapur, K., and Shklar, C.: The effect of complete dentures on alveolar mucosa. J. Prosth. Dent., 13:1030, 1963.

Koper, A.: Difficult denture birds. I. Prosth. Dent., 17:532, 1967.

Kouats. J. T.: Clinical evaluation of the gagging denture patient, J. Prosth. Dent., 25: 613 1971.

Lambson, G. O., and Anderson, R. R.: Palatal papillary hyperplasia. J. Prosth. Dent., 18:528, 1967.

QUESTIONS

1. Why is typical biting with the front teeth difficult for denture patients?

2. What is the most likely cause of hyperemic, painful, and detached areas of epithelium that develop on the slopes of the residual ridges?

3. What could be possible causes for dislodgement of the maxillary denture during function?

4. What denture conditions can lead to commissural cheilitis?

ANSWERS

1. There is no direct support under the incisal edges of the anterior teeth in most instances due to ridge resorption. The long lever arm created by these teeth tends to destabilize the denture when a bolus of food is placed between incisors for shearing.

2. They are usually the result of disharmony of occlusion when the teeth are making unbalanced contact in eccentric jaw positions.

3. Dislodgement during function could be the result of overfilled buccal vestibule; overextension in the hamular notch area; inadequate notches for frenum attachments; excessively thick denture base over the distobuccal alveolar tubercle area—leaving insufficient space for the forward and medial movement of the anterior border of the coronoid process; placing the maxillary anterior teeth too far in an anterior direction; placing the maxillary posterior teeth too far in a buccal direction; or placing the posterior palatal seal too deep causing excessive displacement of soft palate tissues. Lack of occlusal harmony can also cause dislodgement of the denture during function.

4. Commissural cheilitis, inflammation of the angles of the mouth, is frequently attributed to excessive interocclusal distance (reduced vertical dimension of occlusion). However, placing the maxillary posterior teeth too far in a lateral direction eliminates the buccal corridor and, when the crowns of the teeth

are against the cheeks, the saliva collects at the necks of the teeth and makes its escape in the area of the canines. Commissural cheilitis can also develop when the occlusal plane of the lower teeth is too high. This prevents the regular action of the cheek from eliminating the saliva from the lower buccal vestibule, so the saliva will exit through the corners of the mouth.

CHAPTER

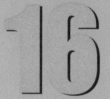

Overview of Single Dentures, Overdentures, and Immediate Dentures

Dr. Dennis Kiernan
Dr. Kevin Plummer

No textbook on complete dentures would be thorough without at least a brief mention of certain special circumstances that demonstrate the versatility of the complete denture prosthesis. The goal of this chapter is to provide a brief overview of the major indications, advantages, and disadvantages of single dentures, overdentures, and immediate dentures. All of these treatment modalities are far more challenging for the dentist and the patient than the fabrication of a conventional set of complete dentures would be. However, if both parties are fully aware of the limitations and have reasonable treatment expectations, the outcome can be very gratifying.

Single Dentures

When only one arch is being restored with a denture, it is called a single denture (Figure 16–1). Single dentures may be fabricated to oppose:

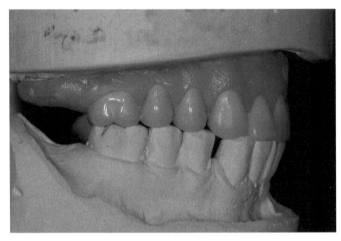

Figure 16–1 Wax set-up of a maxillary single denture; opposing natural teeth on the mandibular arch

1. An arch containing a sufficient number of natural teeth and fixed restorations so as to not require any other prostheses.
2. A partially edentulous arch in which the missing teeth have been or will be replaced by a removable partial denture, fixed partial dentures, or implant-supported prostheses.
3. An existing acceptable complete denture, whether it be mucosal-borne, tooth-supported, or implant-supported.

The conditions leading to the recommendation of treatment by means of a single complete denture can be quite varied. Patient availability, financial ability, desires, and the old prosthodontic principle to "preserve that which remains," may all influence the eventual treatment plan and should be carefully considered during the diagnostic evaluation appointment. A frank discussion of treatment advantages, disadvantages, limitations, and patient expectations of the treatment should ensue. Any alternative treatment

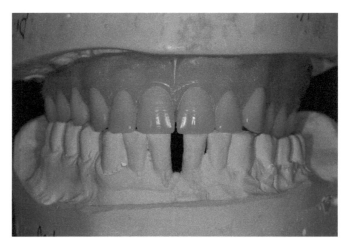

Figure 16–2 Wax set-up of a maxillary single denture; opposing natural teeth on the mandible. Note the occlusal plane discrepancy on the patient's left side. This might result in difficulty balancing the excursive contacts during function of the denture.

regimens should be discussed so that the patient can make the most informed decision possible.

When the dentist and the patient have chosen the single denture as the treatment, both should fully realize that the ability to achieve stability, retention, and support of the newly fabricated single denture is of paramount importance to its success. Because the opposing arch may not be treated, the dentist's ability to obtain an optimum occlusal scheme may be compromised. Therefore, the fabrication of the single denture may be difficult, and the end result from a functional or even esthetic standpoint, may be less than ideal (Figure 16–2).

Maxillary single dentures are often more successful than mandibular dentures for a number of reasons. First, the mandibular arch is the moveable member of the stomatognathic system (mouth, jaws, and related structures), which inherently decreases its stability. Additionally, the proximity of the mandibular denture borders to the tongue and other moveable mucosa may lead to easier displacement. Thirdly, the mandibular edentulous ridge, with its limited amount of attached submucosal tissue, provides less support for the denture base. Therefore, if stability of the single denture is of primary importance for its success, it is clear why patient satisfaction is greater with maxillary single dentures.

Stability and retention of the single denture can be increased by means of adjunctive treatment using dental implants and attachments (Figure 16–3). Dental implants have the added benefit of preserving alveolar bone. This is even more important for the younger patients who, after many decades of support loss, may find themselves unable to tolerate dentures.

Another way of potentially increasing the stability and retention of the single denture is to use anatomic-form posterior denture teeth and a balanced occlusal scheme. By providing bilateral balancing contacts when the patient moves through the eccentric movements, the denture is not subjected to tipping forces that can lead to its dislodgement. If the opposing dentition has been worn flat and is not being restored, a monoplane denture setup may accomplish the same result.

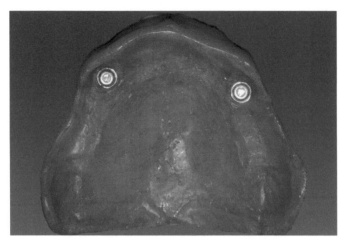

Figure 16–3 Two implant attachments located in the approximate area of the canines provide both retention and stability for the single maxillary denture.

A frequent obstacle to obtaining a balanced occlusion is an irregular occlusal plane of the teeth in the opposing arch, as a result of supraeruption—or tilting of the teeth. A consequence of this irregular plane is an unfavorable distribution of forces. The irregular occlusal plane may also compromise the final esthetic outcome of the single denture. This problem may be resolved by orthodontic repositioning of the opposing teeth or by altering the clinical crowns of the teeth by means of selective grinding or with restorations. Of course, the clinician may be forced to accept good centric occlusion contacts and premature contacts in the eccentric positions. The excessive premature contacts often cannot be eliminated.

Fracturing the denture base of the single denture is a common complication because the denture is often opposed by a full or nearly full complement of natural teeth or fixed restorations. The resulting high occlusal forces on the denture combined with a typical denture base thickness sometimes results in fracture. Careful control over the occlusion or use of a cast metal base are considerations to prevent this problem.

The single denture offers various challenges to the clinician. Careful evaluation and treatment planning are essential to the success of the prosthesis. As long as the dentist and the patient are aware of the treatment limitations and have reasonable expectations, the final outcome can be a very gratifying experience for both.

Overdentures

An overdenture is a removable dental prosthesis that covers and rests on one or more remaining natural teeth, the roots of natural teeth, and/or dental implants. The implants or modified natural teeth provide for additional support, stability, and retention of the overdenture than the edentulous ridges alone can provide (Figures 16–3 and 16–4). This is particularly advantageous in the mandibular arch, where edentulous ridges may resorb at a rate four times greater than that of the maxillary arch.

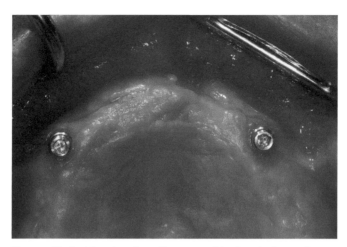

Figure 16–4 Two implant fixtures with simple "snap" attachments help maintain bone, and provide retention and stability for complete dentures.

There are several advantages to the overdenture. Implants or the roots of natural teeth are present to provide stimulation to the alveolar bone, which is conducive to bone repair and maintenance, thus preserving the alveolar ridge. A definite vertical stop is provided, which can be advantageous in situations where hypertrophic soft tissue is present. Horizontal and torquing forces can be minimized, and stability and support are increased, thereby reducing forces of occlusion on the supporting tissues. Finally, a real psychological advantage can be realized in patients who are unwilling to lose the last of their remaining natural teeth.

Overdentures should be considered for any patient facing the loss of the remaining dentition. The younger the patient, the greater the indication for this treatment may be because of the anticipated significant bone loss over many years. If retention is expected to be difficult to obtain or is of primary importance, attachments may be particularly useful. Examples of where attachments would be beneficial include severe cases of xerostomia, minimal alveolar ridge height in edentulous areas, loss of a part of the maxilla or mandible, or congenital deformities such as cleft palates.

Teeth to be prepared for denture abutments are usually reduced to a coronal height of 2–3 mm and then contoured to a convex or dome-shaped surface (Figure 16–5). In order to accomplish this, most teeth usually require endodontic treatment, the teeth are shortened and contoured, and the pulp chamber is simply sealed with an amalgam or composite restoration. Those teeth requiring the replacement of lost tooth structure or contour, often a result of caries, are prepared to receive a cast metal post and coping. Intraradicular attachments may be used as the final restoration when an increase in retention is desirable. These treatments add significant overall cost and time to the treatment plan, and the patient should be adequately informed.

Contraindications of this treatment should be carefully considered. Obviously, increased cost could preclude the patient from accepting this treatment modality. Patients who, for one reason or another, cannot maintain adequate oral hygiene are poor candidates for overdentures; recurrent caries or periodontal disease of the natural tooth abutments would obviously lead to treatment failure. Additionally, problems related to endodontic or periodontic therapy could result in less-than-ideal abutments and should

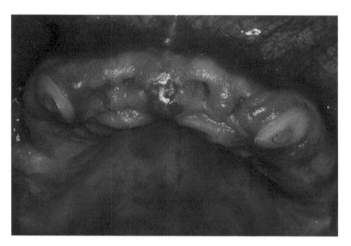

Figure 16–5   Natural teeth that have been prepared to
serve as overdenture abutments

be carefully evaluated for suitability. The absence or inability to obtain a sufficient zone
of attached mucosa around the proposed abutment teeth to guard against inflammation
should be considered a contraindication. Excessive mobility of the abutment teeth may
also be a cause of concern, but mobility may improve as the clinical crown is reduced,
thereby resulting in a more favorable crown to root ratio. The number and position of
the abutment teeth in the arch should be carefully considered when treatment planning
for an overdenture. The ideal situation exists when four or more abutment teeth are
spread out over as wide a rectangular area as possible. This configuration provides for
maximum denture stability. Three widespread remaining teeth will generally provide for
a tripod effect and would be the next-most-favorable arrangement. One or two teeth,
though less than ideal, can be used satisfactorily. Preferably, there should be several
millimeters of space between adjacent retained teeth to minimize compromises in soft
tissue health.

A complication may arise in the positioning of the denture teeth over the abutment
teeth if the available interarch space is limited. Potential weakness of the acrylic resin
denture base over these areas may require fabrication of a cast metal superstructure,
which increases cost and treatment time. Also, any undercuts present on the abutment
teeth will need to be relieved in the denture base (if they were not blocked out during
the impression appointment) in order to achieve complete seating of the overdenture.
Attachments, if used, are secured to the denture base either during processing or chairside at the time of overdenture insertion.

Fabrication of the overdenture follows standard prosthodontic procedures for
complete dentures. These include preliminary impressions, abutment tooth reduction
and recontouring, final impressions, interocclusal records, trial insertion, insertion, and
postinsertion appointments. There can be major exception to the presented sequence of
treatment. Ideally the abutment teeth are prepared prior to the final impression appointment so that the master cast reflects an exact replica of the prepared teeth. Occasionally
the abutment teeth cannot be prepared until the day of insertion. This is usually the
result of a patient needing to retain the abutment teeth because they are also the abutment teeth for an existing removable partial denture that will be replaced by the overdenture. For these patients, the master cast will reflect the natural contour and length of
the abutment teeth prior to preparation. A complete trial insertion is not possible

because the natural teeth are occupying the space of the future denture teeth. However, a trial insertion appointment should be completed to verify that the casts are correctly positioned on the articulator. Following the trial insertion appointment and prior to investing and processing, the abutment teeth are prepared on the master cast to the anticipated and desired height and contour. The remaining denture teeth are then arranged, and the denture is invested, processed, and finished. The insertion appointment will be more time consuming for these patients than for conventional overdenture patients because of the need to prepare the abutment teeth on the day of insertion. Additionally, because the teeth as prepared on the master cast and those prepared intra-orally are invariably different, time must be spent making the denture fit the abutment teeth. Occasionally, the denture must have an autopolymerizing acrylic resin placed to obtain the desired support from the newly contoured abutments. Once the fit of the intaglio surface is verified, the remainder of the insertion appointment is the same as conventional complete dentures.

Immediate Dentures

An immediate denture is defined as any removable dental prosthesis fabricated for place-ment immediately following the removal of a natural tooth or multiple teeth (Figures 16–6A and 16–6B). Immediate dentures may be a single denture in either arch or one denture in each arch. They are often more challenging to fabricate than routine dentures. Because an esthetic trial prior to extracting the teeth is not possible, the patient's expectations of the appearance and fit may not be fully realized at the time of insertion.

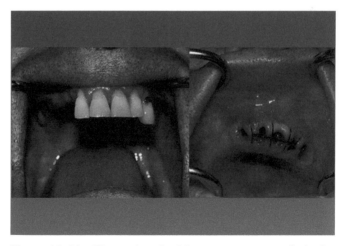

Figure 16–6A The patient in this treatment scenario had posterior teeth missing for a number of years and wore a removable partial denture until the anterior teeth were no longer able to support the prosthesis. Impressions for a maxillary immediate denture were made, and the insertion occurred the same day as the extraction of the remaining teeth.

(Continued)

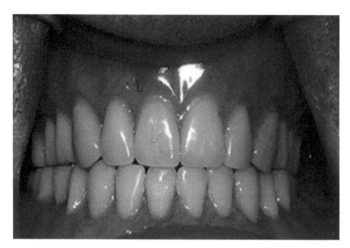

Figure 16–6B   Initial insertion of the immediate dentures following surgery.

Generally, there are two types of immediate dentures. The first is the conventional (classic) immediate denture in which the denture is intended to serve as a long-term prosthesis. Following the completion of the healing phase (usually a minimum or three to six months), the conventional immediate denture may be relined to maintain its basal adaptation to the supporting structures. The second type of immediate denture is the interim (transitional, "throw-away") immediate denture, which is designed to serve for a limited amount of time, usually through the healing phase, after which it is replaced by a more definitive type of prosthesis.

There are many advantages for immediate denture fabrication. Because there is no completely edentulous period, the patient's appearance is maintained, and potential social embarrassment is avoided. The denture base serves as a bandage following tooth extraction to help control bleeding, protect against trauma, and protect the blood clot. Thus, more rapid healing is promoted, and less postoperative discomfort is likely to be encountered. Furthermore, the position of the tongue, lip, and cheeks are maintained, allowing the patient to better adapt to denture service. Without an extended edentulous period, patients often adapt more easily to speech and mastication, and are thus able to maintain good nutritional intake. Additionally, it is easier to replicate the shape and arrangement of the natural teeth (if desired) and to maintain the occlusal vertical dimension.

Despite all the potential advantages, there are a few specific disadvantages of immediate dentures. Because of the difficulty and demanding procedures required, additional and longer appointments are required, which increase cost to the patient. Bone resorption and shrinkage of the healing soft tissues occur at a greater rate compared to already well-healed tissues. These changes often require reline procedures to maintain a well-adapted fit. Moreover, the esthetic arrangement of the anterior teeth cannot be previewed prior to tooth extractions and the denture insertion. Also, the remaining anterior teeth may create an anterior ridge undercut that is difficult to capture with the impression procedure and may necessitate a sectional impression technique.

An additional consideration to this treatment modality includes the necessity of a surgical template whenever alveoloplasties or tuberosity reductions are necessary (Figure 16–7). This template serves as a guide during the surgery and is made from a

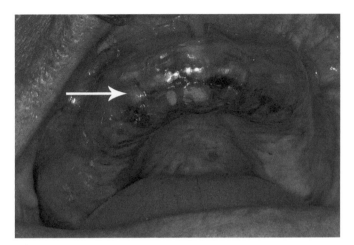

Figure 16–7   A surgical template (duplicates the intaglio surface of the denture) will help to identify severe pressure areas where additional surgical intervention is needed. The arrow indicates blanching of the tissue, which may mean excessive pressure from the denture base.

thin, transparent material that has the form of the intaglio surface of the immediate denture. Use of this template helps ensure that the interim denture will seat as intended and lessens the chances of occlusal discrepancies or postsurgical discomfort.

The impression procedure for immediate dentures depends on the number of remaining teeth. Undercuts and anatomy make border molding very difficult when more than just the anterior teeth remain. For patients with anterior and posterior teeth alginate impressions in stock trays may the procedure of choice. This usually results in overextended final impressions and requires precise information transferred to the impression in order to minimize the potential problems at the insertion appointment.

When only anterior teeth remain, a split tray or sectional impression technique may produce a more suitable master cast. A custom tray is fabricated for the posterior areas and rests on the remaining anterior teeth. The tray is border molded and a wash impression made. The tray is re-seated in the patient's mouth and a heavy body impression putty is used to form the anterior segment capturing both the teeth and to border mold the anterior vestibule. This impression can be separated into two pieces the facilitate removal from the patient's mouth and then reassembled to pour the master cast.

The vertical and horizontal relationships of the maxilla to the mandible are recorded in a similar manner as conventional complete dentures. However, the record base and occlusion rim will only cover the edentulous areas of the residual ridges. Stabilization of these partial record bases can be a challenge during these procedures.

Tooth selection proceeds as described for conventional complete dentures and a trial insertion of the dentures can be accomplished for those areas where the teeth have already been removed. This is rarely an esthetic trial insertion but rather a functional trial insertion to verify the maxillomandibular records.

Following extractions, the denture is inserted. The intaglio surface is adjusted with pressure disclosing paste until a comfortable pressure free fit is obtained. In order not to prolong the insertion appointment, the occlusion is adjusted intra-orally to obtain solid contact in the posterior on the patient's arc of closure. The remount and final adjustment usually occurs one or two weeks after the initial insertion. It is important to have good retention and stability of the immediate denture otherwise the denture may actually prolong post-operative bleeding and discomfort. The patient is instructed to avoid removing the immediate denture for the first 24 hours. Premature removal of the denture can lead to swelling that may prevent the denture's reinsertion for several days. If swelling occurs, but the denture is still able to be reinserted, the number of sore spots will often increase because the fit of the denture has been altered. After 24 hours, the patient should return to the dentist's office for removal of the denture, at which time an inspection of the tissues is performed to identify and adjust irritated areas induced by the denture. The patient is instructed to continue wearing the denture at night for about seven more days, or until the swelling has subsided. During this time, the patient should be instructed to only remove the denture after meals to clean it and rinse out the mouth. The denture should be also removed prior to bedtime to again clean and rinse the mouth. After a week has passed, the patient is instructed to leave the denture out during the night. Further follow-up care may be done on a weekly basis or on request of the patient to address any additional sore spots.

The immediate denture serves quite an important role for the newly edentulous patient. Though technically demanding, when accomplished successfully, the immediate denture can satisfy the requirements of function, esthetics, and emotional support during the healing phase following multiple tooth extractions.

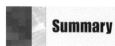

Summary

Single dentures, overdentures, and immediate dentures all pose different challenges to the patient and the dentist providing care. However, despite the extra effort required, when used appropriately, all of these prostheses can lead to a very satisfying result. Careful treatment planning and patient selection are paramount to success. As the current trend of an aging population of longer-living individuals continues, there will be no shortage of edentulous patients who may be in need of these services.

References

Jerbi, F.: Trimming the cast in the costruction of immediate dentures. J Prosthet Dent 16: 1047-1053, 1966.

Pound, E.: Controlled immediate dentures. J South Calif Dent Assoc 38: 810-817, Sep 1970.

Rahn, A. O., and Heartwell, C. M., editors: Textbook of Complete Dentures. 5th Ed. Philadelphia: Lippincott, 1993. Chapters 22, 23, and 24.

Rudd, K., Morrow, R.: Occlusion and the single denture. J Prosthet Dent 1973; 4-10.

Stansbury, C.: Single denture construction against a non-modified natural dentition. J Prosthet Dent 1951; 692-699.

QUESTIONS

1. The primary reason for failures when attempting single maxillary dentures opposing natural dentition is:
   a. Optimum occlusal scheme may be compromised
   b. Retention is impossible to obtain
   c. Poor impression technique
   d. Dentist's errors

2. What is one way to increase stability and retention of single maxillary dentures?

3. Overdentures usually cover and rest on:
   a. Natural teeth
   b. Implants
   c. Roots of natural teeth
   d. All of the above

4. Immediate dentures cannot be accessed for esthetic results prior to the insertion appointment.
   a. TRUE
   b. FALSE

ANSWERS

1. a.

2. Using adjunctive treatment, such as implants and attachments.

3. d.

4. a.

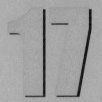

Relining Complete Dentures

Dr John R. Ivanhoe
Dr. Kevin D. Plummer

Patients often present with existing complete dentures that, while still structurally sound, are not retentive or stable because they no longer properly fit the soft tissues and residual ridges. These patients often present with obvious occlusal and/or facial changes. They may exhibit poor esthetics because excessive bone loss under the prostheses has resulted in a loss of face height or repositioning of the anterior teeth. Their occluding vertical dimension (OVD) and their occlusion may also be compromised because the dramatic tissue changes have caused the dentures to lose their proper ridge orientation. The tissue underlying the dentures is frequently abused and irritated. Most of these changes are the result of poorly fitting dentures. If these changes are not too great, and the dentures are still in reasonably good condition, these problems may be corrected by relining the dentures. Relining is a procedure to resurface the tissue (intaglio) surface of an existing denture with new denture base material. Other indications for relining may have to do with flange length problems or nondisplaced fractures of existing dentures.

If conditions have led to abused support tissues, some corrective actions must be taken prior to the relining procedures. A tissue conditioning material is often used in conjunction with other procedures (such as surgery) to return abused oral tissues to a healthy state. Because tissue conditioning material has a short, usable, functional life, both the tissues and material must be examined frequently, with the material being replaced as necessary.

The decision to reline an existing denture is based on a number of factors. The occluding vertical dimension must be correct or it must be able to be corrected during the impression procedure for the reline. The patient's centric relation occlusal position must be stable or correctable through occlusal adjustment. The general appearance of the teeth must be satisfactory to the patient, and there should not be severe occlusal wear (Figure 17–1). Speech patterns should also be satisfactory. As stated previously, the soft tissue must be healthy or correctable.

Making the impression for a reline is much like the conventional final impression technique. However, there are some differences and several additional objectives that must be achieved simultaneously when making the impression for relining a denture, as

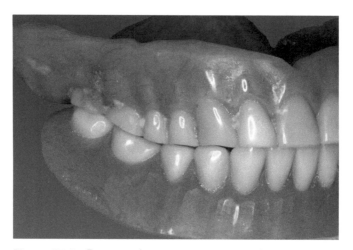

Figure 17–1 Dentures have severe wear and poor general appearance, which may preclude a successful reline procedure.

opposed to a conventional complete denture impression. The most obvious difference is that an existing denture is used in place of the custom impression tray. A second and significant difference is that, when relining a denture, the final impression must be completed while maintaining the correct occlusal vertical dimension and making sure that the patient remains in the centric relation position through the border molding procedures and the final set of the impression material. Maintaining the occluding vertical dimension and the centric relation position is not a consideration when making a conventional final impression. This may be a difficult procedure on some patients, and a poor occlusal scheme may complicate this endeavor (Figure 17–2). An occlusal equilibration of the existing dentures may be necessary before the reline procedure to insure adequate positioning of the dentures during the impression procedures.

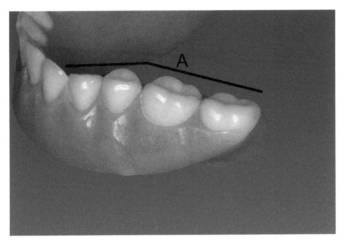

Figure 17–2   A poor occlusal plane (A) that cannot be corrected is a contraindication to a reline procedure.

Dentures demonstrating simple looseness without apparent occlusal disharmony, and without noticeable changes in the vertical dimension of occlusion or appearance, are ideal candidates for being relined. However, because these dentures fit closely to the underlying tissues, an extra step is necessary prior to making the final impression. The viscosity of the impression material can prevent a denture from being properly seated when attempting the impression, if insufficient space or sufficient relief exists for the ipression material. Additionally, even if tissue conditioning was done, some areas of the denture may be placing unacceptable forces on the underlying tissues. Therefore approximately 1.5 mm of resin must be removed from the tissue side of the denture prior to making the impression. This may be difficult or impossible in those dentures whose base may be little more than 1 mm in thickness.

Both the maxillary and mandibular denture for some patients may require relining. When both dentures must be relined, one denture at a time is relined rather than attempting to complete opposing relines simultaneously. When deciding which denture to reline first, usually the less stable of the two is relined first. If there is no significant difference between the stability or retention of the opposing dentures, then the maxillary denture is often selected. Once relined, it will provide a stable opposing arch when relining the mandibular denture.

Dentures may be relined using either a "closed-" or "open-" mouth technique. Because one of the primary objectives of a denture reline is maintaining the proper occlusion, many clinicians select the closed-mouth technique. The primary difference is that with the closed-mouth technique, the patient is required to close and maintain the dentures in proper occlusion at the correct OVD while the impression material sets. With the open-mouth technique, the patient is not allowed to maintain occlusal contact. The open mouth technique usually requires extensive occlusal equilibration at insertion and can even allow the denture to be misaligned in its proper relationship to the residual ridges.

Impression Technique

The denture flanges are reduced so that 2–3 mm of space exists between the flanges and the depth of the vestibules to provide space for the border molding material (Figure 17–3). To allow the laboratory technicians to remove the denture from the master cast during processing, enough resin is removed from the tissue side of the denture to eliminate all resin undercuts on the denture base.

Next, to create space for the impression material, reduce at least one millimeter of the remaining unreduced denture base material over the entire tissue surface (Figure 17–3). At this point, space for the impression material has been created but, the plane of occlusion has been changed and the vertical dimension of occlusion has been overly reduced by approximately 1–1.5 mm. This loss can be regained by adding 4 "stops." Small tissue stops are created with spots of heavy-bodied vinyl polysiloxane material about 3 mm in diameter. The stops are placed in the canine and second molar areas, the denture is gently seated, and the patient is closed into the CR position at the proper OVD (Figure 17–4). A small dot of adhesive will be needed to keep the VPS material in position. If the

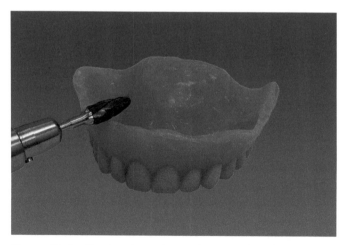

Figure 17–3 Borders have been shortened, and 1–1.5 mm of acrylic resin has been removed from the intaglio surface of the denture.

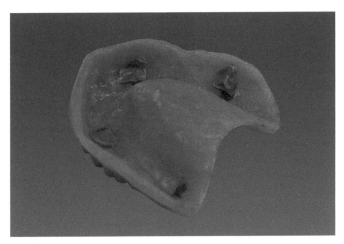

Figure 17–4 Vinyl polysiloxane material has been placed to create tissue stops, to maintain the denture at the proper occluding vertical dimension during the impression procedures.

denture cannot be positioned properly by creating these stops, it may be necessary to reevaluate the reline procedure as a treatment option.

Border molding is now completed, as with a conventional impression, with the exception that the vertical dimension of occlusion and centric occlusion positions must not be compromised (Figure 17–5). The occlusion is continuously evaluated to make sure no changes in denture position have occurred.

Four to six holes are placed into the maxillary denture, spaced approximately 12 mm (half inch) apart through the palate of the denture with a round bur (#6). These holes provide escape vents to minimize hydraulic pressure buildup during the wash impression. Three holes are generally placed following the midline raphe, beginning with one hole at the incisive foramen. Two holes are cut on each side lateral to the

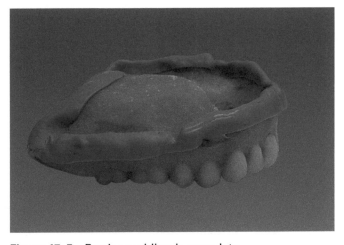

Figure 17–5 Border molding is complete.

midline, in approximately the canine areas. Care should be exercised to avoid making these holes through the existing denture teeth. Generally, unless the denture is very large, no holes are required on the mandibular arch—unless the ridges are massive and there is concern about hydraulic pressures within the impression material that may prevent the complete seating of the denture. When required, holes may be placed approximately 12 mm (half inch) apart.

The impression material is mixed and loaded uniformly inside the denture. For the maxillary denture, the denture is seated onto the ridges by exerting gentle pressure upward and backward. The patient is instructed to close into the centric occlusion position, and the clinician must manipulate the denture until the desired occlusion is achieved at the correct vertical dimension of occlusion (Figure 17–6). While maintaining the correct occlusal position the musculature of the mouth is border molded in same manner as a conventional complete denture impression. Centric occlusion, occluding vertical dimension and denture position are all examined for correctness at this time. The impression material is allowed to set according to the manufacturer's instructions.

After the impression material has set, the denture is removed from the mouth, and the excess impression material is trimmed from the denture and surfaces of the teeth (Figure 17–7). The vertical dimension of occlusion and centric occlusion are reconfirmed. If they are acceptable and retention and stability is adequate, the denture is then ready for the laboratory procedures.

If the clinician or staff pours the final impression in dental stone, it is essential that the denture not be removed from the cast prior to submission to the laboratory. If removed, it may be impossible for the laboratory technician to properly reseat the denture on the cast and the proper cast/occlusion orientation will be lost. The laboratory technicians will invest the denture in a processing flask prior to removing it from the cast. If any resin undercuts were not removed prior to making the impression, it may be impossible for the technician to remove the denture from the cast without breaking the cast. That is why it was important to remove all resin undercuts prior to making the impression. If a posterior palatal seal is required it is usually cut into the cast just before processing the denture.

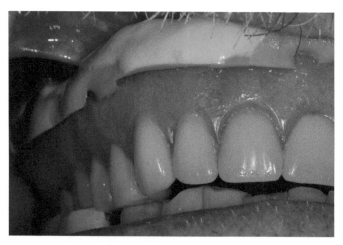

Figure 17–6   The final impression is made with the patient in the proper occlusal position at the proper occluding vertical dimension.

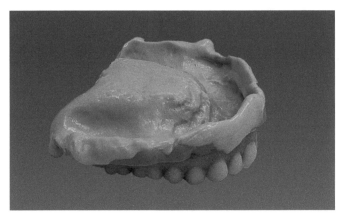

Figure 17–7   Completed reline impression

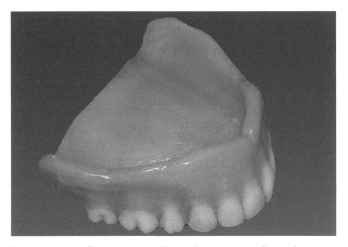

Figure 17–8   Completed reline with new acrylic resin on the intaglio surface

    The denture is returned from the laboratory just as if it were any other new denture (Figure 17–8). Insertion, adjustment, and post-insertion procedures are followed, just as for a conventional denture. Because there was no facebow made, the relined dentures will have remount casts but no index to place the maxillary remount cast/denture on the articulator in the proper relationship to the condyles. A facebow recording and a centric relation record may be necessary for extensive occlusal equilibration.

References

Boucher, C. O.: The relining of complete dentures. J Prosthet Dent. 1973;30:521-6.

Braden, M.: Tissue conditioners. 1. Composition and structure. J Dent Res. 1970;49:145-8.

Nassif, J., Jumbelic, R.: Current concepts for relining complete dentures: a survey. J Prosthet Dent. 1984;51:11-5.

Zarb, G. A., Jacob, R. F.: Prolonging the useful life of complete dentures: The relining technique. In: Zarb, G. A., Bolander, C. L., eds: Prosthodontic Treatment for Edentulous Patients. 12 th ed. St. Louis: Mosby Inc; 2004. pp. 471-480.

QUESTIONS

1. What are some of the clinical features that would indicate that a patient's dentures need to be relined?

2. What pre-reline procedures may be necessary for a patient with abused oral tissues underlying the existing dentures?

3. Not all existing dentures can or should be relined. List several indications for completing a denture reline.

4. What are the two reline techniques, and how are they different?

5. List several differences between a conventional and reline impression.

6. When both dentures must be relined, one denture at a time is relined rather than attempting to complete opposing relines simultaneously. Which denture should be relined first?

7. All resin undercuts on a denture base must be eliminated prior to using the denture to make the final impression. Why is this important?

8. To allow space for the impression material and to minimize direct contact between the denture base and underlying tissues, 1–1.5 mm of resin is removed from the intaglio of the denture prior to making the impression. What features of the denture may become unsatisfactory and must be corrected prior to making the impression?

9. What two methods may be used to create a posterior palatal seal in the denture?

10. Why are four to six holes cut into the maxillary denture following the border molding and prior to making the impression?

ANSWERS

1. Patient presents with some of the following:
   a. Existing complete dentures that, while still structurally sound, are not retentive or stable.
   b. Occlusal and/or facial changes.
   c. Poor esthetics because excessive bone loss under the prostheses has resulted in a loss of face height or repositioning of the anterior teeth.
   d. Compromised occlusal vertical dimension (OVD) and occlusion.
   e. Tissue underlying the dentures is abused and irritated.

2. If the patient exhibits abused support tissues, a tissue conditioning material is often used in conjunction with other procedures (such as surgery) to return abused oral tissues to a healthy state.

3. Dentures demonstrating simple looseness without apparent occlusal disharmony, and without noticeable changes in the vertical dimension of occlusion or appearance that do not abuse the underlying tissues, are ideal candidates for being relined. A denture can usually be satisfactorily relined if the following features are observed:
   a. The occluding vertical dimension is correct or can be corrected during the impression making procedure.
   b. Centric relation occlusal position is stable or correctable through occlusal adjustment.
   c. The general appearance of the teeth is satisfactory to the patient and there is not severe occlusal wear.
   d. Patient's speech patterns are acceptable.
   e. The soft tissue is healthy or can be made healthy.

4. Open- and closed-mouth techniques. With the open-mouth technique, the patient is instructed to come into an initial occlusal contact, so the clinician can achieve the desired vertical and horizontal relations of the dentures, and then open and remain open while the impression material is allowed to set. In the closed-mouth technique, the patient is allowed to maintain light occlusal contacts between the opposing dentures while the impression material is allowed to set.

5. Differences between a reline and conventional impression include:
   a. An existing denture is used in place of the custom impression tray.
   b. The final impression must be completed while maintaining the correct occlusal vertical dimension and making sure that the patient remains in the centric relation position through the border molding procedures and the final set of the impression material.
   c. An occlusal equilibration of the existing dentures may be necessary before the reline procedure to ensure adequate positioning of the dentures during the impression procedures.

6. When deciding which denture to reline first, usually the less stable of the two is relined first. If there is no significant difference between the stability or retention of the opposing dentures, then the maxillary denture is often selected. Once relined, it will provide a stable opposing arch when relining the mandibular denture.

7. When pouring the master cast for a reline procedure, if dental stone is poured into a resin undercut of the denture, it becomes extremely difficult for the laboratory technician to separate the denture from the cast with causing breakage to the cast and/or the denture. To allow the laboratory technicians to remove the denture from the master cast during processing, enough resin is removed from the tissue side of the denture to eliminate all resin undercuts on the denture base.

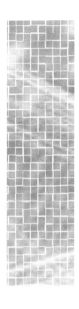

8. The plane of occlusion may have been unacceptably altered, which may be an esthetic problem, and the vertical dimension of occlusion has been overly reduced by approximately 1–1.5 mm. This loss can be reversed by adding 4 "stops." Small stops are created with spots of heavy-bodied polyvinyl siloxane material, about 3 mm in diameter. The stops are placed in the canine and second molar areas.

9. One method is achieved clinically, and the second is achieved as a laboratory procedure. The laboratory procedure involves cutting the posterior palatal seal into the master cast, as is usually done with a conventional denture. Modeling plastic is warmed and formed across the posterior border of the denture in the clinical method.

10. Four to six holes are placed into the maxillary denture—spaced approximately 12 mm (half inch) apart—to allow the escape of excess impression material, thereby minimizing hydraulic pressure buildup, which may prevent the denture from being properly seated, or to displace soft underlying tissues.

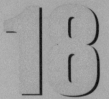

CHAPTER 18

Implant Supported Complete Dentures

Kevin Plummer

Introduction

Implant overdentures are rapidly becoming the standard for denture services, especially for mandibular complete dentures. Implant-retained or implant-supported overdentures are an alternative to both conventional complete dentures and complex fixed-implant prostheses. The implant retained overdenture is secured by either a bar/retainer combination or individual mechanical retention devices fitted to each implant component (Figures 18–1, 18–2, 18–3). These act as both retentive components and stabilizing elements for the complete denture and can often alleviate the "removable" feeling of complete dentures. These overdentures can be easily removed by the patient and, by

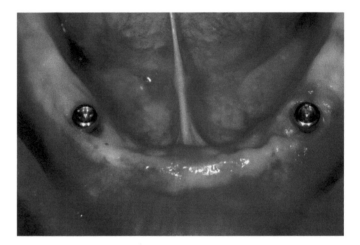

Figure 18–1   Mechanical retentive abutments

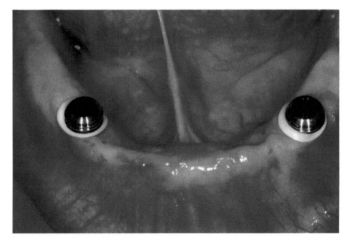

Figure 18–2   Mechanical retention devices in place on the retentive abutments

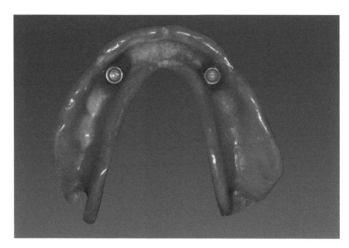

Figure 18–3   Mechanical retention devices after transfer and bonding to the prosthesis

virtue of the implant components' simpler design, hygiene procedures are usually much simpler for the patient to perform.

The scope of this textbook is the realm of removable conventional dentures, and this section will be limited to implant-retained and tissue-supported overdentures. Many times even patients with extreme resorption can benefit from a simple overdenture retained by as few as two implants with uncomplicated retention devices. The improved retention and stability helps to alleviate the typical "sore" spots from more unstable conventional prostheses. Patients report increased function and less discomfort with implant-retained overdentures. Many times the severe resorption patterns seen in denture patients will require the conventional support for function and esthetics provided by flanges and acrylic resin bases that cannot be duplicated by fixed prostheses. The less complex removable overdentures tend to be more economical due to the limited number of implants needed and the lower cost of basic components. Because there are still changes in the supporting structures under the implant-retained tissue-supported overdenture, those elements must be monitored and corrected if the prostheses becomes unstable. Even though the implants themselves stabilize the bone and soft tissue in their immediate vicinity, relines or rebases will be needed on a periodic basis to compensate for the areas that remain "tissue supported."

Treatment Planning

Treatment planning for implant-retained overdentures is no different than for a conventional denture, except considerations for the implant placement and design of the prostheses must be taken into account. In addition to the conventional workup, the patient must be evaluated for implant sites, possible bone augmentation, and the vertical space needed for the implant components. The patient condition (bone anatomy, alveolar nerve position, sinus size and shape, and bone quality) may limit the options for implant placement. The patient's financial ability may also impact the final treatment plan. An emphasis on medical conditions (such as diabetes and other chronic and acute disease states that affect healing potential) and personal habits (smoking etc.) that may affect the success of the implant fixture placement must be evaluated and discussed with the patient.

Often the patient considering implant-supported dentures has been wearing prostheses for a number of years. The benefits of implant overdentures make them an attractive alternative to struggling with conventional complete dentures when the residual ridges no longer offer adequate retention and stability. If patients have existing complete dentures they must be evaluated to see if they will be usable as temporary dentures during the healing process after implant placement. Occasionally the existing dentures meet all the requirements for a final set of implant overdentures and can be successfully retrofitted to the new implant components. Most common will be a set of complete dentures that is adequate from esthetic and functional aspects, and that will allow their use as a guide for implant placement, as temporary prostheses during healing, and a guide for the fabrication of the new implant-supported overdentures. On the other end of the spectrum will be patients whose existing dentures are not useful in any manner due to resorptive changes, loss of vertical dimension, poor esthetics, and the inability to refit those prostheses effectively. These patients may need to proceed with new denture fabrication to the point of the esthetic and functional try-in, in order to establish the proper information for successful implant placement. In some cases, the prostheses should actually be finished and the patient made comfortable with the new dentures before proceeding with the implant placement.

In evaluating existing prostheses, the clinician should evaluate the fit of the intaglio surfaces, esthetic and phonetic contours of the anterior teeth, the occlusal vertical dimension, the type of posterior occlusion (intended function and wear), and the closure position in reference to the centric relation position. The space between the ridges at the patient's proper vertical dimension of occlusion should be evaluated to make sure it is adequate for planned implant components. Any areas that need correction before implant placement should be scheduled for those procedures as soon as possible.

After arriving at the prosthodontic treatment plan and choosing the implant components, the recipient sites must be evaluated for the proper quantity and quality of bone to complete the fixture placement procedures. Conventional radiographs should be made, and careful evaluation of the bone shape and quality made. Where information from conventional radiographs is inadequate to make a definitive diagnosis, more sophisticated procedures such as various views (lateral, frontal, and sagittal) made with standard-sized markers or computed tomograms may be needed to complete the diagnosis. The maxilla will more frequently need the more sophisticated technology due to the nature of the loosely structured cancellous bone and little or no cortical plate. If bone augmentation procedures are contemplated, referral to an implant specialist may be indicated.

The radiographic evaluation should be augmented by a physical examination of the ridge topography and an assessment of the soft tissue in the implant zone. The ability of the soft tissue to support part of the load of the implant-supported overdenture is critical if the number of implants is to be kept at the minimum. If the tissue is not capable of providing this support, the number of implants should be increased to remove the load from the tissue. This is especially important in the mandible. Keep in mind soreness problems with conventional dentures are more likely associated with stability problems than with vertical forces against the ridge. The lateral stability provided by even two single-attachment overdenture connections will make a marked improvement in patient comfort.

After careful assessment of the patient's condition is completed, the treatment plan can be formulated. The treatment may need to be phased in order to evaluate each part of treatment in improving the patient's ability to function with the prostheses. For example, once a mandibular denture is stabilized by an implant overdenture, the opposing arch may also function better for a patient because of increased stability of the mandibular denture. Many treatment plans should begin by addressing the mandible first and then reevaluating the condition of the maxilla.

The mandible requires at least two implants placed in the anterior symphyseal region equidistant from the midline. These implants can be joined by a metal bar or used as single retainers. If more than two implants can be safely placed, a bar with short cantilever arms to the distal is usually used to improve the support provided to the overdenture. With a bar substructure, various clips or other types of retentive components (ERA for example) can be used to provide retention (Figure 18–4). Often the support provided by the extended bar substructure may actually support the overdenture in the

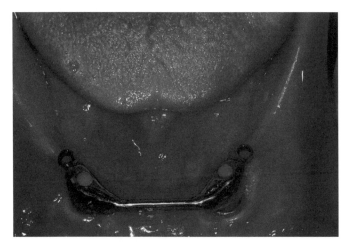

Figure 18–4   Bar substructure with ERA attachments to provide retention of the prosthesis

premolar region, which removes a great deal of load from the tissue (Figures 18–5 and 18–6). If single components are used, they usually have some type of retention/support system like a ball/O-ring, magnets, or other type of design (Figure 18-7). With reasonable tissue support, many patients find the simpler design adequate for their needs (Figures 18–1 to 18–3).

The maxilla is usually treated with three or four implants and a bar substructure for support and retention. However, many patients function very well with unconnected implants using simpler retentive component designs (Figures 18–8 and 18–9). If the retention is sufficient, the palate may be removed from the maxillary denture for patient comfort. If the palate is removed from the maxillary denture, the structure may be weakened, and a metal framework may need to be incorporated into the prosthesis design (Figure 18–10). Whatever method is used, the vertical and horizontal dimensions of the denture must be evaluated to ensure adequate space for the selected components. Obviously, the bar substructure will require more space than single-implant components. There are many manufacturers of implant components, so be sure to have the component dimensions available during treatment planning.

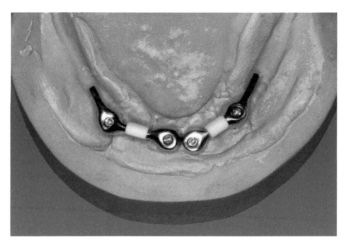

Figure 18–5   Bar substructures with distal cantilever components to provide additional support of the prosthesis (Occlusal View)

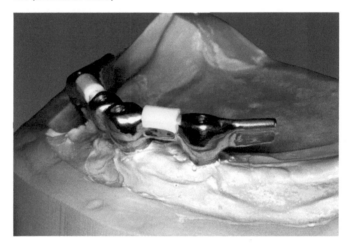

Figure 18–6   Bar substructures with distal cantilever components to provide additional support of the prosthesis (Lateral View)

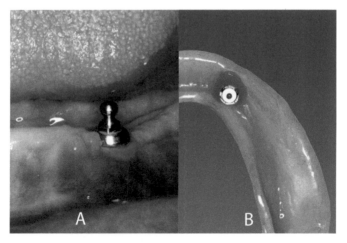

Figure 18–7   A - Ball/O-ring abutment, B – Mechanical retentive device for the ball/O-ring abutment

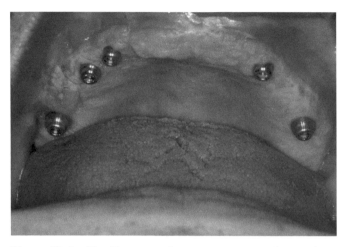

Figure 18–8 Maxillary overdenture support and retention from unconnected mechanical retentive abutments

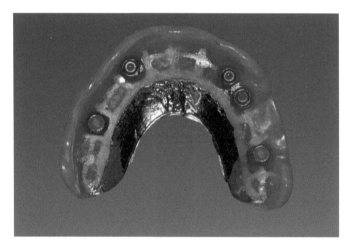

Figure 18–9 Maxillary implant overdenture utilizing single unconnected retentive components. The palate has been removed from this design.

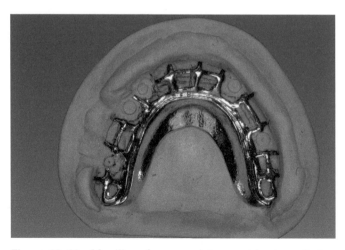

Figure 18–10 Maxillary framework to provide strength for a prosthesis design with no palate

Clinical Procedures

This clinical procedure section is in no way a complete guide to these procedures, but rather an introduction to the clinical steps required to perform these procedures. The authors recommend consulting a reference specific to the type of procedure that is contemplated.

Retrofitting Existing Prostheses

Patients with new prostheses that are optimal in design and function can have those prostheses retrofitted to the new implant components. The prostheses will need a soft liner added to the areas of the fixture surgical sites, and the patient can wear the prostheses during the integration phase of the implants. At the second stage of surgery, the soft liner can be modified to accommodate the selected retentive component or a healing cap depending on the type of retention/support that is planned.

Bar Substructure

Approximately two weeks after the second stage of surgery, alginate impressions are made for use in fabricating custom impression trays for the bar substructure fabrication. Trays have conventional complete denture design with regard to border extension and size and shape. Most abutment components for substructures have screw retention. The tray may be of an open design over the implants to capture impression copings that have guide pin screws. The impression copings emulate the position of the final abutments. A final impression is made, and the impression is removed from the patient's mouth. With the open tray design, the guide pin screws must be loosened prior to removing the impression. If the impression copings that are chosen do not require guide pin screws, the tray will have a closed design with sufficient block-out to avoid contact with the impression copings.

With the open tray design, appropriate analogs are attached to the impression copings by tightening the guide pin screws into the analogs. With the closed tray design, the analogs are snapped into the proper position in the impression. A conventional cast is poured to provide proper soft tissue anatomy for laboratory procedures. A bar substructure is fabricated according to the clinician's instructions and it is returned with the proper retentive devices. The bar substructure will either incorporate the abutment, which fits the implant fixture, or will be designed to fit on an appropriate abutment attached to the implant fixture. If the substructure fits on abutments, the abutments are placed and properly tightened. The bar substructure is tried in and adjusted for a passive fit to the implant components.

Once the bar substructure is in place, the existing denture can be altered to fit over the bar substructure assembly (Figure 18–11). The retentive components are picked up from the bar substructure using an auto-polymerizing resin in a manner similar to a reline procedure (Figure 18–12). During the pick-up procedure, the patient is maintained in the correct occlusal relationship to ensure the proper function of the prostheses.

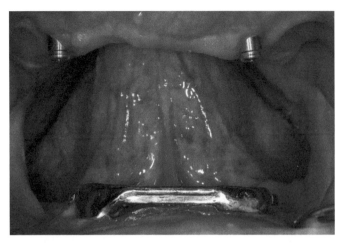

Figure 18–11   Bar sub-structure using a clip and ERA attachments to provide support and retention for a mandibular overdenture

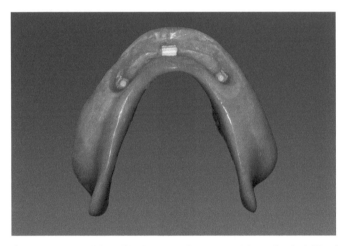

Figure 18–12   Mandibular overdenture with a clip (midline) and ERA attachments to fit on and over an implant bar substructure

The procedure for picking up retentive components requires block-out of areas that might trap auto-polymerizing resin in an undercut on the substructure or abutments.

Another possibility is to perform a reline procedure on the existing denture. The denture is modified to allow a passive fit over the bar substructure. The bar substructure is blocked out using a suitable material, and a closed mouth reline impression is made. The impression is recovered, and the bar substructure is removed from the patient and placed back into the impression after appropriate analogs are attached. The laboratory reline is performed in a routine manner except that the bar substructure is blocked out prior to acrylic resin packing, and the retentive components are added to the bar substructure so they can be incorporated into the new resin. Always follow the manufacturers' instructions concerning laboratory procedures for implant components, as they may be somewhat different from those described above.

Single Component Support

If no bar substructure is planned, the single-implant retentive components can be added to the existing prosthesis quite easily. The retentive abutment is selected to provide the proper tissue support and is placed on the implant and tightened. The existing denture is modified to provide a passive fit over the abutments with clearance for the pick-up resin. The retentive component that will be attached to the denture is placed on the abutment, and the denture is placed to ensure passive fit against the tissue. Proper block-out is performed on the abutments, and auto-polymerizing resin is used to pick up the retentive component in the existing denture (Figures 18–13 and 18–14).

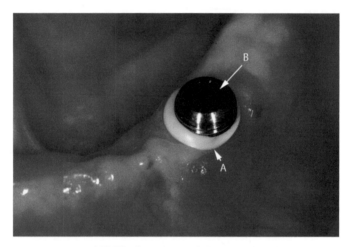

Figure 18–13   (A) Blockout material protecting the over-denture abutment placed under and around the (B) mechanical retentive device to prevent excess acrylic resin from flowing into undesirable undercuts

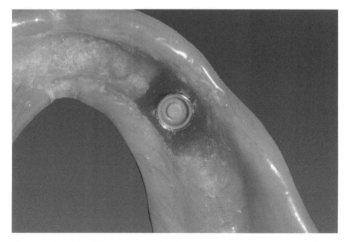

Figure 18–14   The mechanical retentive device secured to the overdenture using auto-polymerizing acrylic resin

New Prostheses

In some cases, if patients do not have adequate existing dentures to use for evaluating the space available for implant components, the dentures will need to be completed through the esthetic and functional try-in stage before selecting the type of retentive system to use. At the maxillomandibular records appointment or the trial insertion appointment there should be sufficient information to decide on the type of retentive components desired for the new dentures. If space permits a bar substructure can be selected or individual retentive components can be used. If there is limited space then single retentive components are chosen. This information can also be determined using mounted diagnostic casts during the treatment planning phase.

Bar Substructure

If a bar substructure is used, the procedure is the same for fabricating that unit as described in the previous section on bar substructures.

Once the bar substructure is in place, the new denture can be altered to fit over the bar substructure assembly. The retentive components are picked up from the bar substructure using an auto-polymerizing resin in a manner similar to a reline procedure. During the pick-up procedure the patient is maintained in the appropriate occlusal position to ensure the proper function of the prostheses. The procedure for picking up retentive components requires block-out of areas that might trap auto-polymerizing resin in an undercut on the substructure or abutments.

Another possibility is to use the final impression with the bar substructure to fabricate the entire denture. The new denture captures the retentive components during that process. The final denture impression also captures the location of the implant fixtures and uses analogs in the master cast to duplicate their location. The record base and occlusion rim are fabricated on the master cast with the bar substructure and can either be blocked out or can have retentive components added to the record base to stabilize the base during the jaw relation record appointment. If the latter is the case, the bar substructure is placed in the patient's mouth during that procedure and used to stabilize the record base. At the trial insertion, the trial denture is modified to allow a passive fit over the bar substructure. The bar substructure is placed on the master cast and blocked out using a suitable material, the denture is processed around the bar substructure, and the retentive components are imbedded into the denture base resin.

Always follow the manufacturers' instructions concerning laboratory procedures for implant components as they may be somewhat different from those described above.

Single Component Support

If no bar substructure is planned, the single implant retentive components can be added to the new prosthesis quite easily. The retentive abutment is selected to provide the proper tissue support and is placed on the implant and tightened. The existing denture is modified to provide a passive fit over the abutments. The retentive component that will become part of the denture is placed on the abutment and the denture is placed to ensure passive fit against the tissue. Proper block-out is performed on the abutments, and auto-polymerizing resin is used to pick up the retentive component in the existing denture.

The components can also be added to the new prosthesis during the processing procedure. The final denture impression is made using impression analogs, and the subsequent master cast is fabricated with abutment analogs placed into the cast. The record base and occlusion rim are fabricated using retentive components to stabilize the record base during the jaw relations appointment. After the trial insertion the processing step is completed after proper block-out of the abutment analogs and the addition of the retentive components to the abutment analogs. The exact procedure may vary by manufacturer, so be sure to check their technical procedure manual.

References

Misch, C. E., ed.: Dental Implant prosthodontics. St. Louis, MO.: Elsevier Mosby, 2005. Chapters 14-18.

Stevens, P. J., Fredrickson, E. J., and Gress, M. L., eds.: Implant Prosthodontics – Clinical and Laboratory Procedures. 2nd edition. Philadelphia, PA.: Mosby, Inc, 2000.

Zarb, G. A., and Bolendar, C. L., editors.: Prosthodontic Treatment for Edentulous Patients. 12th Edition. St. Louis, MO.: Elsevier Mosby, 2004. Chapters 25-30.

ACKNOWLEDGMENT: "Figures for Chapter 18 provided by Dr. Yousef Marafie"

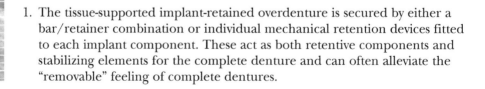

QUESTIONS

1. How are tissue-supported implant overdentures typically secured to the implant fixtures?

2. Do implant-supported overdentures ever need relining or rebasing to maintain proper fit?

3. If a patient has no existing dentures, how can the evaluation for implant overdentures ensure adequate space for all the required components?

ANSWERS

1. The tissue-supported implant-retained overdenture is secured by either a bar/retainer combination or individual mechanical retention devices fitted to each implant component. These act as both retentive components and stabilizing elements for the complete denture and can often alleviate the "removable" feeling of complete dentures.

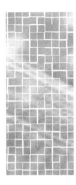

2. Because there are still changes in the supporting structures under the implant-retained tissue supported overdenture, those elements must be monitored and corrected if the prostheses becomes unstable. Even though the implants themselves stabilize the bone and soft tissue in their immediate vicinity, relines or rebases will be needed on a periodic basis to compensate for the areas that remain "tissue supported."

3. In some cases, if patients do not have adequate existing dentures to use for evaluating the space available for implant components, the dentures will need to be completed through the esthetic and functional try-in stage before selecting the type of retentive system to use.

Clinical and Technical Procedures

Preliminary
Impressions

Mandibular Impression

Figure A1–1   The edentulous mandibular arch must be thoroughly evaluated prior to making the preliminary impression. The properly made preliminary impression will be used to fabricate a diagnostic cast. The cast must be as accurate a representation of the ridges and undistorted surrounding tissues as possible because this cast will be used to fabricate a custom impression tray, which will be used to make the final impression.

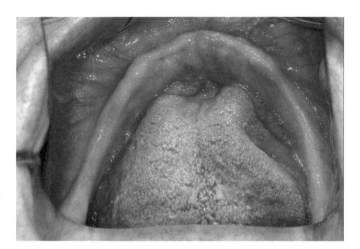

Figure A1–2   It is extremely important to capture the retromolar pad in the preliminary impression. This is a critical area of support for the completed denture.

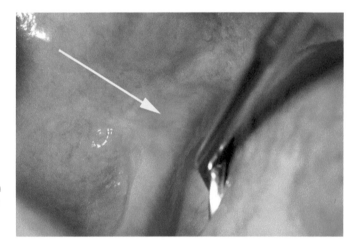

Figure A1–3   The masseter muscle area will often exhibit a fatty pad or roll of tissue partially covering the retromolar pad. The diagnostic cast will not be an inaccurate representation of this area if this tissue roll is captured in the impression.

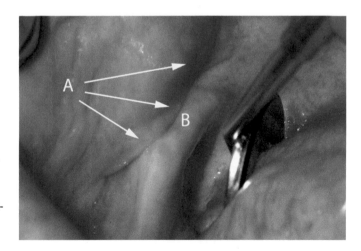

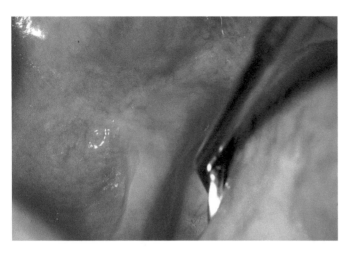

Figure A1–4 The cheek must be gently stretched away from the area during the impression making procedure. When properly stretched, the fatty roll is eliminated from the impression area.

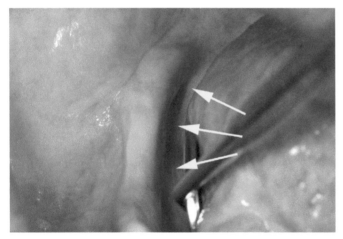

Figure A1–5 The retromylohyoid area is located lingual to the retromolar pad area. A custom impression tray will be fabricated as the next procedure and must be properly extended into this area to obtain an acceptable final impression. Fabrication of a properly extended custom tray won't be possible if the entire extension of this area is not captured in the preliminary impression.

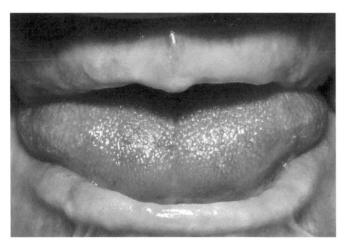

Figure A1–6 An excessively enlarged tongue can make all steps in the fabrication of completed dentures very difficult. Practice inserting the trays and have the patient close slightly during impression procedures to keep the tongue as relaxed as possible

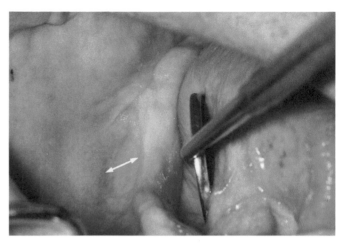

Figure A1–7   The buccal shelf area is extremely important in the fabrication of mandibular complete dentures because it is the primary stress-bearing area of the mandibular arch. A very accurate impression of this area, not artificially overextended, is also important.

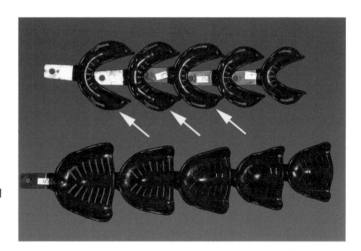

Figure A1–8   Many brands of stock impression trays are available, but some are poorly shaped and make obtaining excellent preliminary impressions almost impossible. These are examples of well-shaped edentulous impression trays. (Border-Lock Impression Tray, Accu-Liner Products, Woodinville, WA). Note particularly that the masseter muscle areas of the trays have no sharp corners. The flange of these trays cover the buccal shelf area and then approach and cross the retromolar pad into the mylohyoid areas as a smooth continuous border.

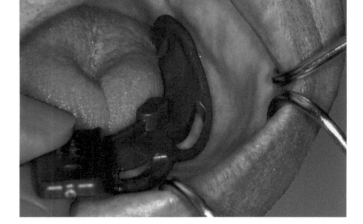

Figure A1–9   A stock tray of the generally correct size is selected and then must be evaluated in all vestibular areas and posteriorly.

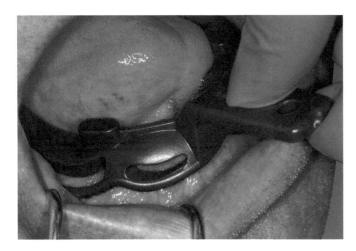

Figure A1–10   Properly desired extension of the tray in the anterior. A well-fitting tray should provide approximately 6 mm of space between the flange and undistorted vestibule.

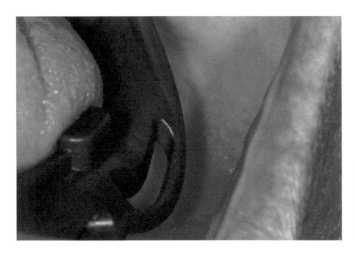

Figure A1–11   A properly fitting impression tray must not be overextended and should not distort the soft tissues. This tray follows the vestibule in the buccal shelf area very nicely.

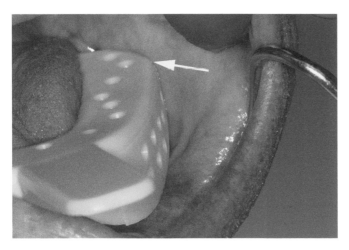

Figure A1–12   This impression tray is too long and improperly shaped for this distobuccal area.

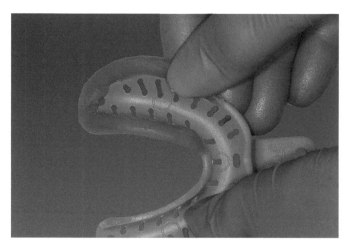

Figure A1–13   Once the "best fit" trays are selected, they must usually be modified with periphery wax. A properly fitting tray must have approximately a 6 mm space between the tray and the tissues. If a larger space exists or if the extension of the tray must be increased, periphery wax is indicated.

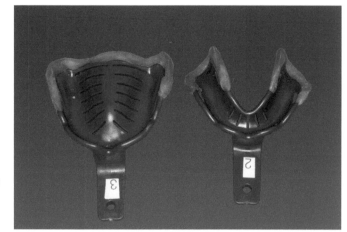

Figure A1–14   Typical required tray modification. Do not add wax unless needed! Wax is occasionally necessary to protect the soft tissues, if the trays have sharp flanges.

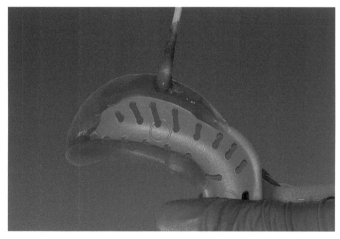

Figure A1–15   The appropriate adhesive for the impression material selected should be placed on any added periphery wax. When making preliminary impressions for complete dentures, placing adhesive on the impression tray itself may not be necessary if the tray has retention holes or rim locks.

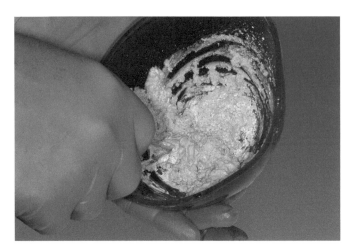

Figure A1–16 Irreversible hydrocolloid impression material is an ideal material for making preliminary impressions. It is inexpensive, provides acceptable working times, and makes excellent impressions. Using the water-to-powder ratio suggested by the manufacturer is recommended, varying the ratio slightly is acceptable to modify the viscosity of the impression material in order to meet the desires of the clinician. Most manufacturers recommend adding the powder to the water in the mixing bowl to minimize the capturing of bubbles within the mixture. However, proper mixing technique will minimize the problem.

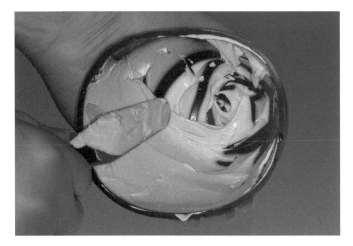

Figure A1–17 When properly mixed, the irreversible impression material should be completely smooth. There should be no dry powder remaining when the mixing is completed!

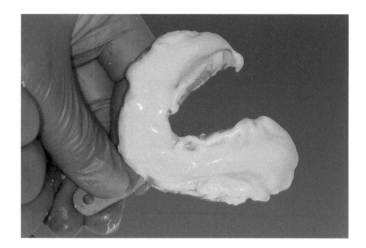

Figure A1–18   The impression tray should be loaded only approximately three-quarters full.

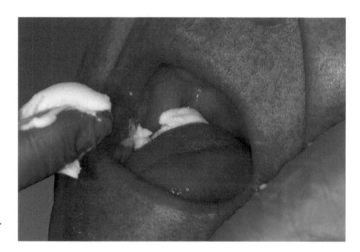

Figure A1–19   Using fingers or a large syringe, a small amount of impression material should be placed in areas that may be difficult to capture in the impression. These areas often include the retromylohyoid areas.

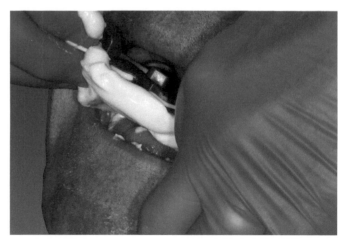

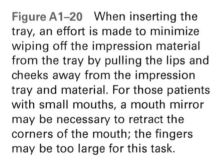

Figure A1–20   When inserting the tray, an effort is made to minimize wiping off the impression material from the tray by pulling the lips and cheeks away from the impression tray and material. For those patients with small mouths, a mouth mirror may be necessary to retract the corners of the mouth; the fingers may be too large for this task.

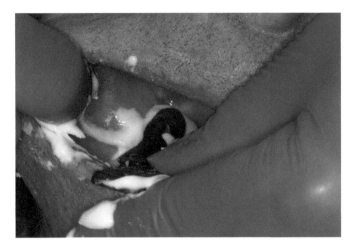

Figure A1–21   As the tray is seated, the cheeks and lips are stretched away from the ridge crest. This will allow the impression material to totally fill the vestibular areas and captured air bubbles to be expelled. This is especially important in the masseter muscle area, where the fatty tissue roll will often be captured in the impression if care is not taken.

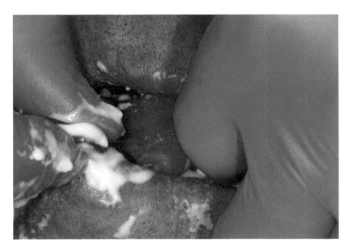

Figure A1–22   Once the tray is completely seated, the patient is instructed to lift and extend the tongue to form the lingual surface of the impression. The patient should not make any exaggerated movements. The tongue should only be protruded to just beyond the lips. It can also be moved laterally until the tip gently touches the inside of the cheeks.

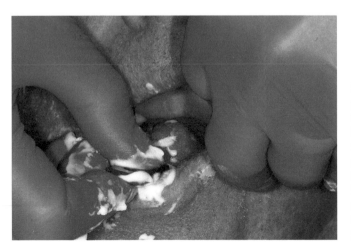

Figure A1–23   The cheeks are lifted gently at about a 45-degree angle upward and outward and manipu- lated anteriorly and posteriorly to reduce overextension of the borders of the impression. This manipulation can be continued until the working time of the material has been reached. Manufacturer's instructions will indicate the working time of the material being used.

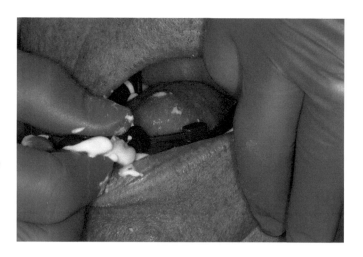

Figure A1–24 Once all manipulation has been completed, the impression is prevented from moving by gently maintaining its position. Basically the clinician is simply preventing the impression tray from being lifted away from the ridge until the impression material has reached its setting time. Lifting the cheek to break the seal around the impression will make removal easier.

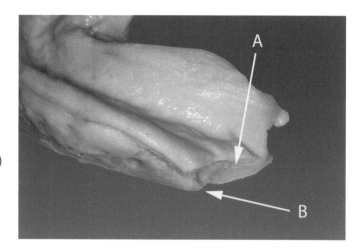

Figure A1–25 Note that this impression captured the fatty tissue roll in the masseter muscle area. (A) Note also that this impression tray had a corner in this area. (B) This is not an ideal tray for the mandibular arch. This impression should be remade.

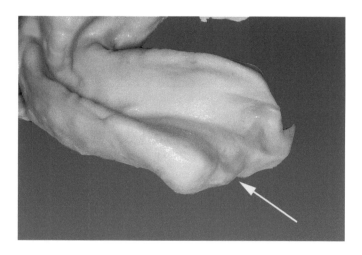

Figure A1–26 This masseter muscle area is accurately captured.

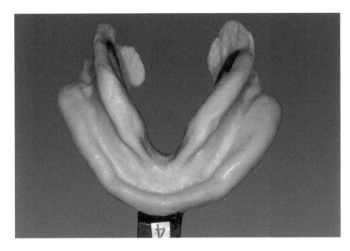

Figure A1–27   A well-made mandibular preliminary impression. Note that all vestibules and posterior extensions have been captured without grossly overextending the impression. Minimal bubbles and voids have been captured in the impression. A well-made preliminary impression should closely resemble a well-made final impression.

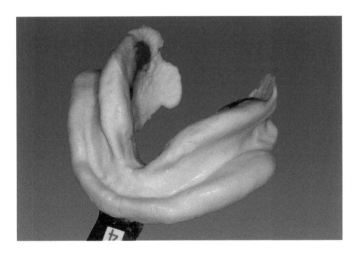

Figure A1–28   A well-made mandibular preliminary impression. This impression should immediately be taken to the laboratory and poured with a dental stone.

Maxillary Impression

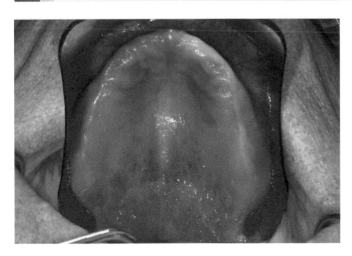

Figure A1–29   The edentulous maxillary arch must be thoroughly evaluated prior to making the preliminary impression.

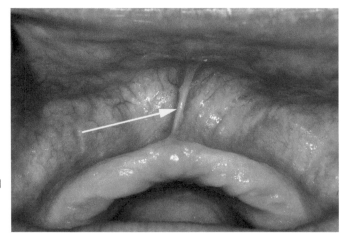

Figure A1–30 Multiple areas of the arch must be evaluated before and during impression making. The labial frenulum area is often prominent and easily displaced. Care must be taken when making an impression of this structure.

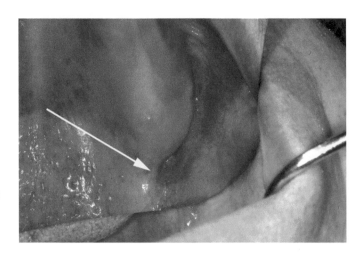

Figure A1–31 The hamular notch area. This is a critical area that must be accurately and completely captured in both the preliminary and final impression.

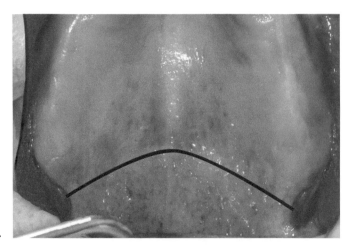

Figure A1–32 The vibrating line area must be visualized. This is also an area that must be accurately captured in both the preliminary and final impression, therefore the impression tray must cover this area.

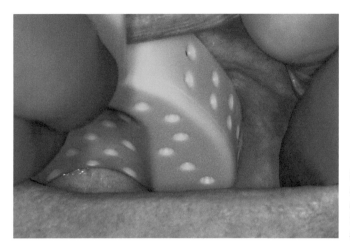

Figure A1–33   As in the mandibular arch, a stock impression tray is selected to "best fit" the arch. This is a reasonably well-fitting impression tray.

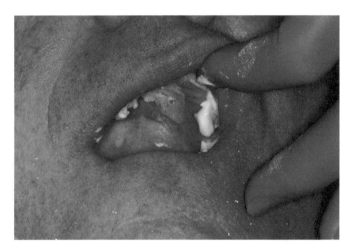

Figure A1–34   As in the mandibular arch, small amounts of impression material are placed by finger in areas that may be difficult to capture in the impression.

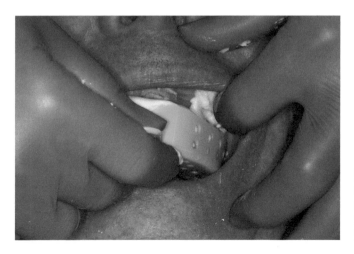

Figure A1–35   Care must be taken when initially inserting the impression to capture all desired areas of the arch and yet minimize discomfort to the patient.

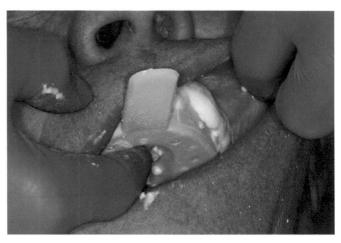

Figure A1–36   Seat the posterior of the tray first, rolling the anterior portion into position while displacing the cheeks to allow air to escape in front of the impression material. The cheeks are then manipulated to reduce overextension of the impression.

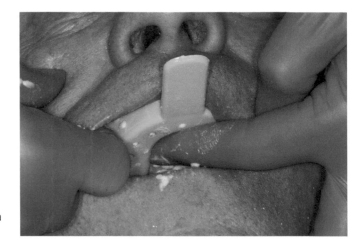

Figure A1–37   The impression tray must not be allowed to move during the setting of the impression material.

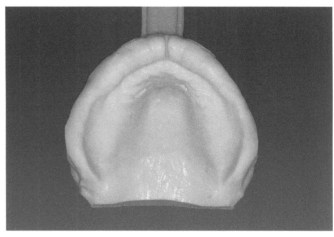

Figure A1–38   Even though the impression material on the flanges is slightly thicker than desired, this is a well-made maxillary preliminary impression. Note that the incisal frenulum, hamular notches, and vibrating line area are all captured with minimal bubbles and blebs. This impression should immediately taken to the laboratory and poured with a dental stone.

Creating Diagnostic Casts

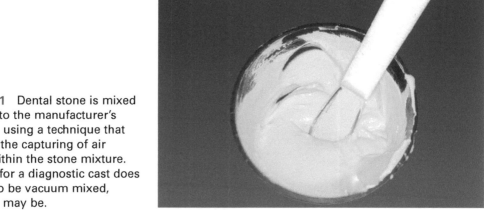

Figure A2–1 Dental stone is mixed according to the manufacturer's instruction using a technique that minimizes the capturing of air bubbles within the stone mixture. The stone for a diagnostic cast does not need to be vacuum mixed, however it may be.

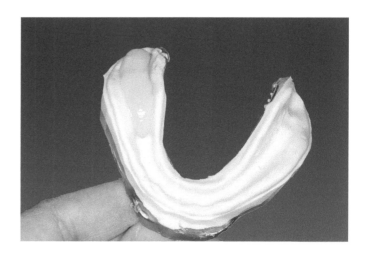

Figure A2–2 The preliminary impression is carefully and slowly filled generally beginning in one posterior area and continuing to flow the material around the impression using gentle vibration.

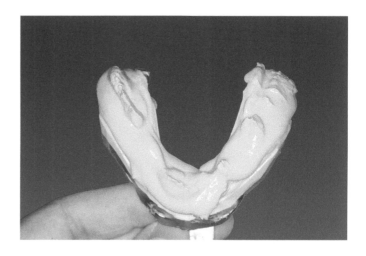

Figure A2–3 This slow fill is followed until the stone completely fills the impression. This first pour of stone must cover all anatomical surfaces of the impression without extending onto the impression tray.

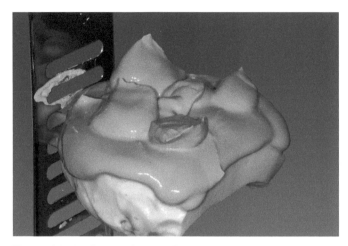

Figure A2–4   Separating the impression and tray from the diagnostic cast can be very difficult if stone is allowed to be in contact with the tray. Care should be taken to restrict the stone to covering only the impression material. Note that nodules were placed on the stone surface. These nodules will aid in bonding and strength between this first and the second base pour of stone.

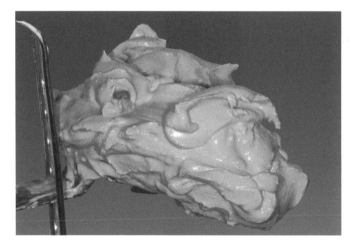

Figure A2–5   Excessive stone has been allowed to flow over the sides of this impression. The impression tray will be captured in the stone, and separation of the cast from the impression will be very difficult.

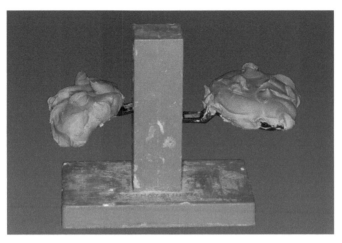

Figure A2–6   Once an impression has been made, care must be taken to prevent distortion of the impression material. This may happen through loss of water or physical displacement from the tray. Typically unsupported impression material will extend beyond the posterior of the impression tray and, if allowed to contact the bench top, physical displacement may cause distortion. This potential is increased once the weight of the stone is added to the impression. Therefore, once the initial pour of stone is completed, the impression tray and material should not be allowed to contact the bench top until at least the initial setting of the stone has occurred.

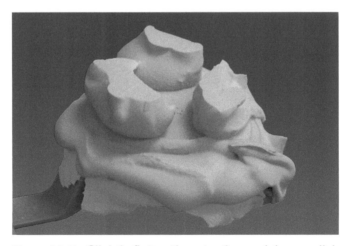

Figure A2–7   Slightly flatten the retention nodules parallel with the crest of the ridges. This will stabilize the first pour when it is inverted into the stone for the base of the cast.

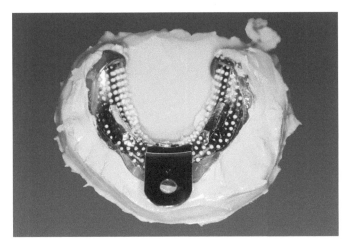

Figure A2–8 Following the initial setting of the stone, a second pour of stone is prepared and piled to a height of about 5 cm. The impression/cast is inverted and placed onto this base, making an attempt to visualize and make the crest of the ridges parallel to the bench top.

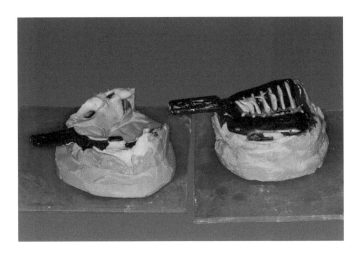

Figure A2–9 An attempt is made to remove excessive stone to minimize trimming at the next step. The stone is allowed to set according to the manufacturer's instructions.

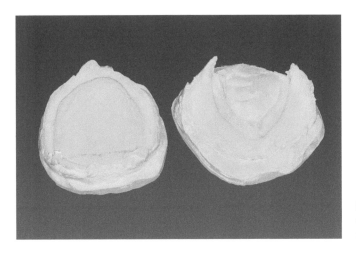

Figure A2–10 Once the stone has set, the impression is carefully removed from the stone cast.

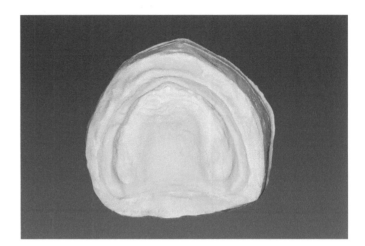

Figure A2–11   Example of a nicely poured maxillary diagnostic cast before trimming.

Figure A2–12   Even though an attempt was made to have the crest of the ridges parallel to the bench top during the making of the base of the cast, this goal is seldom achieved. The necessary trimming must be visualized. In this example, it is obvious that the cast is thicker on one side that the other. Therefore, the ridge crests are not parallel to the bench top. When trimming the cast, the first objective will be to correct this thickness discrepancy and make the ridges parallel to the bench top. Remember this may be an anterior-posterior problem also.

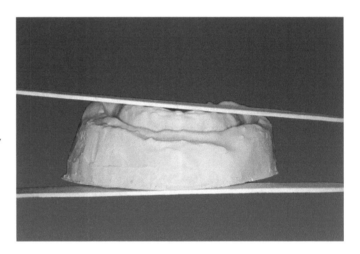

Figure A2–13   Prior to trimming the cast, it should be thoroughly dampened by soaking in water for approximately five minutes. Soaking longer than this can damage the surface of the cast. The purpose of wetting the cast is to prevent "slurry" material from sticking to a dry cast. See Figure A2-15 on next page.

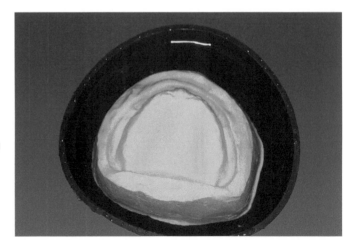

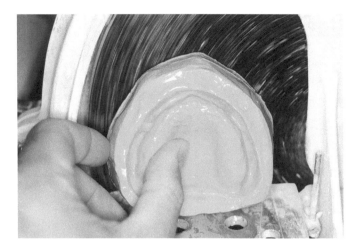

Figure A2–14   Using a model trimmer, the initial trimming of the cast will be to the *bottom* of the cast and will be to correct inconsistent and/or excess cast thickness. Remember to always have water running when using a model trimmer and to rinse off all stone slurry once the trimming is completed.

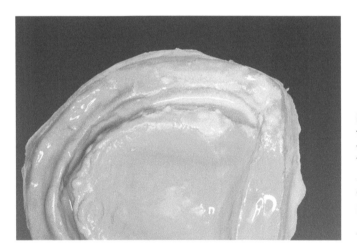

Figure A2–15   As the cast is trimmed, the stone mixes with water and forms a slurry mixture. This mixture will stick to a dry cast and can make a cast unusable. This cast was thoroughly dampened prior to beginning to trim the cast in an attempt to prevent the slurry from sticking to the cast.

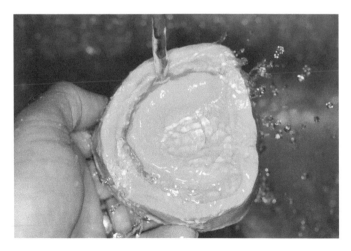

Figure A2–16   The cast must repeatedly be rinsed to remove all slurry mixture.

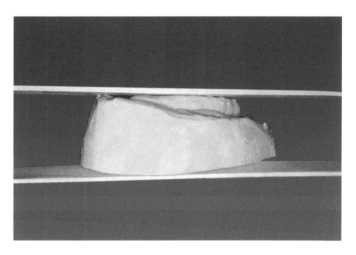

Figure A2–17   The bottom of the base of this cast has now been trimmed so that it is not too thick or thin and is reasonably parallel to the crest of the ridges. See Figure A2-18 X. Remember, a cast must be sufficiently thick to prevent breakage, but excessive thickness is undesirable. Excessive thickness becomes significant when creating master casts because those casts must fit in a flask when processing the denture.

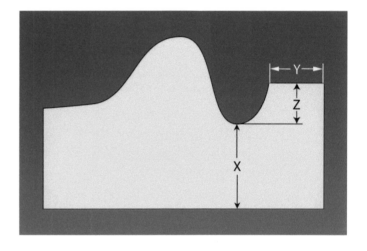

Figure A2–18   Diagramatic view of desired dimensions of a trimmed diagnostic or master cast. X: thickness of cast (12–18 mm in thinnest area). Y: width of land area (2–3 mm). Z: depth of vestibules (2–3 mm).

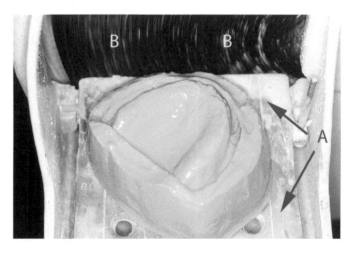

Figure A2–19   Once the bottom of the base of the cast is corrected, the sides of the base can be trimmed using the model trimmer. See Figure A2-18 Y. Prior to trimming the sides of the base, always verify that the platform of the model trimmer (A) is perpendicular to the trimming wheel (B).

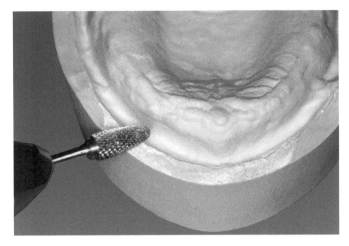

Figure A2–20 Once the land areas on the dry cast are the correct width, an acrylic bur can be used to reduce the height as necessary to create the approximate desired depth of the vestibules. This is necessary, particularly on master casts, so that the laboratory technician has access to all areas of the cast and also reduces the possibility of cast breakage during laboratory procedures. See Figure A2-18 Z.

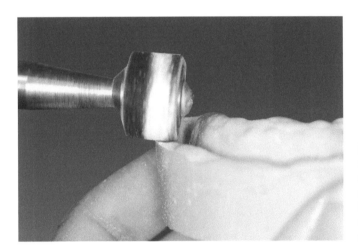

Figure A2–21 An arbor band can also be used to reduce the land areas to create the approximate desired depth of the vestibules. See Figure A2-18 Z. Once again, the cast must be dry prior to using an arbor band.

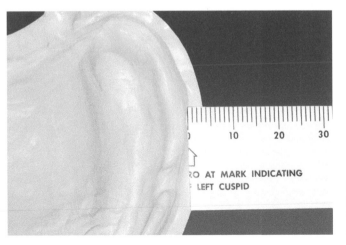

Figure A2–22 These land areas have been trimmed to the correct width, and any excess vestibular depth has been eliminated.

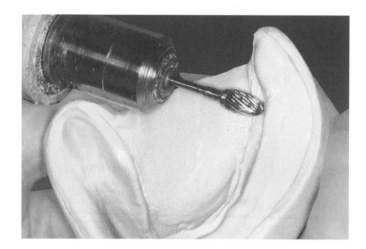

Figure A2–23   On the mandibular cast, the tongue area should also be contoured so that the vestibules are the correct depth and the stone is either flat or gently curves from one side to the other.

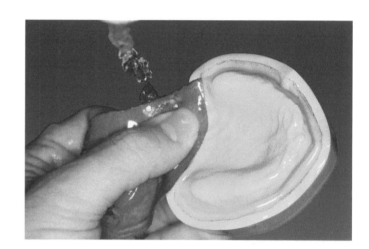

Figure A2–24   Once the cast is properly trimmed, wet and dry sandpaper can be used to smooth the trimmed portions of the cast.

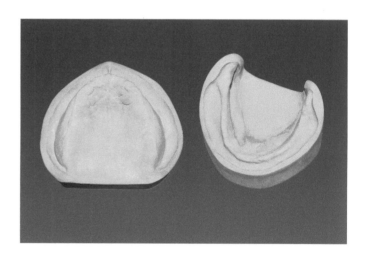

Figure A2–25   Examples of excellent diagnostic casts

Custom Impression Trays

Mandibular Custom Tray

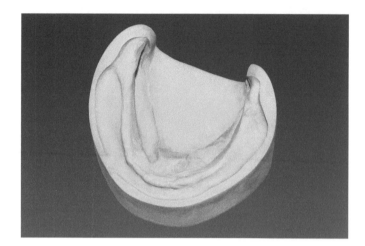

Figure A3–1 A mandibular diagnostic cast properly trimmed and ready for custom impression tray fabrication.

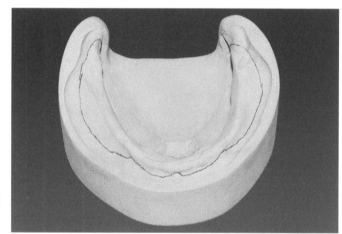

Figure A3–2 The desired tray extension has been drawn on the cast. Generally the extension is approximately 2–3 mm above the depth of the vestibule, if the vestibule was not artificially overextended during the making of the impression.

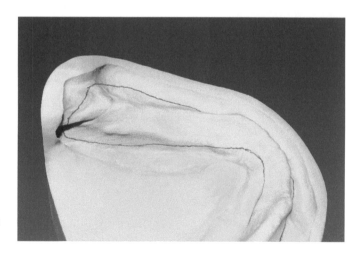

Figure A3–3 Desired tray extension properly indicated on the lingual

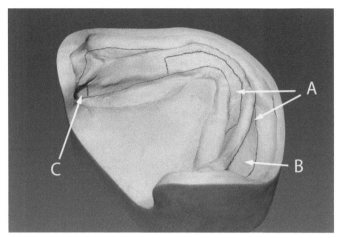

Figure A3–4   The nonstress-bearing areas have been delineated on the mandibular cast. Note that relief wax will not be extended to the buccal and lingual of the anterior ridge (A) because they are considered secondary stress-bearing areas. Note also that the buccal shelves will not have relief wax because they are the primary stress-bearing areas (B). The retromylohyoid areas receive minimal wax relief (C) in order to have good adaptation of this area. This area must receive enough block-out wax so that the impression tray can be removed from the cast.

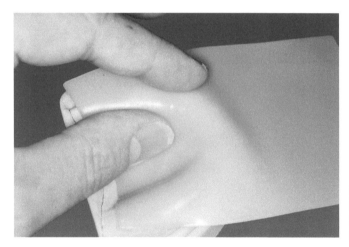

Figure A3–5   A half sheet of warmed baseplate wax being adapted to cast, to form the layer of relief wax (1.5 mm thick).

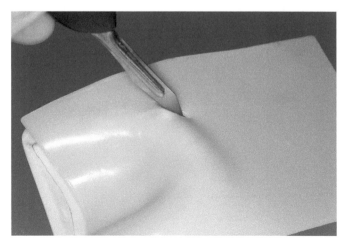

Figure A3–6   The relief wax is trimmed back to the desired outline. It should be lightly tacked to the cast by melting very small areas of the wax to the cast, about every 12 mm.

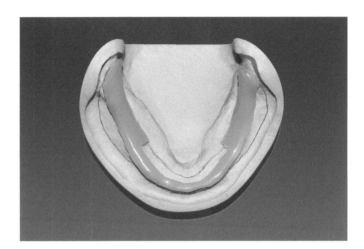

Figure A3–7 The mandibular cast with relief and block-out wax placed.

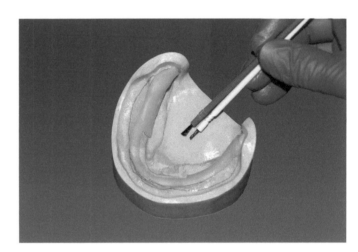

Figure A3–8 A separating medium must cover all exposed areas of stone even extending somewhat down the sides of the cast. Vaseline is commonly used in a very thin film.

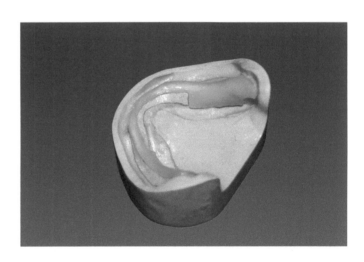

Figure A3–9 Separating medium properly extended on mandibular cast. Note that the material is only a very thin film. It is not used as a block-out material.

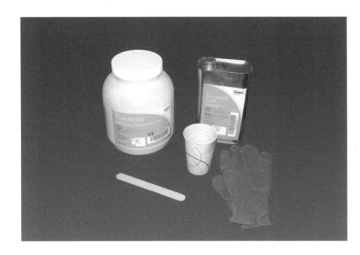

Figure A3–10   Autopolymerizing resins are commonly used as impression tray materials.

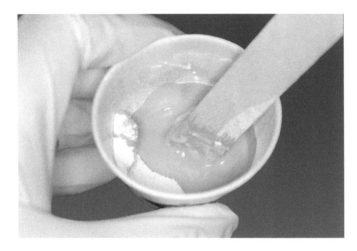

Figure A3–11   The resin is mixed in a paper cup with a tongue blade, using the manufacturer's directions. The powder-to-liquid ratio is often 3 to 1.

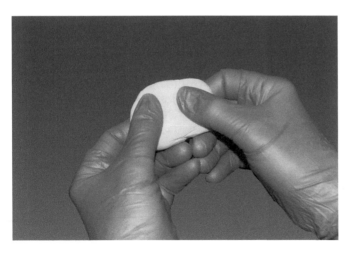

Figure A3–12   Once completely mixed, the resin is allowed begin to polymerize until it can be handled without sticking to gloves. The tray material must be thoroughly blended using the fingers.

Figure A3–13 The tray material must be thinned to approximately 3 mm in thickness. This will provide sufficient strength to the tray while not being excessively thick. Two glass slabs can be used to create a sheet of resin of the correct thickness. Vaseline should be used as a separating medium on both glass slabs. The material can be shaped to resemble the mandibular arch using a sharp knife. Three small pieces of the trimmed resin are retained to make one anterior and two posterior handles.

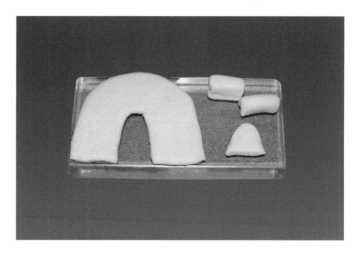

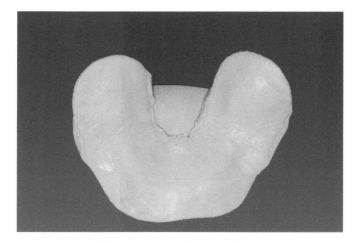

Figure A3–14 The resin is initially carefully placed on the cast and then properly extended almost to the depth of the vestibules and posteriorly completely through the retromylohyoid area. An effort is made not to thin the material. Excess material should be trimmed back to the lines indicating the desired extensions with a sharp knife, while the material is still in a softened state. This will make further shaping much easier. While still workable, the tray handles are added. See Figure A3-18 for the shape of the handles. The anterior handle should be perpendicular to the arch and approximately 16 mm in height, 12 mm in width, and 6 mm in thickness. The posterior handles should be approximately 10 mm in height, 14 mm in length, and 6 mm in thickness.

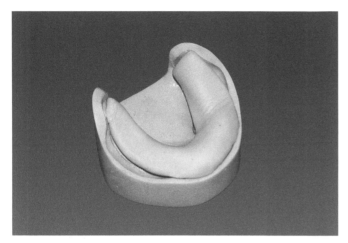

Figure A3–15 Once the material is completely polymerized, it is removed from the cast. Often removal is difficult, and the tray should be removed by first attempting to lift one side with a laboratory knife before switching to the opposite side. This is continued until the tray is removed. Because the retromylohyoid areas are often significantly undercut in relation to each other, if insufficient block-out was completed, it will very difficult to remove the tray, and the cast may be broken.

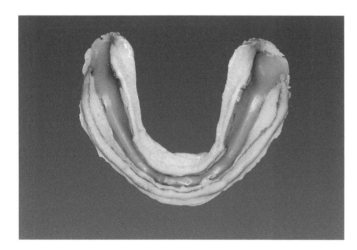

Figure A3–16 Often the pencil lines placed on the diagnostic cast delineating the desired extension of the tray will be visible on the tray. If present, these lines are used to properly shape the impression tray.

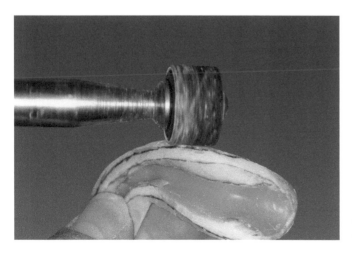

Figure A3–17 Using an arbor band or large resin trimming bur, all overextension is eliminated.

Figure A3–18   When completed, the tray should extend to within 2–3 mm from the depth of the vestibules and to the most posterior extent to the retromylohyoid area. All excessively thick areas of the tray are thinned to approximately 3 mm in thickness. Sharp areas are smoothed.

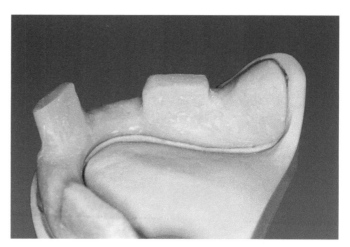

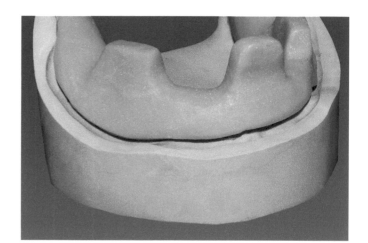

Figure A3–19   Mandibular tray length properly reduced

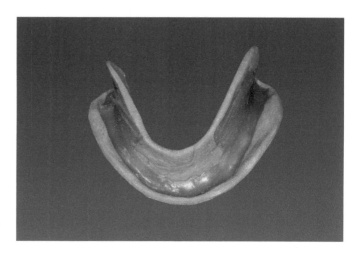

Figure A3–20   Completed mandibular impression tray as seen from the tissue side

Maxillary Custom Tray

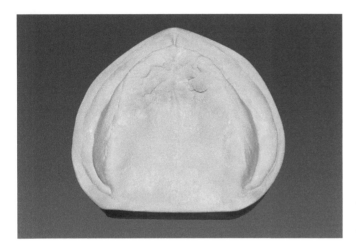

Figure A3–21   A maxillary diagnostic cast properly trimmed and ready for custom impression tray fabrication.

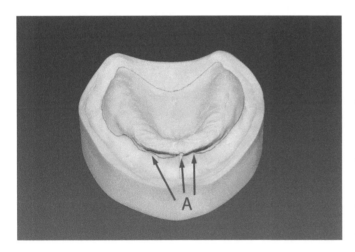

Figure A3–22   A maxillary diagnostic cast with desired tray extension marked. Even though the desired extensions are generally approximately 2–3 mm short of the depth of the vestibules, in this situation the anterior lines are placed approximately 6 mm short of the depth of the vestibule (A). This placement is caused by muscle attachments close to the ridge crest.

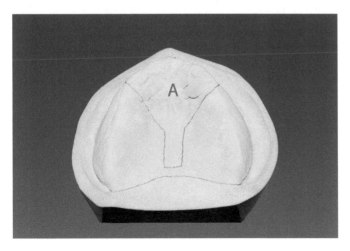

Figure A3–23   The nonstress-bearing area is indicated for a layer of relief wax on the maxillary arch. Note its mushroom-shaped appearance (A). This area is neither a primary nor secondary stress-bearing area. This area extends from approximately 5 mm short of the anticipated distal-most extension of the impression tray and extends anteriorly staying 3 mm on either side of the midline suture. It then turns diagonally toward the ridge crest just posterior of the rugae area.

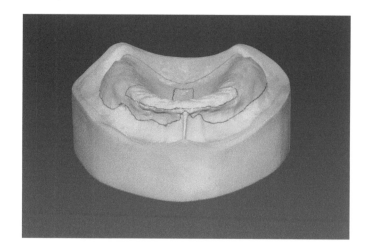

Figure A3–24   The mushroom-shaped area extends just over the crest of the ridge.

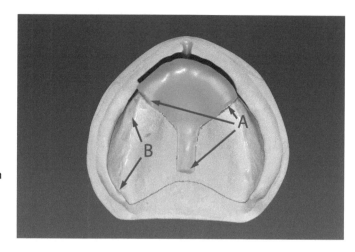

Figure A3–25   Relief wax adapted to the maxillary cast. Note that it is tacked down in several areas by simply melting a small area of wax onto the cast (A). Also note that irregular areas of the cast have been additionally blocked out with thin layers of wax (B). Note also that the labial frenum has been blocked out to prevent breakage.

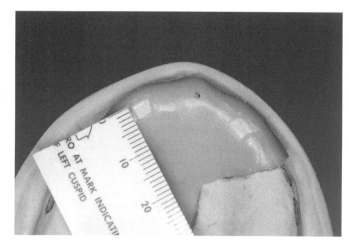

Figure A3–26   Two holes are prepared in the relief wax. Resin will be placed in these holes to create tissue stops. They should be placed 12 mm from the incisive papilla area. They should be approximately 3 mm x 3 mm. These tissue stops are necessary in case the relief wax must be removed during the border molding step of the final impression.

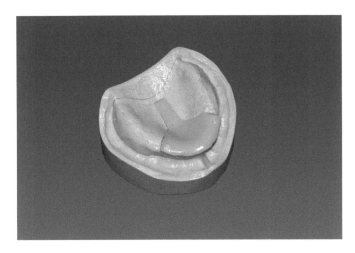

Figure A3–27   A very thin film of separating medium is placed on the maxillary cast.

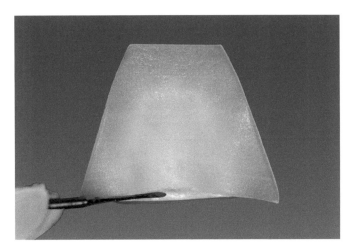

Figure A3–28   The maxillary impression tray is made in the same manner as the mandibular tray. In this example a light polymerizing resin is demonstrated. When this material is selected, a separating medium is placed on the cast as recommended by the manufacturer. In this example, a sheet of colorless resin (Triad Trutray, Dentsply International Inc., York, PA) has been initially positioned on the maxillary cast, and excess material is being removed. The excess material is retained to make a handle for the tray.

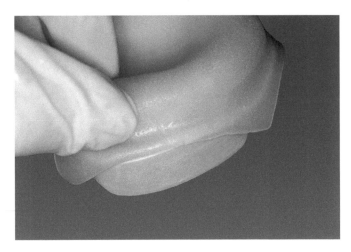

Figure A3–29   When properly adapting the tray, care should be taken to not overly thin the material.

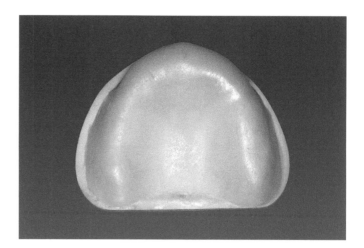

Figure A3–30   The tray material is properly extended on the maxillary cast.

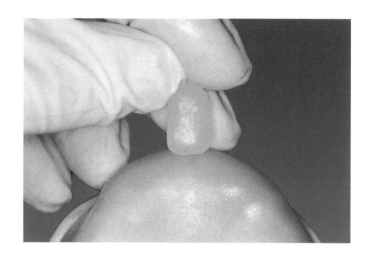

Figure A3–31   The handle is made from the excess material trimmed initially.

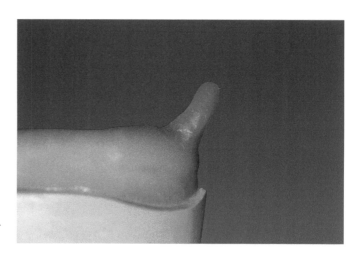

Figure A3–32   When completed, the handle should be approximately 12 mm in length and width, and 6 mm in thickness. It should angle toward the anterior to approximate the central incisors.

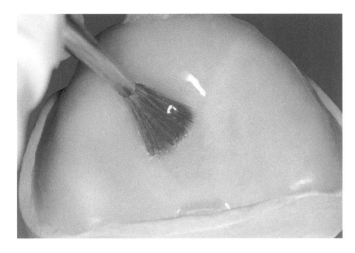

Figure A3–33   All areas of the light polymerized resin are coated with an air-inhibiting material that prevents oxygen from contacting the resin and allows more thorough polymerization.

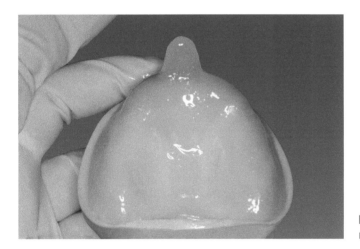

Figure A3–34   The light polymerized resin can now be polymerized.

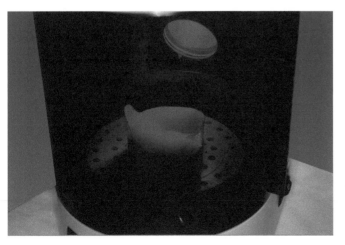

Figure A3–35   The cast and tray are placed in a light polymerization unit (Triad 2000 Light Curing Unit, Dentsply International Inc., York, PA) and polymerized according to the manufacturer's recommendations. The tray is removed from the cast, the internal surface is covered with an air barrier coating, and again polymerized with the internal surface facing upward.

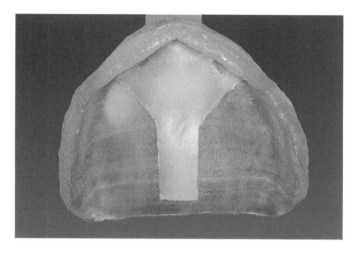

Figure A3–36 . The impression resin tray has been removed from the cast. In this example the relief wax has not been lost from the heat of polymerization of the light polymerized resin. However, because of that potential, two tissue stops were created. Prior to further procedures, it is absolutely necessary to thoroughly remove the air barrier coating from the impression tray following polymerization. his requires thorough cleaning under running water.

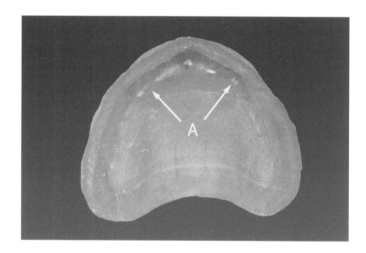

Figure A3–37   The relief wax was lost from this tray, and the tissue stops are visible (A) in the canine areas. The impression tray is trimmed similar to the mandibular tray, with the exception of the tray being trimmed to the vibrating line in the posterior.

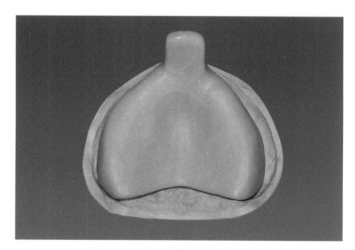

Figure A3–38   A maxillary autopolymerized acrylic resin impression tray neatly trimmed

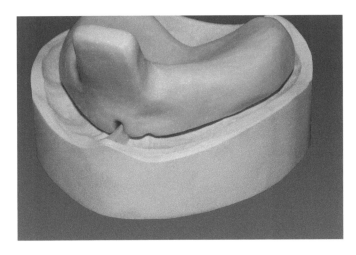

Figure A3–39 This tray has been trimmed 2 mm short of the depth of the vestibules.

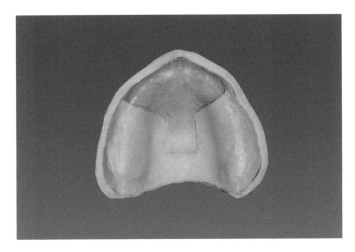

Figure A3–40 A well-fabricated maxillary custom impression tray, as viewed from the tissue side

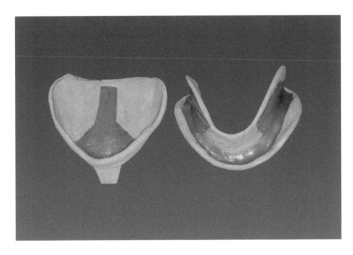

Figure A3–41 The completed maxillary and mandibular custom trays

Final Impressions

Maxillary Impression

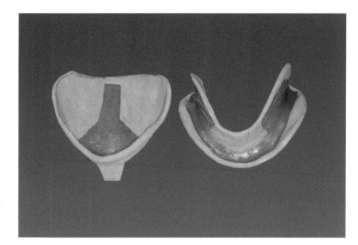

Figure A4–1 Examples of maxillary and mandibular custom impression trays.

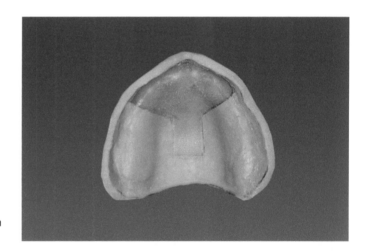

Figure A4–2 Maxillary acrylic resin custom impression tray.

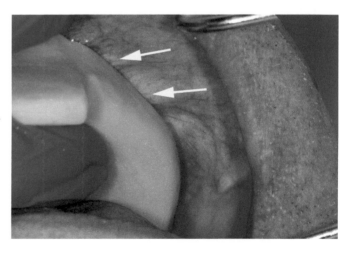

Figure A4–3 The trays must be evaluated for fit and extensions. Ideally a tray should cover all tissues to be impressed and have an even spacing of approximately 2 to 3 mm between the tray flanges and the depth of the vestibules. The borders of this tray are impinging on the soft tissues of the vestibule.

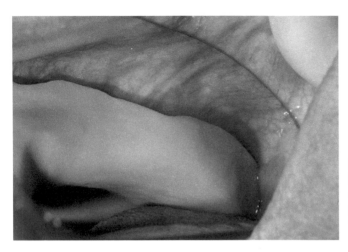

Figure A4–4   The flange length has been corrected. The evaluation and correction is continued around the periphery of the tray to include the posterior length trimmed just slightly longer than the vibrating line.

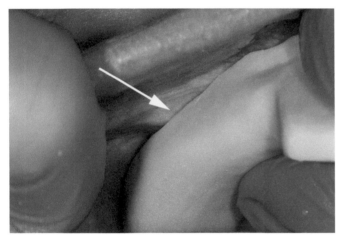

Figure A4–5   The opposite side is also overextended and must be corrected.

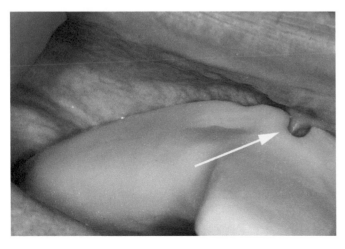

Figure A4–6   Special care must be taken to create space in the labial frenulum area because this tissue has no muscle fibers and is very easily displaced. More relief is needed on this tray.

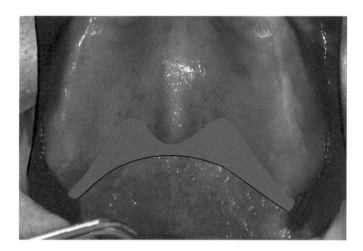

Figure A4–7 The posterior palatal seal area must be visualized when trimming the tray.

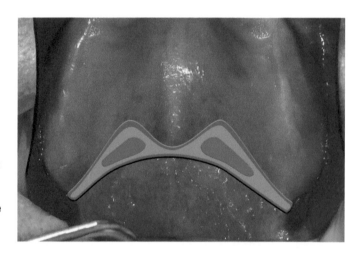

Figure A4–8 Additionally, although evaluated during the initial diagnosis of the patient, the depth of the displaceable tissues must be reviewed because this information will be used when forming the maxillary master cast. The orange/red areas indicate places in which the tissues can be depressed approximately 1 to 2 mm. The green area indicates that the tissue can be depressed approximately 0.5 to 1 mm. The blue area indicates that the tissues can be depressed up to 0.5 mm.

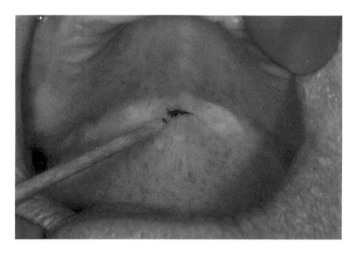

Figure A4–9 The vibrating line is located. The vibrating line is the junction between the reasonably unmovable tissue of the hard palate and the movable tissue of the soft palate. The mark in the figure indicates the beginning slope of the soft palate just distal to the vibrating line. The tray will be slightly longer than the vibrating line in order to record the anatomical detail needed for this landmark.

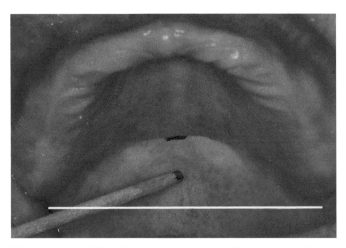

Figure A4–10   This line has been properly placed on the vibrating line. This line could be extended bilaterally through the hamular notches but generally is unnecessary because, for most patients, the vibrating line is a gently curved line that extends from this midline mark through the hamular notches. This is a very typical vibrating line. Note that it is a curved line that is concave toward the anterior as compared with the line drawn straight from one hamular notch to the other. A vibrating line drawn straight across the palate is almost never correctly drawn!

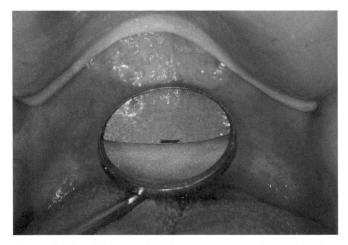

Figure A4–11   This tray has been correctly trimmed back close to the vibrating line. Once again, note that the posterior of the tray is concave in shape toward the anterior. This tray is now ready to be border molded.

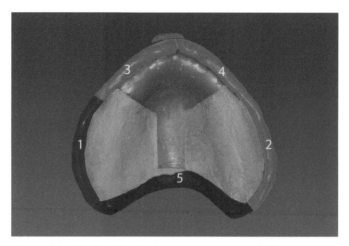

Figure A4–12 For illustration purposes, modeling compound will be used when border molding the maxillary arch. Vinyl polysiloxane will be used for the mandibular arch. Either material could have been used for the maxillary or mandibular arch. The recommended sequence of border molding is indicated in this picture when using modeling compound. Had vinyl polysiloxane been used, longer sections, up to half the tray, can be completed at one time.

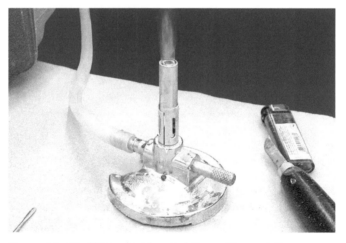

Figure A4–13 When border molding with modeling compound, several pieces of equipment and supplies must be used. A primary requirement is a Bunsen burner.

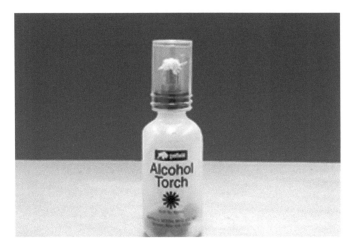

Figure A4–14 A second piece of equipment required is an alcohol torch. An alcohol torch is used to reheat the modeling compound when necessary. It is not used to initially heat the modeling compound because the flame is not hot enough. A significant amount of time will be lost in trying to use the alcohol torch to initially heat the modeling compound.

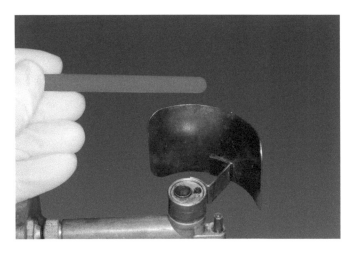

Figure A4–15 The modeling compound is slowly rotated during heating to thoroughly heat the material. It should be removed from the flame when it begins to slump.

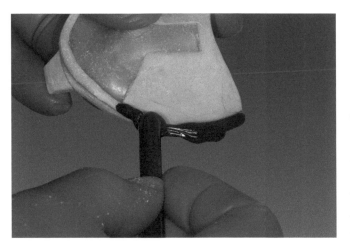

Figure A4–16 The modeling compound is thoroughly heated until to flows freely and is added in small increments to the impression tray following the sequence suggested in Figure A4-12 above. About 2-3 mm of material is needed because that is how much the flange of the tray was shortened from the depth of the vestibules.

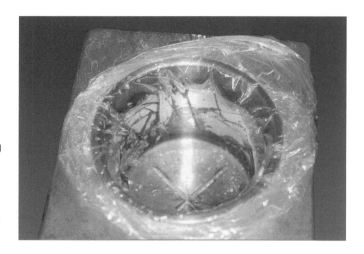

Figure A4–17 Prior to inserting a tray into the mouth with heated modeling compound, the material must be tempered in a hot water bath set to 60⁰ C (140⁰ F). Tempering cools the material to a level that is comfortable to the patient while maintaining the temperature at a level that keeps its viscosity low enough to freely flow. Working time now becomes an important issue.

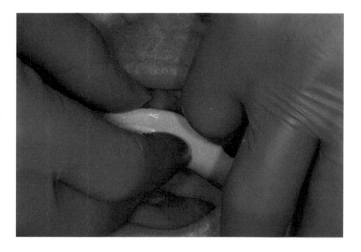

Figure A4–18 The impression tray and modeling compound is inserted being careful not to wipe the material off on the cheeks, tongue, etc. Modeling compound becomes unacceptably rigid in several seconds, the clinician must be quick to insert the tray properly and perform the border molding muscle movement.

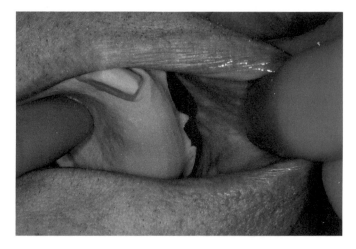

Figure A4–19 Once inserted, the clinician has only about a 10 second working time before the modeling compound becomes too rigid to be usable. While the material is still flowing, the border molding procedures are quickly but thoroughly completed.

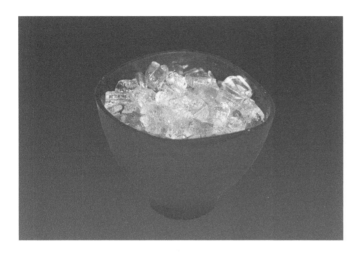

Figure A4–20   Once removed, the tray/compound is immediately inserted into a bowl containing water to increase rigidity and minimize possible distortion. Five seconds in the iced water is sufficient.

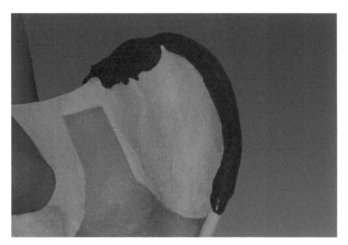

Figure A4–21   The border molded area can now be evaluated. Any excess modeling compound, either inside the tray or in thickness, is removed with a sharp knife. If necessary, additional compound can be added, and the area border molded again if the initial attempt was unacceptable. This procedure is repeated as necessary until this particular area is totally acceptable. Do not begin a second area until the initial area is totally acceptable. This applies through the entire border molding procedure.

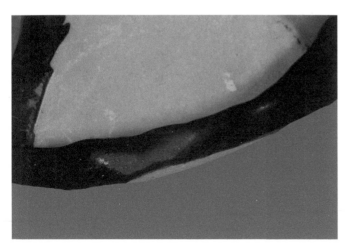

Figure A4–22   When acceptable, the compound should have a smooth but matte (dull) appearance to its surface, it should not be shiny.

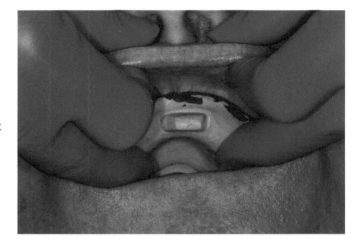

Figure A4–23 A particularly difficult area to border mold can be the labial frenulum. Because this frenulum is very flaccid, it must be thoroughly manipulated, and the compound sufficiently warmed to be workable during the border molding procedure.

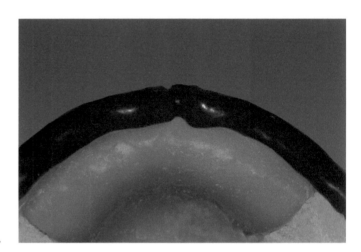

Figure A4–24 Example of a nicely border-molded labial frenulum area.

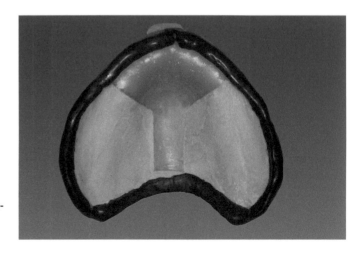

Figure A4–25 The border molding is complete. Notice that the compound does not extend much beyond the tray in the posterior palatal seal area. The tray was cut to the proper extension so the material should be close to the same length as the tray in this area.

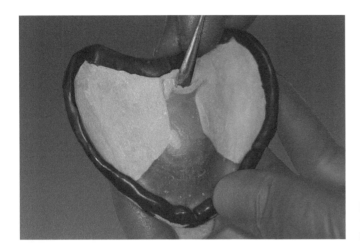

Figure A4–26   The relief wax is now removed to create the relief chamber.

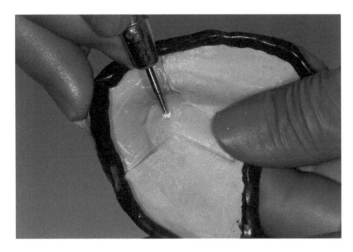

Figure A4–27   Five to six holes can be placed in the relief chamber using a #8 round bur. These holes will allow the impression material to escape as hydraulic forces build during the impression procedure.

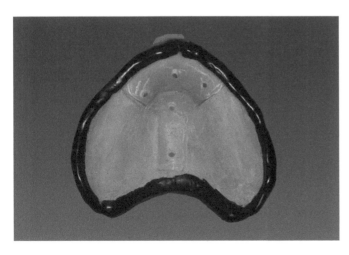

Figure A4–28   The wax has been removed and the holes have been prepared.

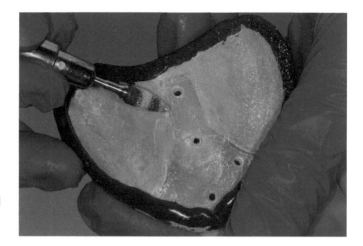

Figure A4–29 Any sharp areas at the wax/resin interface are removed with an acrylic bur. Note the holes that have been prepared.

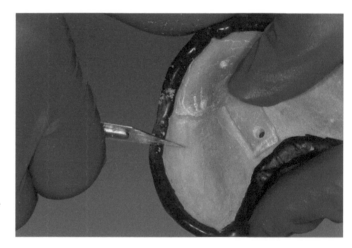

Figure A4–30 Some clinicians remove approximately 0.5 mm of the modeling compound to allow space for the final impression material. With the low viscosity materials available, this is probably not necessary if the border molding was accurate.

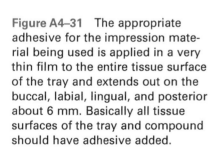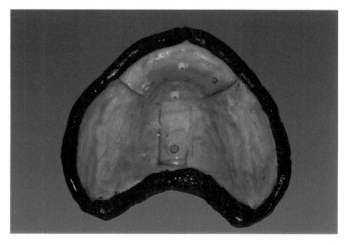

Figure A4–31 The appropriate adhesive for the impression material being used is applied in a very thin film to the entire tissue surface of the tray and extends out on the buccal, labial, lingual, and posterior about 6 mm. Basically all tissue surfaces of the tray and compound should have adhesive added.

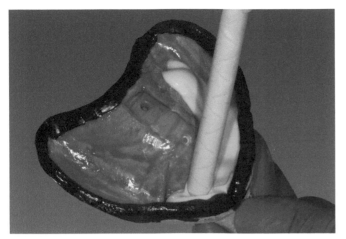

Figure A4–32   There are a myriad of final or "wash" impression materials available. With many choices of working and setting times available, vinyl polysiloxane impression materials are commonly used. Most of these materials use a "gun"-type mixing device to express the impression material. Care is taken when loading the impression material into the tray to preclude the capturing of air bubbles within the material.

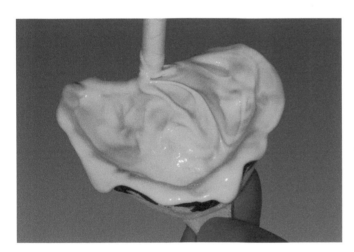

Figure A4–33   The entire tissue side of the tray and compound should be covered with impression material. However only enough material should be placed to cover the tray with a 3mm thickness of material. Slightly more material may be placed in the relief chamber areas. The entire border-molding material should be covered for at least 6 mm on the buccal, labial, and lingual.

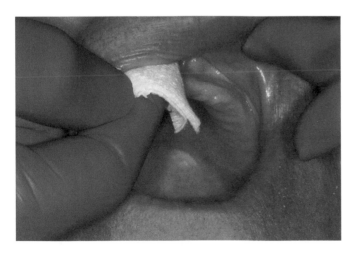

Figure A4–34   Most impression materials are hydrophobic. Prior to inserting the impression material into the mouth, the patient should swallow to remove excess saliva. Any remaining saliva should be dried with gauze.

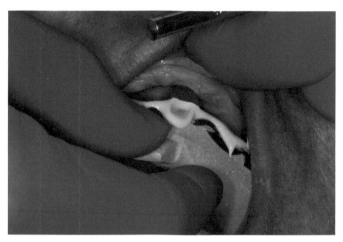

Figure A4–35   Care should be taken when inserting the tray/material to minimize any contact with lips, cheeks, and tongue, as this may wipe material off the tray resulting in a poor impression. The patient should be instructed to totally relax the lips, cheeks, and tongue.

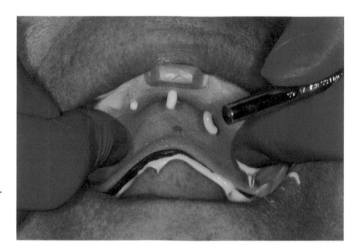

Figure A4–36   Once inserted, all necessary border molding is completed and the tray/material is then secured until the material sets. Manufacturer's information should be consulted concerning working and setting times. Generally a material with a two and a half- to three-minute working and setting time is excellent. It provides sufficient working time and yet minimizes loss of clinical time while waiting for the material to set.

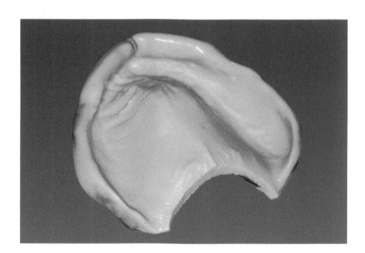

Figure A4–37   Example of a well-made and trimmed maxillary final impression

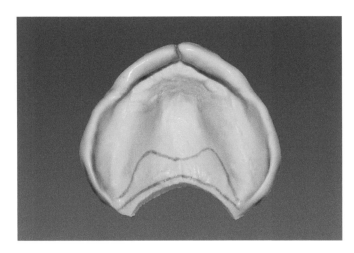

Figure A4–38   Note that the posterior palatal seal area has been drawn on this impression. This is important in order to transfer the outline to the master cast. An indelible marker can be used to outline the area in the mouth, and the impression can be placed back in the mouth. With this technique, when washing and disinfecting the impression, much of the outline may be washed off the impression and must be redrawn.

Mandibular Impression:

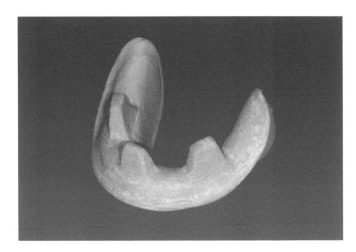

Figure A4–39   Mandibular custom impression tray

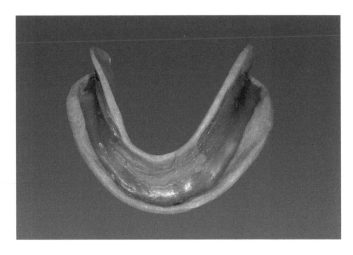

Figure A4–40   Note that the nonstress-bearing areas of this tray were blocked out with relief wax, which will be removed following border molding.

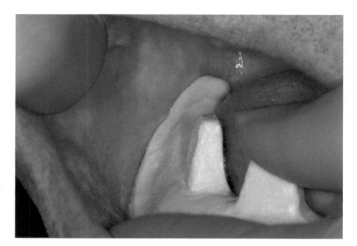

Figure A4–41 As was done with the maxillary tray, the mandibular tray must be evaluated and extensions corrected.

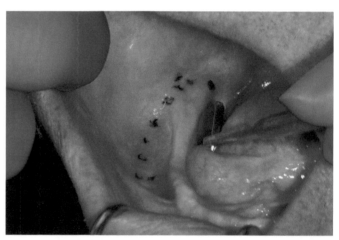

Figure A4–42 Because it may be a difficult area to visualize, the desired extension in the buccal shelf area and masseter muscle areas have been marked with an indelible marker. If using this technique, the tissues should be reasonably dry prior to marking to minimize the spreading of the material throughout the entire area.

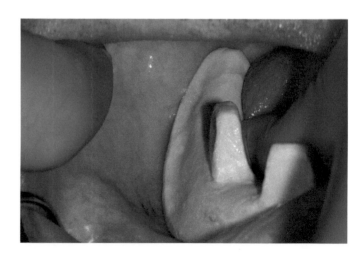

Figure A4–43 The tray is replaced.

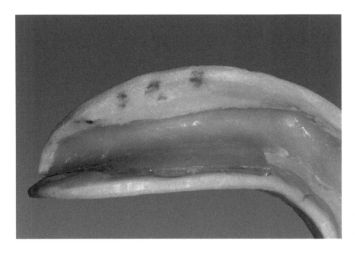

Figure A4-44   The marks have transferred to the tray.

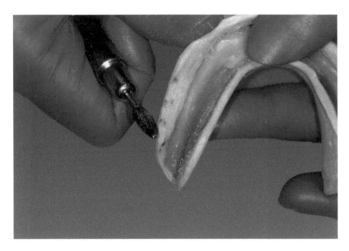

Figure A4-45   The marks were placed in the depth of the vestibules, so the tray must be cut back 2 mm short of the marks to provide space for the border molding material.

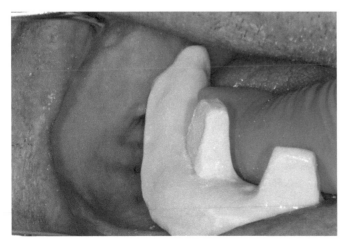

Figure A4-46   The tray is sufficiently reduced in the buccal shelf area, However, it still must be reduced in the masseter muscle area.

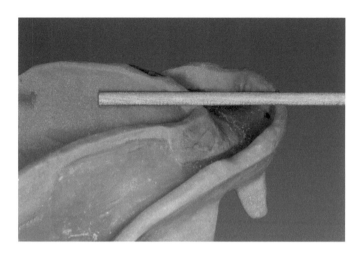

Figure A4–47   For most patients, a correctly trimmed mandibular impression tray will exhibit several characteristics. First, unless the patient has had some type surgical extension of the vestibule, the buccal and lingual flange lengths in the anterior should be approximately the same length.

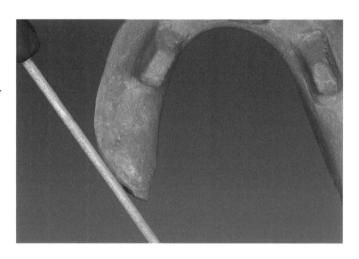

Figure A4–48   Second, the masseter muscle extension of the tray should approach the crest of the ridge at a gradual 45^0 to 60^0 angle and flow smoothly into the retromylohyoid area. There are no sharp corners in these areas. A denture made from an impression with sharp corners will cause severe discomfort to the patient because it will abrade the tissues rather rapidly.

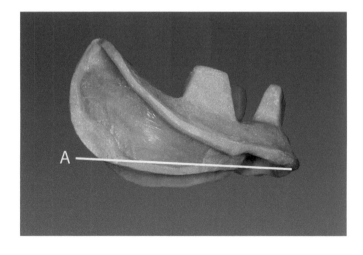

Figure A4–49   Third, the lingual flange should begin approximately even with the buccal flange in the incisal area and then gradually get longer than the buccal flange as it goes posteriorly. The lingual flange should form an almost straight line with minimal curvature. (A)

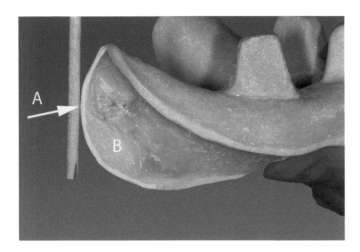

Figure A4–50 Finally, the most distal extent of the impression tray is going to be in the retromylohyoid space area (A), just lingual to the retromolar pad. The retromylohyoid extension should exhibit a smooth curvature from the retromolar pad area to the lingual flange area. (B)

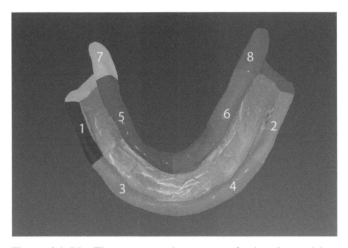

Figure A4–51 The suggested sequence for border molding, if modeling compound is to be used. If vinyl polysiloxane is to be used, generally the entire buccal and then lingual flanges can be completed and then each retromylohyoid area is border molded. Generally, because of the size and strength of the tongue, even though the entire vestibular extension can be obtained in the retromylohyoid areas using vinyl polysiloxane, the thickness of the material will not be acceptable on the first attempt. It will often be knife edged. On subsequent insertions with additional border molding material added, the area can be more easily thickened if the patient closes slightly as the tray is positioned and asked to moisten their lips with the tongue gently to accomplish the border molding.

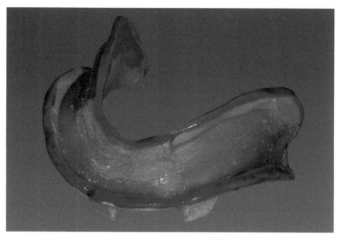

Figure A4–52 Prior to border molding, the correct adhesive for the impression material is applied to the flanges and about 6 mm inside and outside the tray. It is allowed to dry according to the manufacturer's instructions. Do not place the adhesive on the entire internal surface of the impression tray at this time.

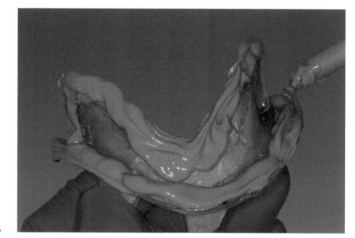

Figure A4–53 A layer of heavy-bodied impression material is applied to the flanges making an attempt to minimize excess material.

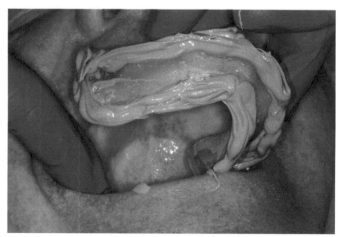

Figure A4–54 Care is taken when inserting the tray for border molding to minimize loss of material onto the cheeks, lips, tongue, etc.. The cheeks should be gently stretched outward while inserting and seating the tray/material to avoid wiping the material from the tray, to remove the fatty roll of tissue in the masseter muscle areas, and to allow any captured air bubbles to escape. It may be necessary to use a mouth mirror to stretch the corner of the mouth if the fingers are too large.

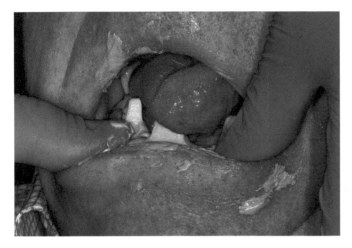

Figure A4–55 Once completely seated, the border molding can begin. The patient should protrude the tongue to form the retromylohyoid areas, move the tip of the tongue from cheek to cheek to form the posterior lingual areas, and then gently protrude the tongue to form the anterior lingual area. Some patients will attempt to exaggerate the tongue protrusion, but the tongue should only be protruded to a normal functional range.

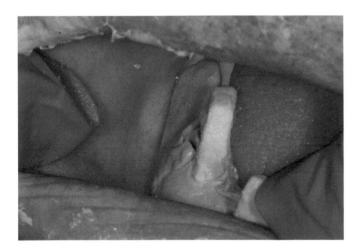

Figure A4–56 The buccal shelf and masseter muscles should be carefully evaluated.

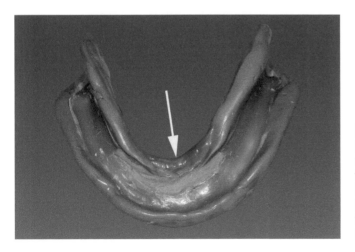

Figure A4–57 This entire tray was border molded in a single attempt with reasonably good results. Other than some minor areas of pressure (show through) the major problem is in the lingual anterior area. Areas that show through the border molding will need correction.

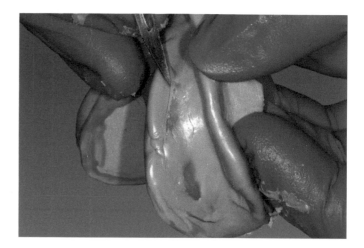

Figure A4–58 Prior to correcting problem areas, all excess material is removed with a sharp knife. It should be easy to remove if the adhesive was properly placed.

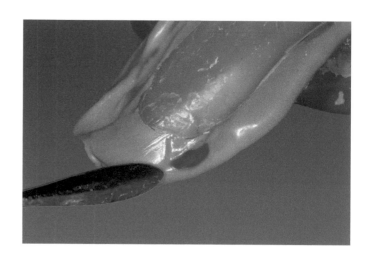

Figure A4–59 Excessive pressure areas to be corrected are noted.

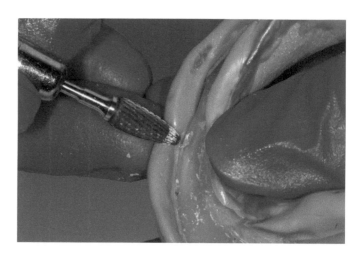

Figure A4–60 All areas of pressure are removed with an acrylic bur.

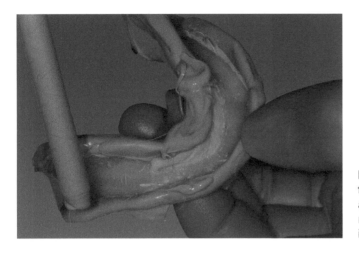

Figure A4–61   Adhesive is added to any newly exposed resin and allowed to dry, heavy-bodied material is again added, the tray/material is reinserted, and border molded.

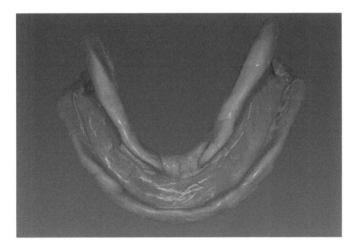

Figure A4–62   This impression tray is acceptably border molded.

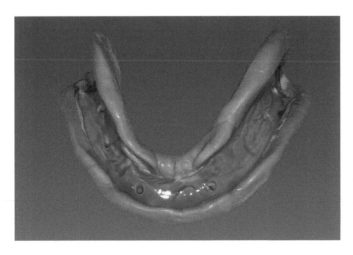

Figure A4–63   Relief holes are placed approximately every 12 mm using a #6 or #8 round bur. Adhesive is applied to all internal resin surfaces; the tray is properly filled with light-bodied impression material; tray/material is inserted, and border molding is completed.

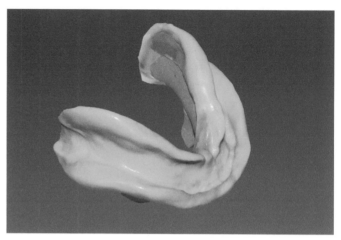

Figure A4–64 Acceptable mandibular final impression. Note the approximately 45⁰ angle in the masseter muscle area, and smooth continuous flow of material from the masseter muscle area across the retromolar pad into the retromylohyoid area. Note also the excellent coverage of the buccal shelf areas.

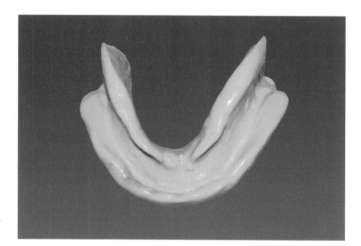

Figure A4–65 Acceptable mandibular final impression

Creating Master Casts

Figure A5–1 Prior to attempting to pour the final impressions, a form should be created around the impressions to simplify the procedure and to give the proper size and shape to the master casts by confining the dental stone while the impressions are poured. This procedure is called beading and boxing the impression. Multiple materials can be used to bead and box an impression, including combination of dental stone and pumice, irreversible hydrocolloid, etc. In this example, Play-doh is being used to bead the impression.

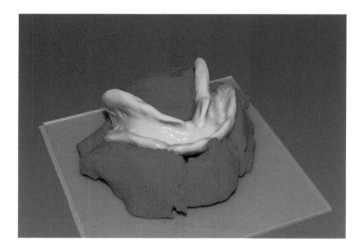

Figure A5–2 The Play-doh should be built up approximately 7.5 cm in height and extended at least 3 mm beyond all border of the impression. This will support the impression and provide for a proper land area on the master cast. In this example, a resin support is being used but is not necessary. All borders of the impression are exposed by approximately 2 mm so as to provide for sufficient depth to the vestibule in the master cast.

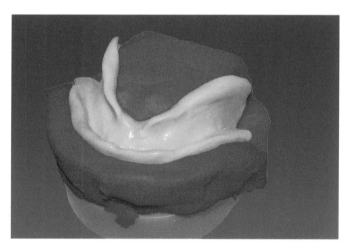

Figure A5–3 On the mandibular arch, the tongue area is flat from one side to the other. Note that the entire roll has been exposed in the masseter muscle, retromolar pad, and retromylohyoid areas. On the maxillary arch, it is also necessary to expose the entire roll at the posterior border of the impression.

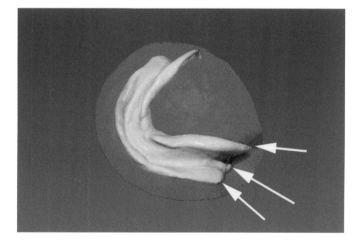

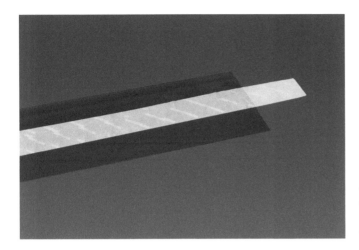

Figure A5-4 The material will be boxed with two pieces of red boxing wax. They should be joined together with the tape. Approximately 7.5 cm of tape is left extended beyond the wax on one end.

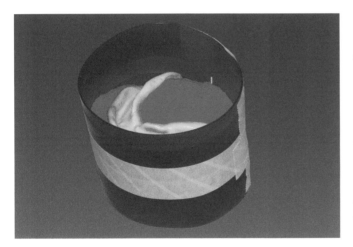

Figure A5-5 The boxing wax is closely adapted to and encloses the beading material, forming a chimney-like form that will retain the dental stone during pouring. Care must be taken not to compress the beading material or collapse the wax chimney. If either occurs, it may be impossible to form a properly shaped and sized base of the master cast. One end of the wax overlaps the other end of the wax, and the tape is used to seal the two ends together.

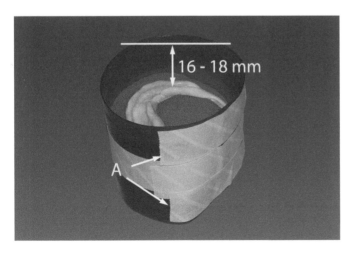

Figure A5-6 To allow for sufficient thickness of stone, the boxing wax chimney should extend 16 to 18 mm above the highest surface of the impression (usually a flange). Two additional pieces of tape (A), one above and one below the first piece, are used to totally seal the form.

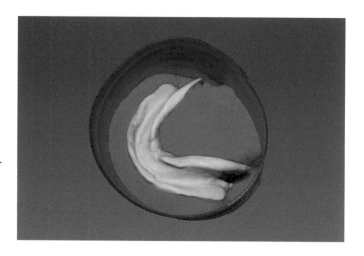

Figure A5–7 When properly completed, the boxing wax should completely seal the impression and beading wax. Additionally, the beading wax must not be compressed nor should the walls of the chimney collapse. Example of a well-beaded and boxed mandibular final impression.

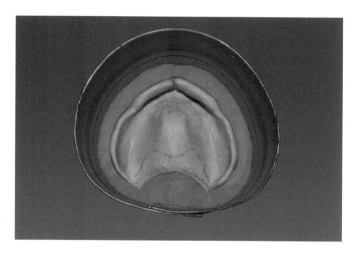

Figure A5–8 A well-beaded and boxed maxillary final impression. The posterior palatal seal area has been marked with an indelible marker. This will usually transfer to the master cast, making it easier to create the posterior palatal seal in the master cast.

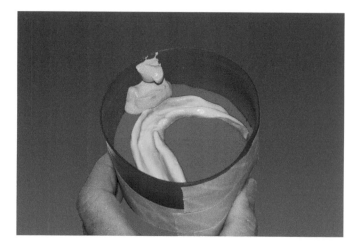

Figure A5–9 The dental stone of choice is prepared according to the manufacturer's instructions and vacuum mixed to minimized air bubbles from becoming entrapped in the mix and being transferred to the master cast. A small initial fill is started, and the stone is flowed into the impression using a vibrator set to a low to moderate level. The vibrator should be set to a level sufficient to slowly flow the stone around the impression.

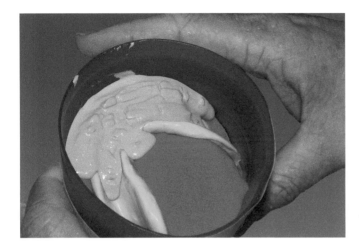

Figure A5–10   Stone is slowly added in small increments. This will allow the stone to slowly fill all impressed areas and minimize trapping bubbles within the master cast.

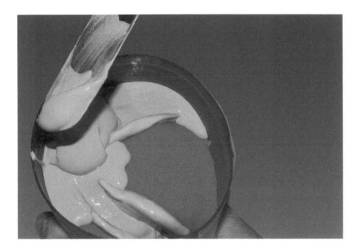

Figure A5–11   The importance of slowly adding small increments of stone to the boxed impression cannot be excessively emphasized. The technician must observe that the stone flows over and covers all impressed surfaces.

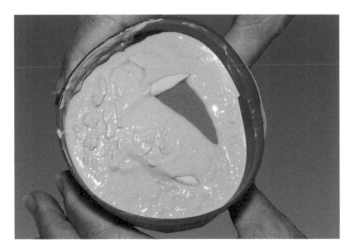

Figure A5–12   The slow fill is followed throughout the pouring of the impression.

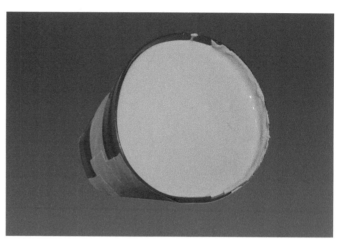

Figure A5–13 Sufficient stone must be added so that the base of the cast will be at least 16 to 18 mm in thickness. This will provide sufficient thickness for necessary strength during laboratory procedures and yet not be excessively thick. Once completely filled, the stone is allowed to set until cooled.

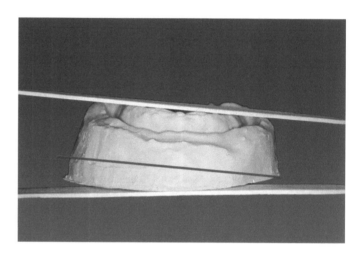

Figure A5–14 The impression is carefully removed from the stone cast and, just as for the diagnostic cast, the base of the cast is evaluated to determine the model trimming necessary to make the ridge crests parallel to the bench top. In this example, the purple line indicates the trimming necessary.

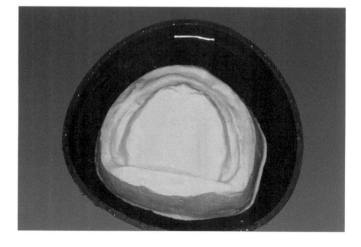

Figure A5–15 To prevent slurry from sticking to the cast during model trimming, the cast should be soaked in water for three minutes.

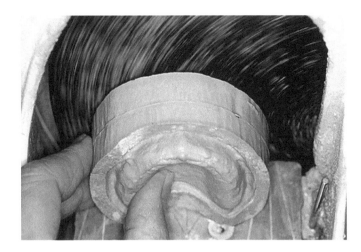

Figure A5–16 The bottom of the base is the first part of the cast trimmed. It should be trimmed as necessary to make the bottom of the cast reasonably parallel to the crest of the ridges.

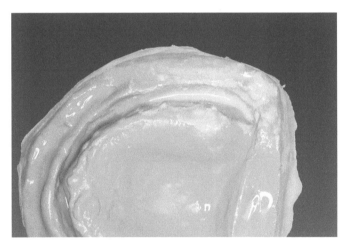

Figure A5–17 Remember to continually check the cast for any slurry mixture.

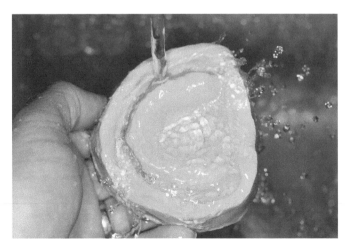

Figure A5–18 Immediately rinse off all slurry mixture from the cast.

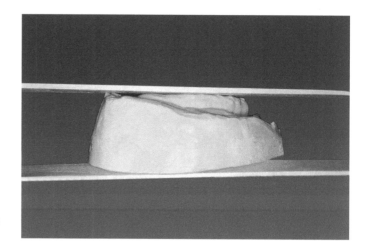

Figure A5–19 The bottom of this base has been trimmed so that it is parallel to the crest of the ridges.

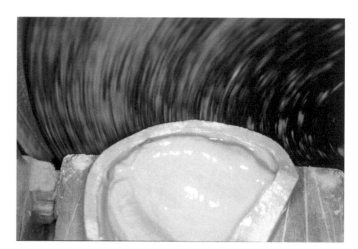

Figure A5–20 Next the width of the land areas is trimmed as necessary.

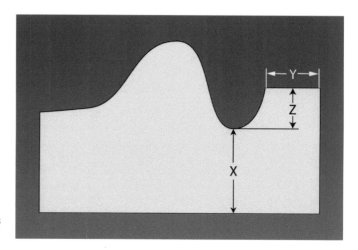

Figure A5–21 Ideally the bottom of the base of the cast should be 12 to 18 mm thick in the thinnest area (X). The land areas should be trimmed so that the width of the land areas is 2–3 mm (Y).

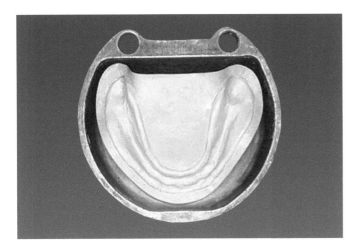

Figure A5–22 When properly trimmed, the casts should fit within the flasks used during processing. They should be evaluated in the flasks, and any necessary additional trimming should be completed.

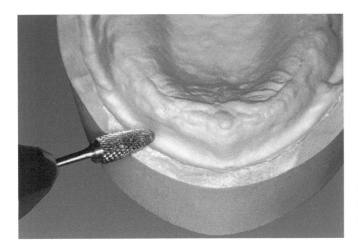

Figure A5–23 The cast should be allowed to thoroughly dry and then, using either an acrylic bur or an arbor band, the land areas should be trimmed so that the depth of the vestibules is 2–3 mm.

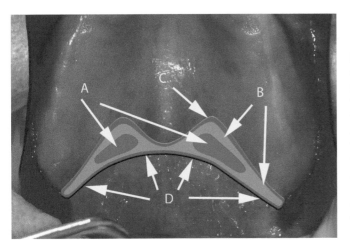

Figure A5–24 The posterior palatal seal (PPS) area must now be prepared into the cast. Intraorally the orange area (A) indicates areas that were able to be compressed approximately 1 mm in the mouth; the green area (B) indicates tissues that were able to be compressed approximately 0.5 to 1 mm; the blue areas (C) indicate areas that were compressible for 0 to 0.5 mm. The vibrating line (D) is the posterior limit of the PPS.

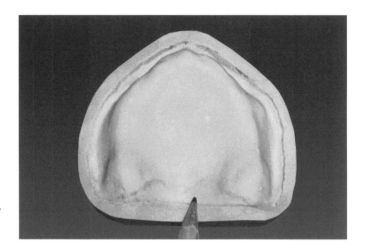

Figure A5–25 In this example, the PPS area was transferred to the master cast using an indelible marker and can be easily visualized. If necessary it can be drawn in with a pencil.

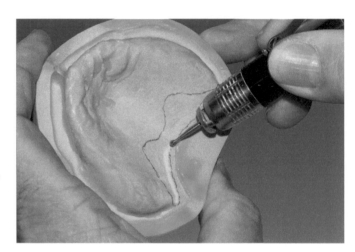

Figure A5–26 The posterior limit of the PPS, the vibrating line, can be delineated with a #6 round bur. It will be approximately 0.5 to 1 mm in depth.

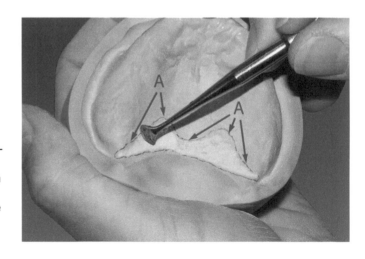

Figure A5–27 All other depths are created into the master cast as indicated by the compressibility of the tissues. See Figure A5-24. All rough areas are then smoothed using a large cleoid/discoid instrument. The anterior border of the PPS should be feathered (A).

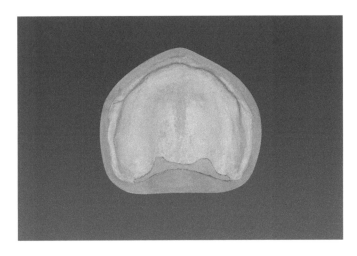

Figure A5–28   The completed PPS

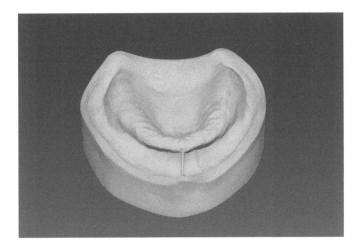

Figure A5–29   Example of an excellent maxillary master cast

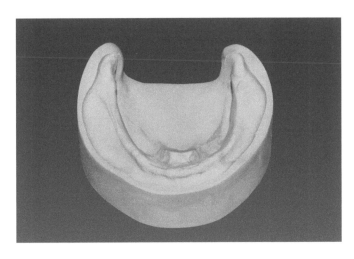

Figure A5–30   Example of an excellent mandibular master cast

Record Bases and Occlusion Rims

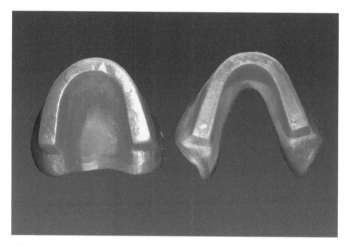

Figure A6–1 Record bases and occlusion rims will be needed for basically all of the remaining steps in the fabrication of the complete dentures. These are examples of well-formed maxillary and mandibular record bases and occlusion rims.

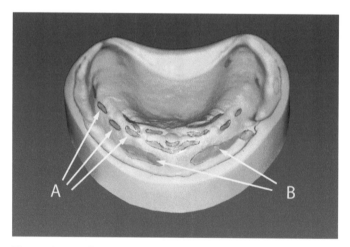

Figure A6–2 Because autopolymerizing acrylic resin will be used to create the record base, all irregularities and undercuts on the master cast are blocked out with baseplate wax. The resin will flow into these areas and polymerize into a rigid unit. If these areas are not blocked out, the master cast can be broken in attempting to remove the record base. All small irregularities are simply filled with wax even with the surrounding surfaces (A). The block-out wax in undercut areas of the cast may be reasonably thick at times. Enough wax must be placed to eliminate the undercut in relation to the path of withdrawal of the record base from the cast (B).

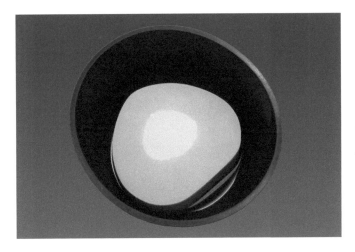

Figure A6–3   The cast should be inverted in a bowl of water to help eliminate air bubbles that could rise from the cast into the autopolymerizing resin and result in porosity. The bottom of the cast should be above the water line; this will allow air to more easily escape as opposed to having the entire cast under water. The cast should be soaked for three to five minutes.

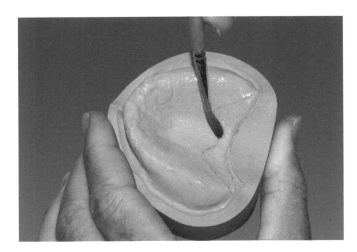

Figure A6–4   The cast is removed from the water and, once the surface of the cast has no standing water, the anatomical portion of the cast and surrounding land areas are coated with a separating medium.

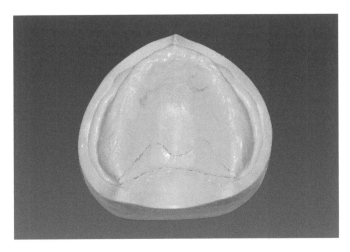

Figure A6–5   This cast has been coated with a separating medium. The separating medium was also extended onto the sides of the cast.

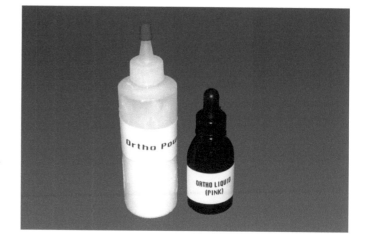

Figure A6–6 An autopolymerizing acrylic resin is used to form the record base using the "sprinkle-on" technique. The powder has been placed in a squeeze bottle, and the liquid has been placed in the bottle with an eye dropper.

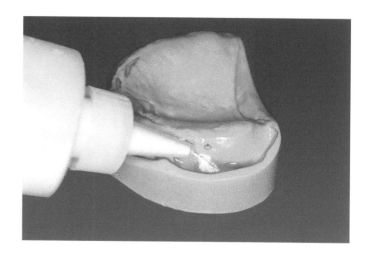

Figure A6–7 With the sprinkle-on technique, first a small area of the cast is wetted using the monomer; then the polymer is sprinkled onto this wetted area. All polymer must be wetted with the monomer to minimize porosity.

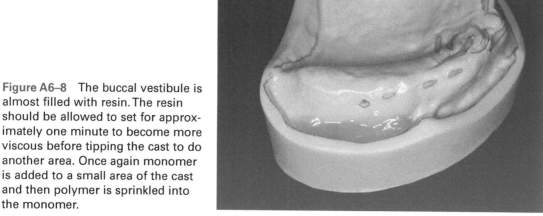

Figure A6–8 The buccal vestibule is almost filled with resin. The resin should be allowed to set for approximately one minute to become more viscous before tipping the cast to do another area. Once again monomer is added to a small area of the cast and then polymer is sprinkled into the monomer.

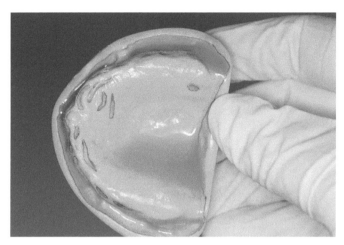

Figure A6–9 When adding the resin, the cast should be tipped so that the surface you are working on is parallel to the bench top. This will help maintain the resin on the desired surface until it has become viscous.

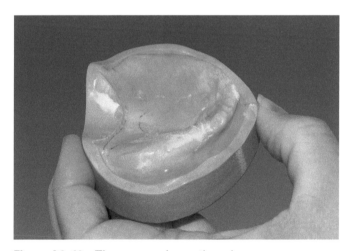

Figure A6–10   The process is continued.

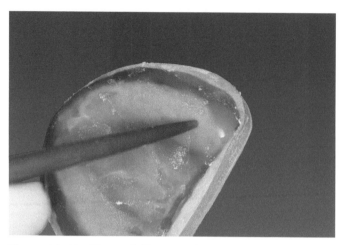

Figure A6–11 The sprinkle-on technique is continued until the tissue surface of the cast is covered and the resin is approximately 3 mm in thickness. Excessively thin areas can be thickened following polymerization of the record base. All necessary resin should be added prior to separating the record base from the cast. Once the record base has been removed, if more thickness is desired, it must be reseated on the cast and new resin added.

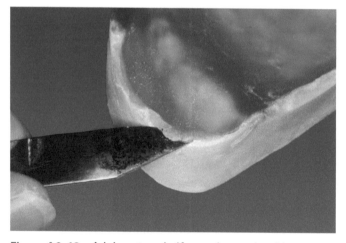

Figure A6–12 A laboratory knife can be wedged between the resin and cast on the land areas, and used to gently lift the record base from the master cast. Care is taken not to damage either the record base or the master cast. The knife should be positioned on one side, then the other, and then in the anterior slowly working the record base off the cast. Additionally an effort is made to lift the record base vertically from the cast in the direction of the anterior ridge as opposed to rotating it off. Attempting to rotate the record base off the cast will often break the master cast.

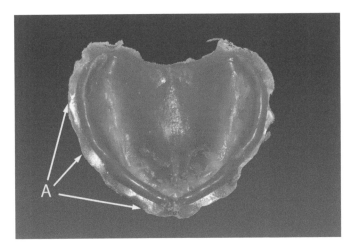

Figure A6–13   When properly fabricated, the record base can be removed from the master cast with no breakage and there should be minimum porosity. The record base should be completely extended to cover all anatomic portions of the cast and should have a minor amount of "flash" (A) extending onto the land areas.

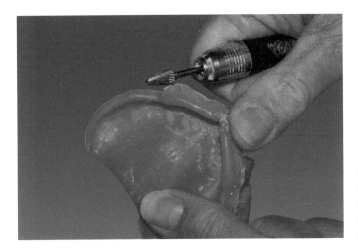

Figure A6–14   The flash can be removed with either an acrylic bur or arbor band. Care should be exercised to avoid the sharp edges of the flash material.

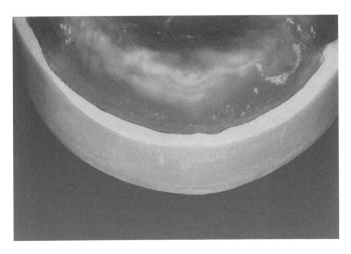

Figure A6–15   When properly trimmed, the record base should fit completely on the master cast with minimal effort, and the flanges should fit flush with the land areas. If the record base is not completely stable on the master cast at this time, it must be remade.

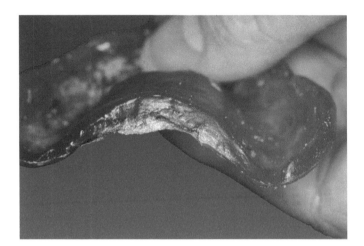

Figure A6–16   The record base should be checked for proper thickness. Two to three mm is ideal.

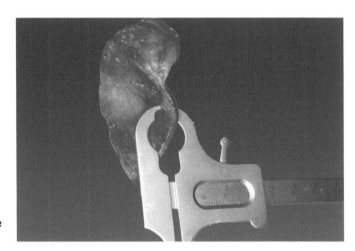

Figure A6–17   A boley gauge can be used to check the palatal thickness.

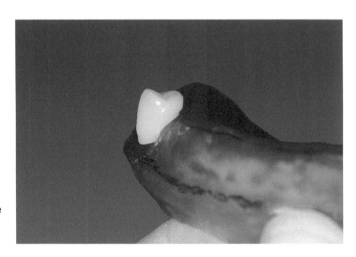

Figure A6–18   Denture teeth will be set on this record base. Therefore, the areas that will eventually receive denture teeth should be very thin, less than 1 mm.

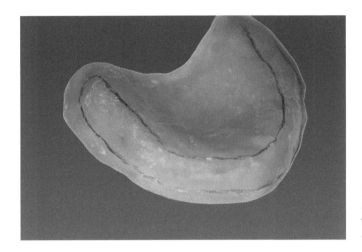

Figure A6–19   The area to eventually receive denture teeth during the tooth arrangement procedure is outlined on this record base.

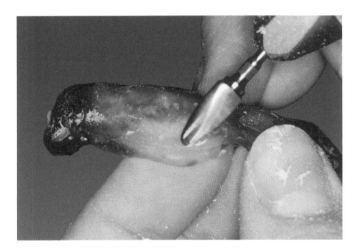

Figure A6–20   This area must be thinned using an acrylic bur until it is less than 1 mm thick. When thinning this area, a finger can be placed opposite the area being trimmed and the finger will feel the resin start to flex just before a hole is created. A small hole is no problem because it can be covered with baseplate wax at the next stage. However, a large hole may require repair with new resin.

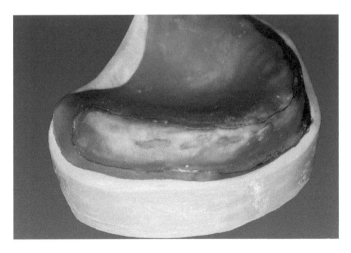

Figure A6–21   This record base has been properly thinned in the area that will receive denture teeth.

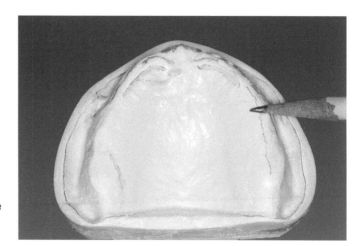

Figure A6–22   The next step will be the fabrication of the occlusion rim. The occlusion rim should be centered over the posterior ridges. A pencil should be used to mark the crest of the posterior residual ridges.

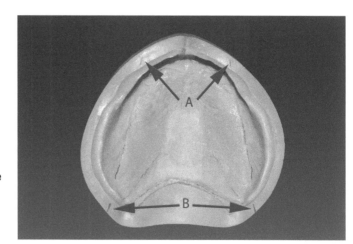

Figure A6–23   The crest of the ridge of this cast has been marked and a straight edge was used to extend the mark to the anterior and posterior land areas (A and B).

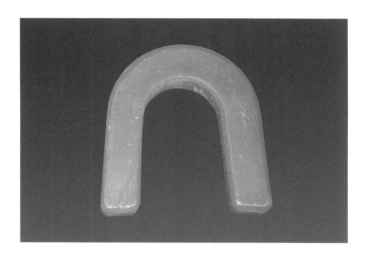

Figure A6–24   A preformed wax pattern can be used to form the occlusion rim.

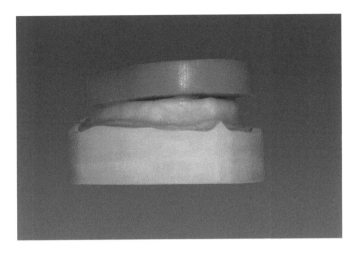

Figure A6–25   The occlusion rim is softened in hot water or over a flame and positioned on the record base. It is shaped by hand until it is centered on the posterior ridges and extends labially in the anterior.

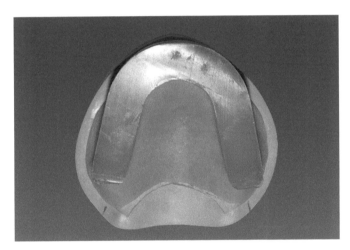

Figure A6–26   Before it is bonded to the record base, the preliminary position of the occlusion rim is checked to verify that it is centered on the residual ridges in the posterior and overextends slightly in the anterior. If the position is not correct, the occlusion rim is removed and repositioned.

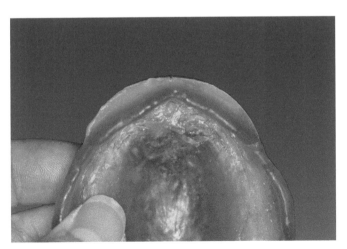

Figure A6–27   When viewed from the tissue side of the record base, the occlusion rim should be symmetrically positioned, and a small amount of occlusion rim visible extending beyond the flange of the record base. It should extend outward by approximately 2 to 3 mm. This same positioning should be present when fabricating the mandibular record base and occlusion rim.

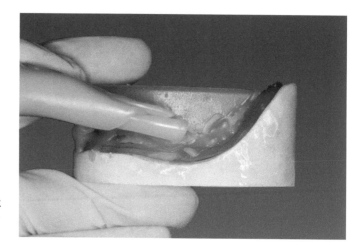

Figure A6–28 Once properly positioned, the occlusion rim is firmly attached to the record base with hot baseplate wax. All voids and irregular areas should be filled.

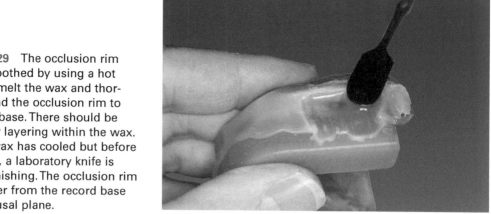

Figure A6–29 The occlusion rim can be smoothed by using a hot spatula to melt the wax and thoroughly bond the occlusion rim to the record base. There should be no voids or layering within the wax. Once the wax has cooled but before it gets cold, a laboratory knife is used for finishing. The occlusion rim should taper from the record base to the occlusal plane.

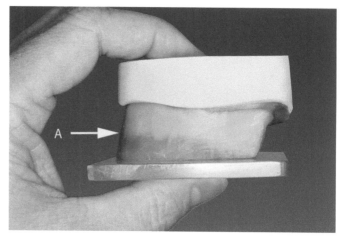

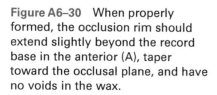

Figure A6–30 When properly formed, the occlusion rim should extend slightly beyond the record base in the anterior (A), taper toward the occlusal plane, and have no voids in the wax.

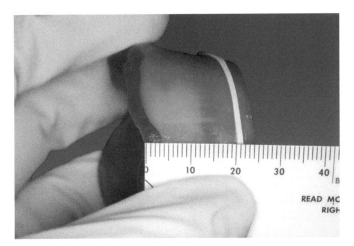

Figure A6–31   The height of the occlusal plane should now be corrected and made basically parallel to residual ridges. Ideally the wax will approximate the desired occlusal plane height intraorally with minimal correction by the clinician. Generally the length of the anterior occlusion rim should be approximately 20 to 21 mm from the notch indicating the labial frenulum on the maxillary arch and 18 to 20 mm on the mandibular arch. A rubber band can be placed at the desired length to help when correcting the height of the plane.

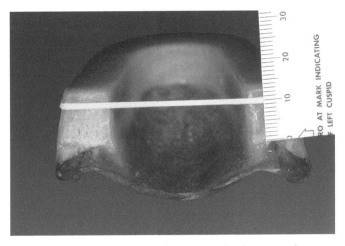

Figure A6–32   The height of the plane in the posterior is generally 9 to 10 mm on the maxillary arch and at the level of the top of the retromolar pad on the mandibular arch.

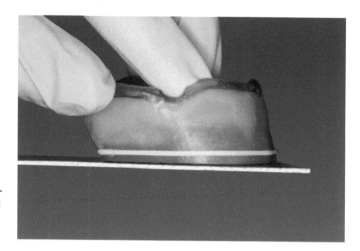

Figure A6–33   A large, flat, hot spatula can be used to form the occlusal plane. A well-formed occlusion rim has a single, smooth occlusal plane.

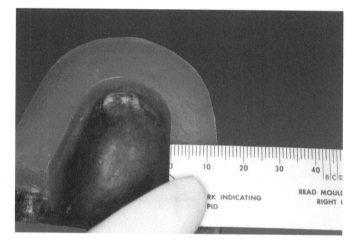

Figure A6–34   The occlusion rim should now be trimmed to be centered on the posterior ridge and be approximate the width of the teeth that will be positioned at a later step. This will feel reasonably normal to the patient. The completed width of the occlusion rim should be 8 to 10 mm in the posterior and 6 to 8 mm in the anterior.

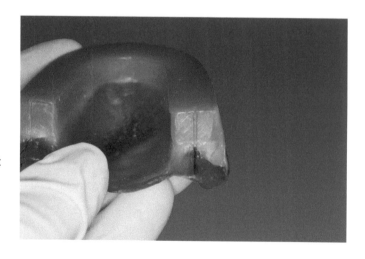

Figure A6–35   Using the marks that were originally placed on the land areas of the master cast, indicating the center of the residual ridges, a line can be drawn on the occlusion rim in the posterior.

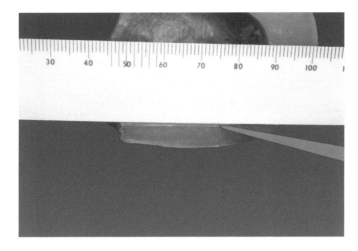

Figure A6–36 Using that line and the line that was placed on the master cast in the anterior, a posterior center line can be drawn into the occlusion rim indicating the crest of the ridge.

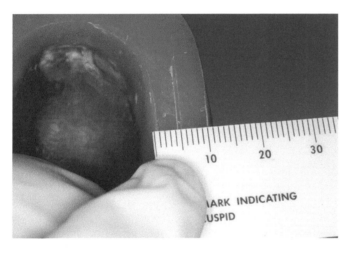

Figure A6–37 The posterior width of the occlusion rim is now formed by using a spatula to remove excess wax from the medial and lateral surfaces. Four to five mm of wax should remain on both sides of the center line.

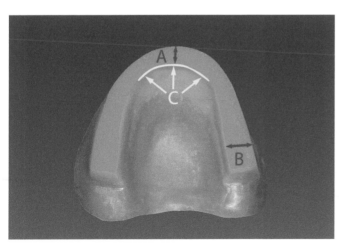

Figure A6–38 An occlusal view of a well-formed maxillary occlusion rim. Note that it is 6 to 8 mm in the anterior (A) and 8 to 10 mm wide in the posterior (B). The desired labial support was created when initially positioning the occlusion rim on the record base so the anterior width is corrected by removing wax from the lingual surface only! (C)

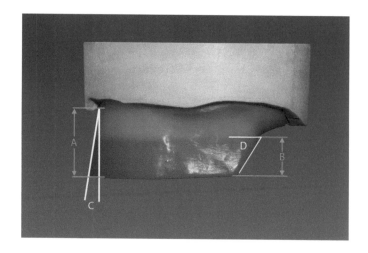

Figure A6–39 A properly completed maxillary record base and occlusion rim. The height of the rim in the anterior should be approximately 22 mm (A). The posterior height should be approximately 10 mm (B). The anterior of the rim should protrude at approximately a 15^0 angle (C), and the posterior of the rim should be tapered at approximately a 45^0 angle (D).

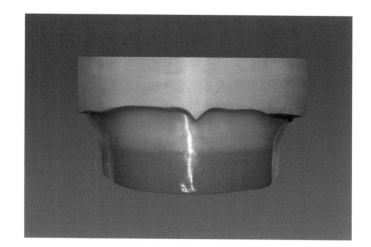

Figure A6–40 Anterior view of a properly finished maxillary record base and occlusion rim

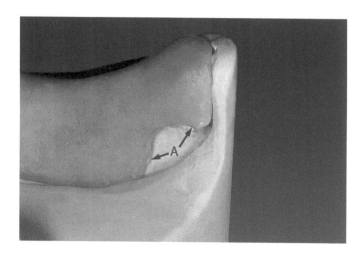

Figure A6–41 Small differences exist between the maxillary and mandibular record base. Here a small area has been removed from the mandibular record base. This portion of the record base is not necessary for the stability of the record base. Removing this area will make inserting the record base into the retromylohyoid area easier during the interocclusal records appointment. The cutout should be in the diagonal corner of the record base and should be approximately 12 to 14 mm wide at its base (A).

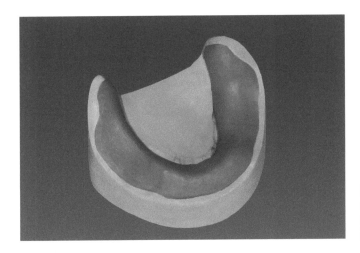

Figure A6–42 Just as for the maxillary arch, the mandibular record base must properly fit the mandibular master cast and be stable.

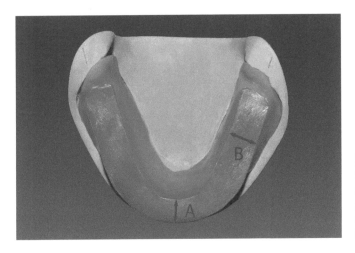

Figure A6–43 A well-formed mandibular record base and occlusion rim. Note that the width of the occlusion rim in the anterior is approximately 6 to 8 mm (A) and 8 to 10 mm in the posterior (B).

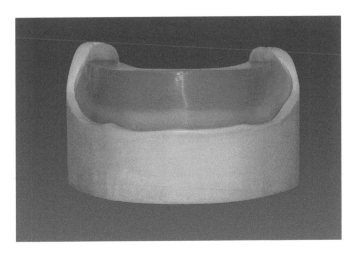

Figure A6–44 A well-formed mandibular occlusion rim as seen from the anterior.

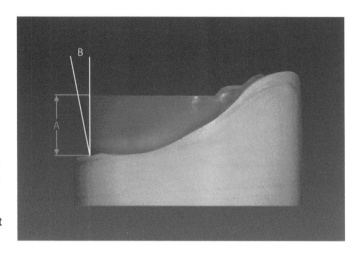

Figure A6–45   A properly completed mandibular occlusion rim. The height of the rim in the anterior is approximately 18 mm (A) and, although not visible, and at the level of the top of the retromolar pad in the posterior. The anterior of the occlusion rim should protrude at approximately a 15^0 angle (B).

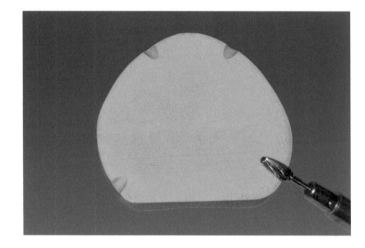

Figure A6–46   The last procedure prior to the maxillomandibular records appointment is to prepare four small remount indices into the bottom of the base of the cast. A medium-sized acrylic resin bur can be use.

Maxillomandibular Records

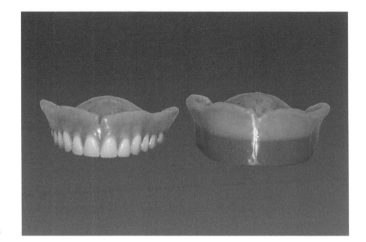

Figure A7–1   Contoured record bases and occlusion rims (RBOR) are used to aid the technician in tooth placement, provide a guide for facial support estimates, determine the occlusal plane, and make both vertical and horizontal records

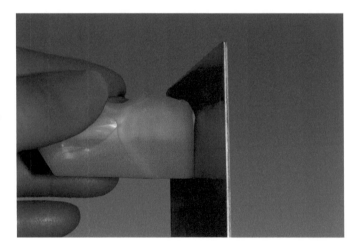

Figure A7–2   The maxillary RBOR is most commonly contoured first. Proper facial contours and the correct occlusal plane are determined using various methods. Heated spatulas and plates are commonly used to melt wax and change contours and planes on the occlusion rims.

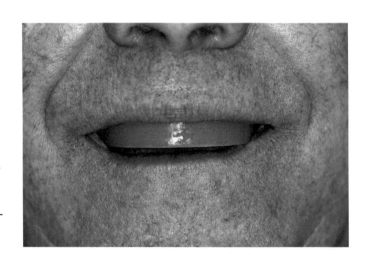

Figure A7–3   The proper facial contour and length of the maxillary RBOR is established using both phonetic and esthetic indicators. This figure represents the initial try-in of the maxillary RBOR, which requires adjustment.

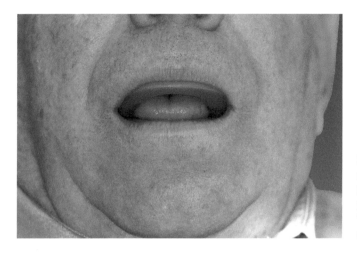

Figure A7–4 The anterior contour and length is determined by the normal esthetic placement of teeth, phonetic sounds, such as "f" and "v," and other functional and esthetic determinants.

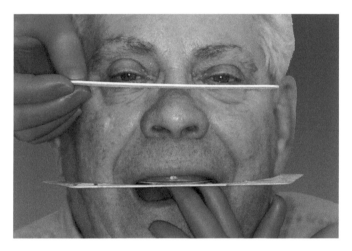

Figure A7–5 The lateral incisal plane can be determined using a Fox Plane Guide and the patient's interpupillary line. A tongue blade can also be used during this determination.

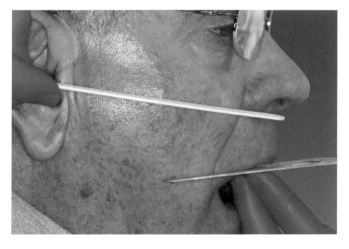

Figure A7–6 The initial evaluation of the anterior-posterior occlusal plane of the maxillary RBOR reveals a discrepancy from the normal anatomic determinants of the proper maxillary occlusal plane. The occlusal plane is often parallel to the ala-tragus line (Camper's Plane).

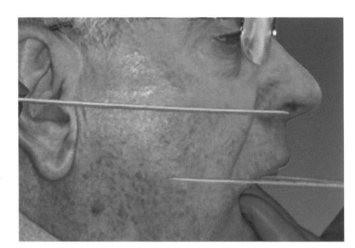

Figure A7–7   Correction of the anterior-posterior occlusal plane on the maxillary RBOR using the Ala-Tragus line (Camper's Plane) as the initial guide.

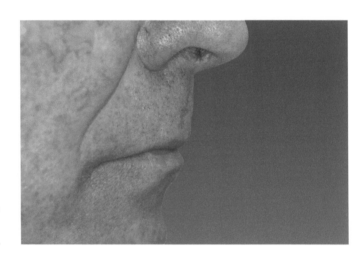

Figure A7–8   Proper lip support for esthetics is evaluated with the contoured maxillary RBOR in place.

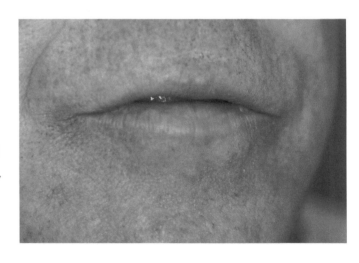

Figure A7–9   Phonetic checks are used to verify the incisal length and anterior edge of the maxillary RBOR. In this figure, the "f" and "v" sound produce contact of the vermillion border of the lower lip with the incisal edge of the maxillary RBOR.

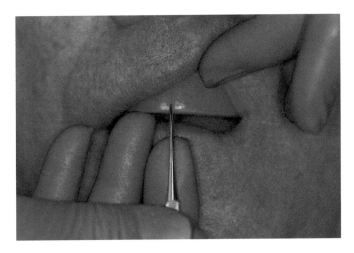

Figure A7–10 Midline marked on the maxillary RBOR. The philtrum of the lip, mid-face line, and other esthetic determinants contribute to the decision of where to place the midline junction between the central incisors.

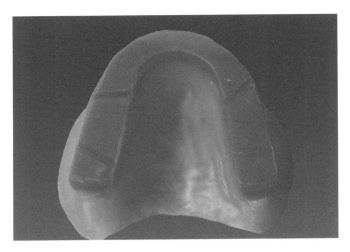

Figure A7–11 Index grooves are placed in the surface of the contoured RBOR for attaching a facebow fork and eventually to be used during the centric relation record making procedure.

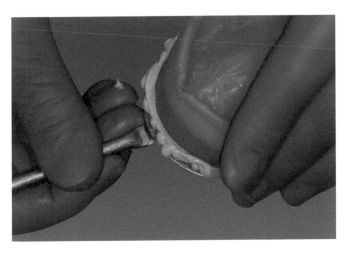

Figure A7–12 Maxillary RBOR is attached to a facebow fork using vinyl polysiloxane (VPS) record material. Consult the facebow manufacturer's instructions for this procedure.

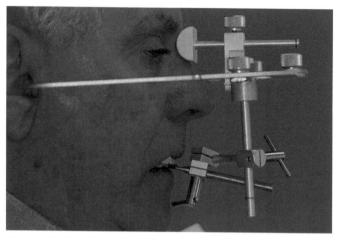

Figure A7–13   A facebow record is made to facilitate placing the maxillary master cast/RBOR on the clinician's choice of articulator.

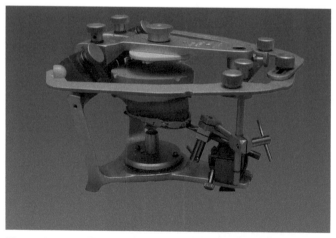

Figure A7–14   The facebow record is used to attach the maxillary master cast to the articulator of choice. This records the relationship of the maxilla to the condylar complex and refines the arc of closure as it relates to the posterior teeth.

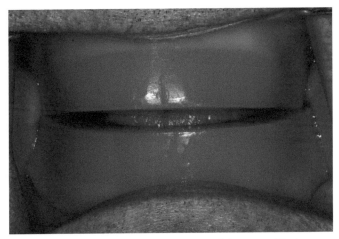

Figure A7–15   The initial placement of the mandibular RBOR. This figure shows the initial placement with premature contact in the posterior, and the patient at an open vertical position. The two RBORs will now be used to determine the proper Occluding Vertical Dimension (OVD) for the patient as well as to record the proper horizontal position of the mandible for denture fabrication. Most adjustments at this point will be made on the mandibular RBOR because the maxillary RBOR is establishing the lateral and anterior-posterior occlusal plane from previous adjustments.

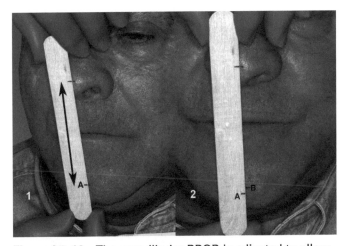

Figure A7–16   The mandibular RBOR is adjusted to allow simultaneous contact of the rim surfaces at the correct occluding vertical dimension. The resting vertical dimension is determined for the patient by using various methods. The interocclusal space requirements are determined, and the final occluding vertical dimension is established. (1A) Resting Vertical Dimension, (2B) Occluding Vertical Dimension, (2 A→B) = Interocclusal Distance. See Chapter 10 (Maxillomandibular Records and Articulators) for more detailed information) on this procedure.

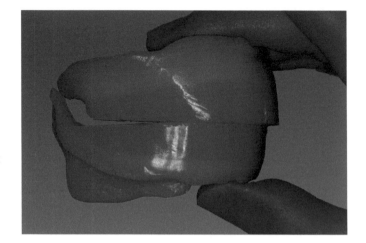

Figure A7–17   Care is taken during this procedure to ensure no contact of the acrylic resin record bases occurs in the posterior. Contact of the record bases can lead to improper vertical and horizontal positions.

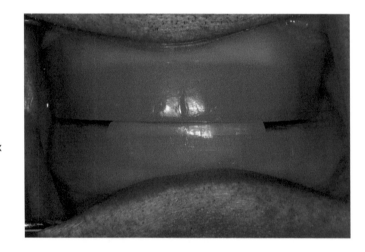

Figure A7–18   After contact of the RBORs at the correct OVD is established, approximately 2 mm of wax is removed from the mandibular RBOR in the posterior to provide space for recording material to capture the patient's mandible in the centric relation position at the correct OVD.

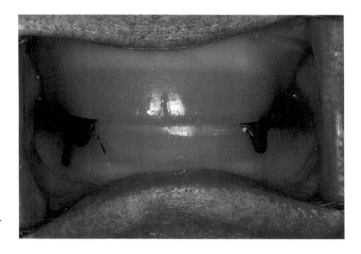

Figure A7–19   A record is made between the maxillary RBOR and the mandibular RBOR at the correct OVD and in the centric relation position. See Chapter 10 (Maxillomandibular Records and Articulators) for more detailed information) on this procedure.

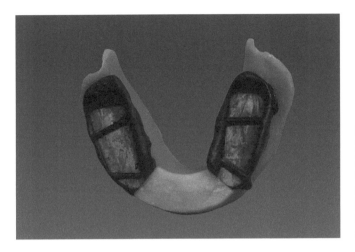

Figure A7–20 The centric relation record should be stable and should record the detail of the notches made in the maxillary RBOR. The recording material could also have been a vinyl polysiloxane material or any material that meets the requirements for stable records.

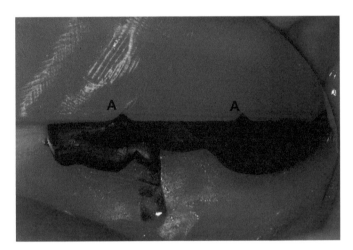

Figure A7–21 After trimming the record, it can be returned to the patient to verify that the mandibular record arcs correctly into the notches (A) on the maxillary RBOR in the centric relation position. The mandibular cast is now positioned on the articulator. See Chapter 10 (Maxillomandibular Records and Articulators) for more detailed information) on this procedure.

Tooth Selection

Clinical and Technical Procedures

Figure A8–1 To select denture teeth, the following information is necessary: height, width, and shape of the crown of the central incisor; and the measurement from the distal of one canine to the distal of the second (as measured on the labial of the anterior teeth). This information is obtained from the patient and used along with a mold guide to select the teeth. Mold guides are in either a paper form or a physical form. The paper mold guide has pictures and information about the teeth. This is an example of a mold guide.

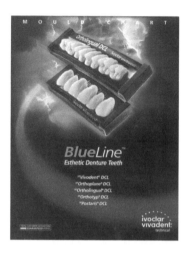

Figure A8–2 This portion of a page from a mold guide provides examples of anterior tooth molds available. The information is generally the mold itself, the width and height of the central incisors, and the measurement of the maxillary six anterior teeth as measured from the distal of one canine to the distal of the opposite canine. In this example, the shape of the tooth is also indicated. This information is used to select the desired denture teeth.

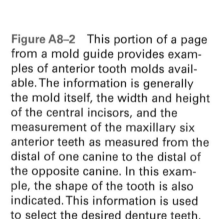

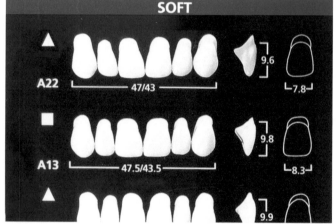

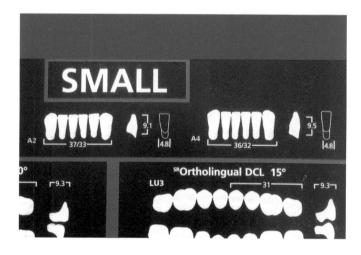

Figure A8–3 There is usually similar information on the mandibular anterior teeth.

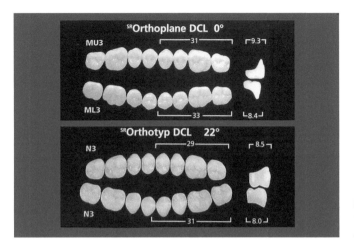

Figure A8–4 Information on the posterior tooth forms available is also presented.

ANTERIOR TEETH			POSTERIOR TEE		
		Maxillary	Mandibular	SR Orthoplane® DCL (monoplane)	SR Ortholingual® DCL (lingualized)	SR Orth (semi-a

			Maxillary	Mandibular	SR Orthoplane® DCL (monoplane)	SR Ortholingual® DCL (lingualized)	SR Orth (semi-a
SMALL	SOFT	SHORT	A22	A3	MU3/ML3	LU3/LL3	N3
			A13	A3/A5	MU3/ML3 MU5/ML5	LU3/LL3 LU5/LU5	N3
			A41	A3	MU3/ML3	LU3/LL3	N3
		LONG	A24	A4/A5	MU3/ML3 MU5/ML5	LU3/LL3 LU5/LU5	N3
	BOLD	SHORT	A11	A3	MU3/ML3	LU3/LL3	N3
			A44	A3	MU3/ML3	LU3/LL3	N3
			A42	A3/A5	MU3/ML3 MU5/ML5	LU3/LL3 LU5/LL5	N3
		LONG	A24B	A4/A5	MU3/ML3 MU5/ML5	LU3/LL3 LU5/LL5	N3
	T	SHORT	A32	A3	MU5/ML5	LU5/LL5	N5
			A36	A7	MU5/ML5	LU5/LL5	N6

Figure A8–5 Suggestions are often made for recommended combinations of anterior and posterior teeth. Remember, these are only recommendations and may be altered as necessary for a specific patient's needs.

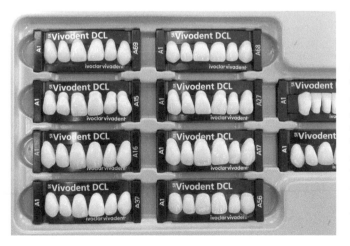

Figure A8–6 The physical mold form has actual denture teeth displayed. However, the teeth are of one shade only and are usually not of the same material quality as the teeth to be used in a denture. They should not be used in a denture. The teeth may be removed from this guide and placed next to the patient's face or when attempting to match a tooth in an existing denture.

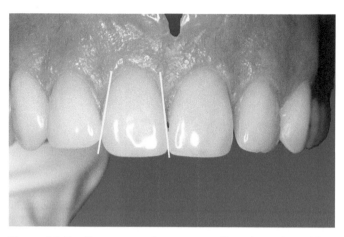

Figure A8–7 Denture teeth are generally selected to either match the mold and/or shade of the teeth on an acceptable existing denture or, when no acceptable existing denture exists, they are selected using multiple guides and measurements made from the patient. In this example, the patient has presented with an existing denture and wishes that the mold and shade of the anterior teeth be matched. The importance and/or shape of an anterior denture tooth are strictly empirical and subject to debate. In this example, the tooth might be considered to be tapering, although some may find it ovoid, and others square-tapering. A tentative selection for the shape should be made. The patient should be informed that different denture tooth manufacturers use different molds and shades; therefore an exact match may not be possible.

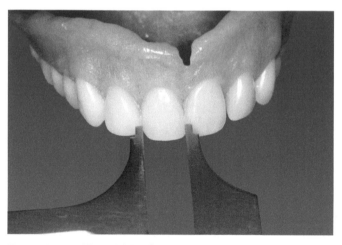

Figure A8–8 The width of the crown of the anterior tooth can be closely estimated by measuring. The exact direct measurement of the crown is not possible because of the proximal teeth.

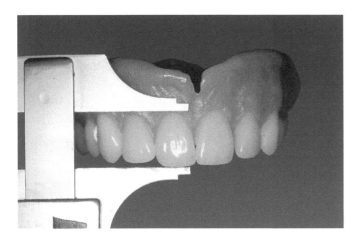

Figure A8–9   The height of the crown can be reasonably accurately measured.

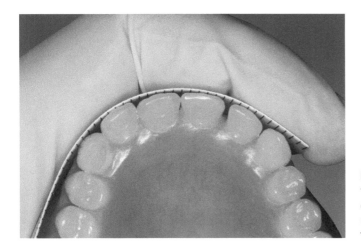

Figure A8–10   The measurement from the distal of one canine to the distal of the opposite canine is measured on the labial surface of the anterior teeth.

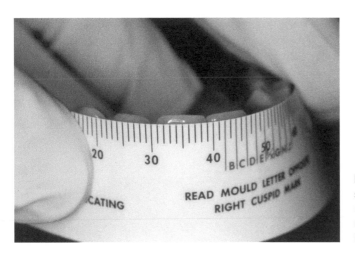

Figure A8–11   The flexible ruler should be positioned so that the ruler rests against the teeth, and the measuring marks are along the incisal edges.

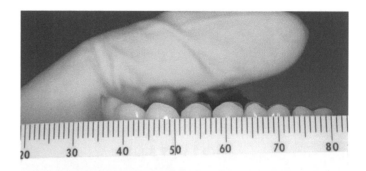

Figure A8–12   Once again, this is not an exact direct measurement but is acceptably accurate. In this example the measurement is 51 mm.

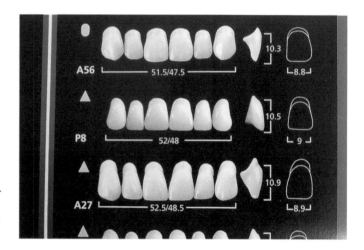

Figure A8–13   With the tooth measurements and information provided in the paper mold guide, a tentative mold selection can be made.

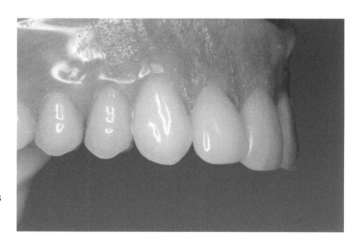

Figure A8–14   Because several molds may very closely match the measurements obtained, sometimes the shape of the canine is the deciding factor.

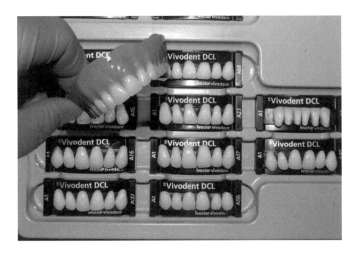

Figure A8–15 The physical mold guide can now be used to view the potential mold or molds selected.

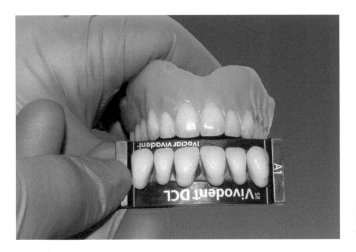

Figure A8–16 The individual teeth in the mold guide can be compared to the existing denture.

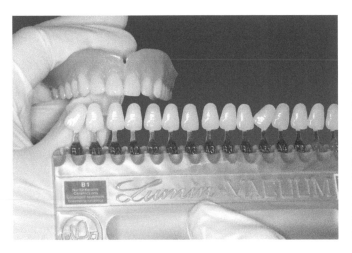

Figure A8–17 Once a mold is selected, then a shade guide can be used to match the existing teeth. The patient should be informed that different tooth manufacturers may use different shade guides; therefore an exact match may not be possible. It can be seen from the previous figures that matching the teeth in an existing denture can be simple and quickly completed.

Figure A8–18   The second and most often-used method of selecting denture teeth is that of using multiple guides to establish an original mold and shade. Using a photograph to provide general size and shape of the natural teeth can sometimes be helpful. A common problem with this guide is that patients will often bring pictures that are too small, may not show teeth, etc.. The teeth of siblings may also provide useful information. Existing casts with the natural teeth present may be extremely beneficial.

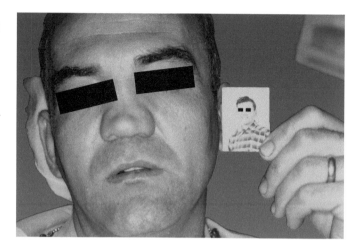

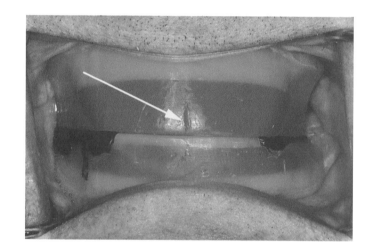

Figure A8–19   Once the occlusion rims have been properly shaped, the midline mark is the starting point for tooth selection.

Figure A8–20   Next, the width of the six anterior teeth can be estimated. This measurement can be obtained in several different ways. A conventional method is to use the relaxed corners of the mouth to indicate the middle to distal edges of the canines. Marks are made on the maxillary occlusion rim indicating this relaxed position. Getting some patients to relax may be difficult, but this is an important landmark, so effort should be made to obtain accurate marks.

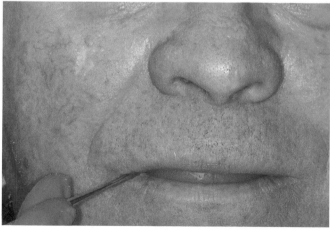

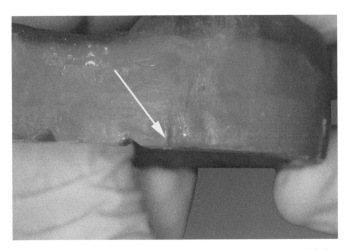

Figure A8–21   A measurement is made around the labial of the occlusion rim between the two marks, just as was done when making the measurement on the existing denture. A measurement should be made from one mark to the midline mark, and a measurement repeated for the opposite side. If the two measurements differ by more than 2 mm, the relaxed corners of the mouth should be remarked and the measurements made again. Once the corners are correctly marked and measured, some clinicians would suggest adding 3 to 5 mm to this measurement. It is more common that this method will produce a slightly smaller measurement than normal and adding the 3-5mm may help make a more natural looking tooth selection.

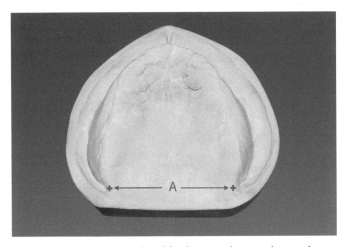

Figure A8–22   A second guide that can be used to estimate the canine-to-canine measurement is to measure between the centers of the left and right hamular notches (A) and add 10 mm. This is a very easy, quick, and an acceptably accurate estimate for most patients. However, it is always advisable to use multiple methods to arrive at this size estimate

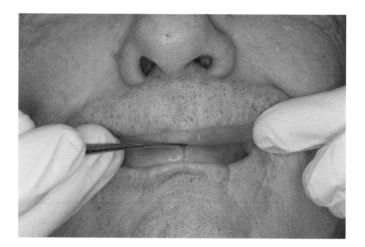

Figure A8–23 Method that may prove useful in estimating the desired height of the central incisor is to have the patient smile and mark the bottom of the upper lip on the maxillary occlusion rim. This mark is called the "high smile line".

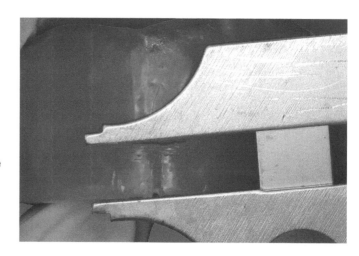

Figure A8–24 A direct measurement between the "high smile line" and the occlusal plane can be made to indicate the desired height of the crown of the central incisor. The addition of 1 to 3 mm may be necessary to provide a meaningful measurement.

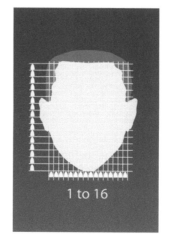

Figure A8–25 Another guide that has proved very useful for many years is that of using anthropometric averages to indicate the height and width of the central incisor. Studies indicate that a relationship exists between the height and width of the face and central incisor. A ratio of 16 to 1 is the accepted standard.

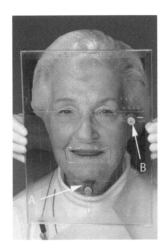

Figure A8–26   A "Trubyte Tooth Indicator" may be used to estimate the height and width of the central incisors. The device is centered on the face, and adjustable arms are moved into contact with the face. The lower arms (A) will indicate a height, and the upper arm (B) will indicate a desired width of the central incisors. Additionally, parallel lines drawn on the indicator may be used to determine the face shape (square, tapering, ovoid, etc). This shape may be used to select a tooth shape. This patient has a square to square-tapering face.

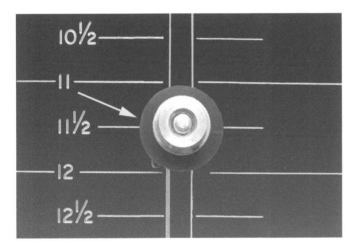

Figure A8–27   The position of the lower arm on this patient indicates that the desired height of the central incisors should be approximately 11.25 to 11.5 mm.

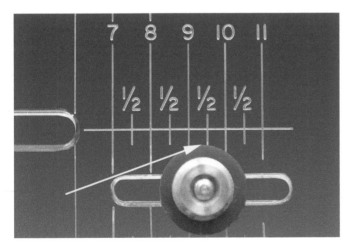

Figure A8–28   The position of the upper arm indicates that the desired width of the central incisors should be approximately 9 to 9.5 mm.

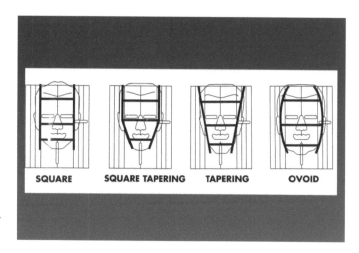

Figure A8–29 Example of using face shape to select a central incisor shape

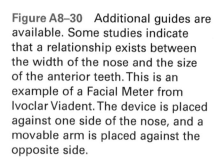

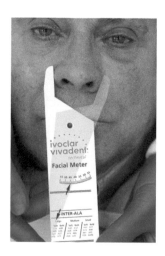

Figure A8–30 Additional guides are available. Some studies indicate that a relationship exists between the width of the nose and the size of the anterior teeth. This is an example of a Facial Meter from Ivoclar Viadent. The device is placed against one side of the nose, and a movable arm is placed against the opposite side.

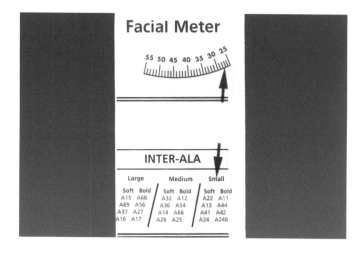

Figure A8–31 An arrow indicates a range of possible molds.

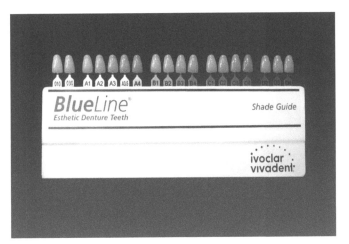

Figure A8–32   Finally, a shade must be selected. Again, take note of the fact that different denture tooth manufacturers use different shade guides. This is an example of a shade guide from Ivoclar Vident. The teeth are grouped into differing shades. When matching existing denture teeth, this shade arrangement is useful. It may, however, be less useful when selecting a new shade.

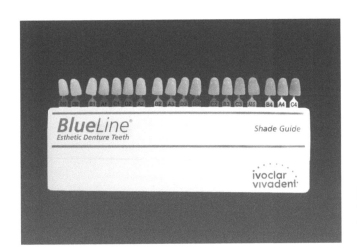

Figure A8–33   A suggestion is made to arrange the teeth from the lightest to the darkest when selecting a new shade.

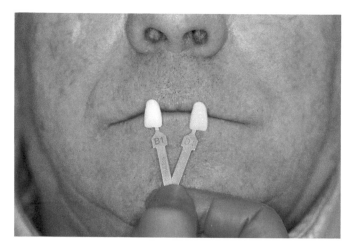

Figure A8–34   When selecting a shade, the object is to select a shade which, while being satisfactory to the patient, blends in with the patient's skin tones and does not stand out as being too light or dark. Showing the entire shade guide to a patient is not recommended. Many patients will automatically select the lightest shade without regard for any other factors. The clinician should select two or three shades and then allow the patient to make the final decision. In starting to eliminate obviously unacceptable shades, with the shade guide arranged from lightest to darkest (Figure A8-33), the two extremes are placed next to the patient's face. In this example, the shades are obviously too light and too dark.

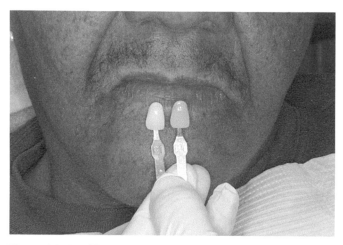

Figure A8–35   The same holds true for this dark-skinned patient.

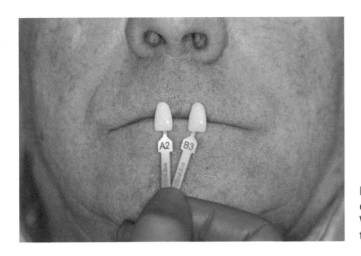

Figure A8–36 Less light and less dark shades have been selected. While the light shade is very close, the dark shade is still too dark.

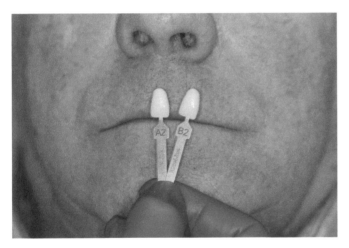

Figure A8–37 Finally, two acceptable shades have been selected. This is the clinician's recommendation, however the patient and any "significant other" must be consulted and the shade approved. Approval of the mold selection may be important, but not as much as the shade.

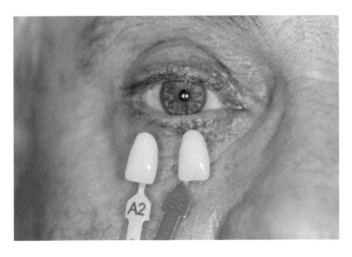

Figure A8–38 At times, attempting to match the sclera of the eye may be of some value.

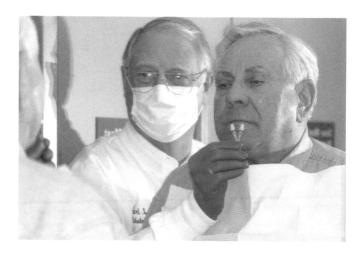

Figure A8–39   The patient should view the recommended shades standing before a mirror ideally at a conversational distance. Input from the spouse or relative or someone close to the patient should be sought. No matter the clinician's recommendation, the desires of the patient should be followed. An acceptable tooth mold and shade has now been chosen.

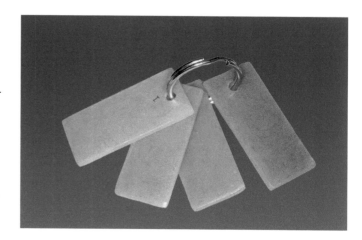

Figure A8–40   This is also an excellent time to make one final shade selection. Some patients have mild to heavy pigmentation of their gingiva. If available, a gingival shade guide should be used to attempt to match the gingival shade of the patient. Dental laboratories may be able to provide this type of shade guide to their clients.

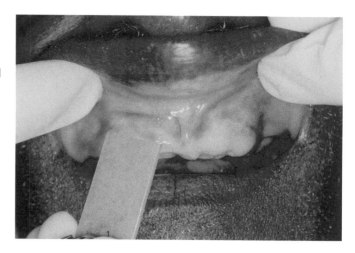

Figure A8–41   Matching the gingival shade can be difficult because the entire gingiva is not one single shade and in fact often varies dramatically from one part of the mouth to another. The shade that best blends with the overall gingival tone should be selected. This shade will be used during the preparation of the denture base material for the packing and processing of the denture.

Esthetic and Functional Trial Insertion

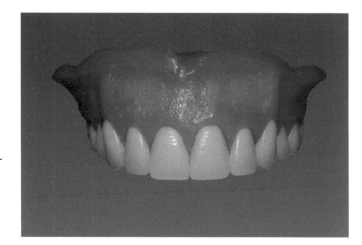

Figure A9-1 The esthetic and functional try-in allows the clinician and the patient to carefully examine the proposed prostheses from both a functional and an esthetic perspective. Maxillary trial set-up.

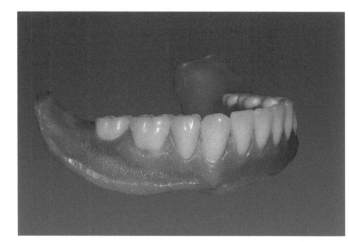

Figure A9-2 The esthetic and functional try-in allows the clinician and the patient to carefully examine the proposed prostheses from both a functional and an esthetic perspective. Mandibular trial set-up.

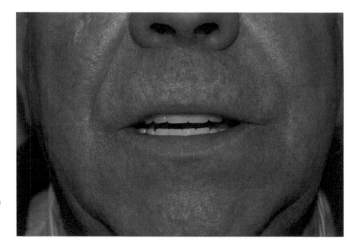

Figure A9-3 The trial dentures are assessed for proper facial support, esthetics, phonetic function, proper occluding vertical dimension and centric relation occlusion using the same criteria that was used during the maxillomandibular records appointment. The basic requirements for speech and esthetics must be balanced with patient desires and expectations. This is an ideal time for both the patient and a "significant other" to approve of the appearance of the dentures before they are processed.

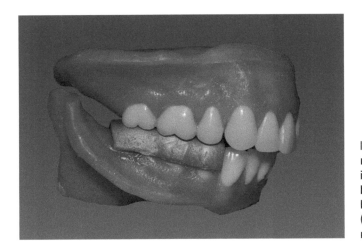

Figure A9–4 A new centric relation record is made during the trial insertion appointment to verify the horizontal position of the mandibular cast is correct. See Chapter 13 (Trial Insertion Appointment) for more detailed information.

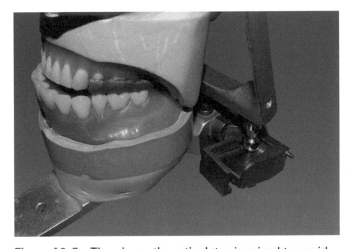

Figure A9–5 The pin on the articulator is raised to avoid interference with seating the dentures into the record correctly. The centric holding device is unlocked to ensure the teeth may occlude into the record without influence from the condylar elements. The dentures are firmly seated into the records, and the fit into the records is checked. At this point, the condylar elements are evaluated to make sure they have remained in the centric relation position with regard to the condylar housing. If they are correctly positioned, the new record verifies the centric relation position already recorded on the articulator.

Figure A9–6   If the new record does not verify the position of the original record, a third record is made just in case the second record may be in error. If the third record matches the first record it verifies the original record. If the third record fits similar to the second record, the mandibular cast is removed and remounted in the new position. The teeth may need to be re-set if the records were incorrect from the original maxillomandibular recording.

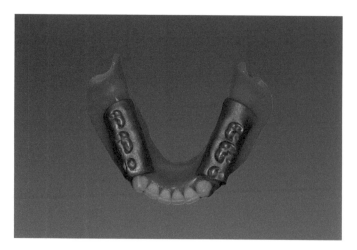

Figure A9–7   If the occlusal scheme requires setting the horizontal condylar guidance (a balanced type occlusion), a protrusive record is made to adjust the articulator.

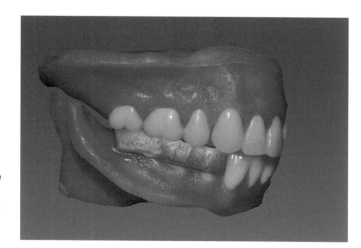

Figure A9–8   If gingival shade guides are available for customized shade selection, this is the last chance to make these selections and communicate this information to the laboratory technician.

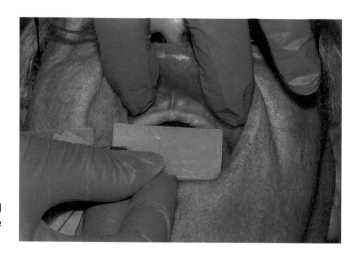

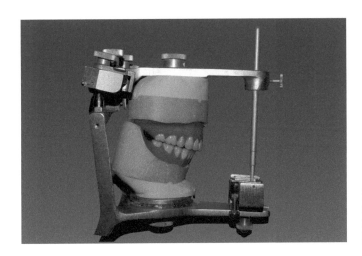

Figure A9–9   After evaluation, adjustments, and patient consent, the final prostheses are sent to the laboratory for processing.

Insertion

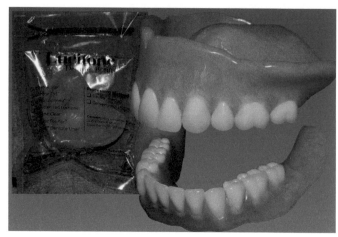

Figure A10–1   Clinicians should open and inspect the processed dentures prior to patient arrival. Obvious corrections can be made to sharp edges, blebs, and other such problems. The prostheses can then be disinfected and will be ready for the initial insertion procedures.

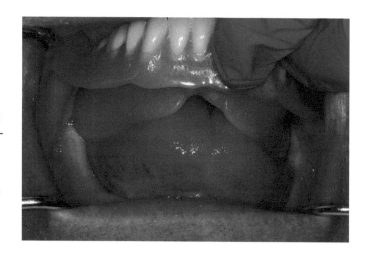

Figure A10–2   The dentures should be gently seated, and severe undercuts that limit placement should be adjusted. The dentures should seat easily with no discomfort reported by the patient. Any severe pressure or areas of extreme discomfort should be eliminated prior to proceeding.

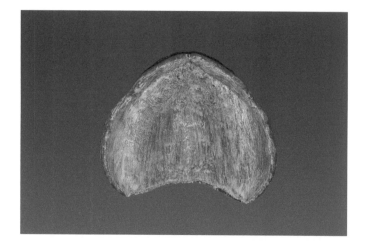

Figure A10–3   Pressure Indicating Paste (PIP) or Pressure Disclosing Paste is placed uniformly on the intaglio surface of the denture.

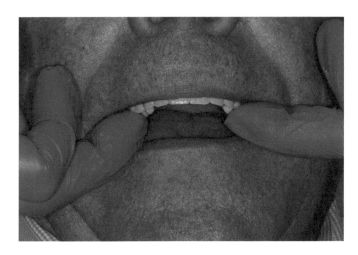

Figure A10–4 The denture is seated with firm pressure. Do not place both dentures and have the patient "bite." This may introduce errors in the PIP from occlusal discrepancies.

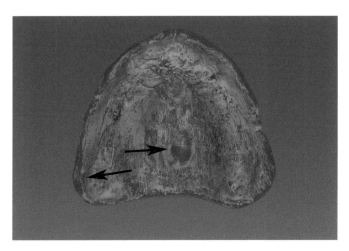

Figure A10–5 Pressure areas should be identified and eliminated by judicious grinding. The most common initial pressure areas will be bony prominences and the medial surfaces of the posterior buccal flanges. Excess pressure prevents the denture from fully seating and may cause soreness and poor retention until the excess pressure is eliminated.

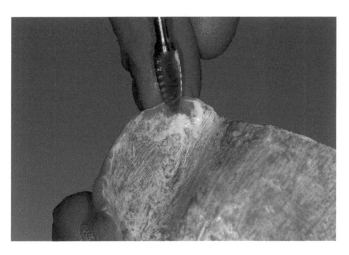

Figure A10–6 Acrylic burs in a slow speed hand piece are the ideal method for eliminating these problem areas.

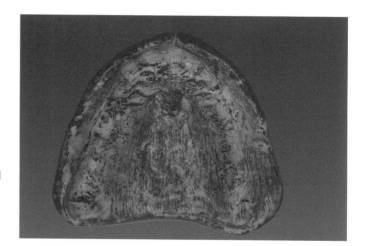

Figure A10–7   Repeated testing and elimination of pressure areas will produce a uniform appearance to the PIP after seating pressure is applied.

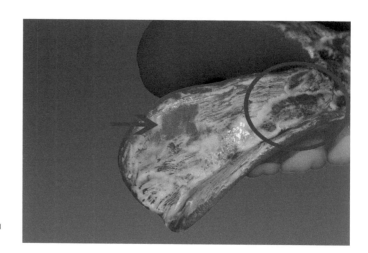

Figure A10–8   The mandibular denture is evaluated with the PIP in a similar manner.

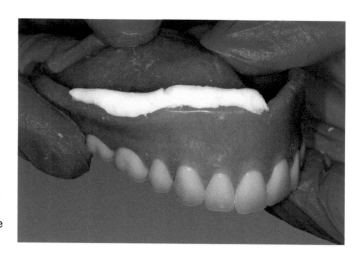

Figure A10–9   Border extension can be evaluated both visually and with Disclosing Wax™ to located possible problem areas.

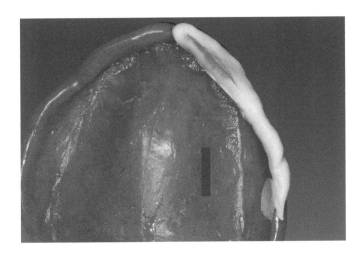

Figure A10–10 Overextended borders will show through the disclosing wax after the wax reaches mouth temperature. They can be adjusted with an acrylic bur.

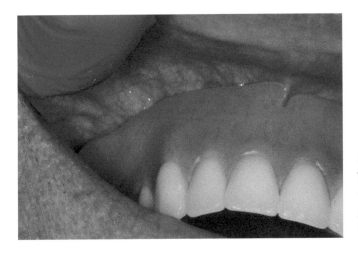

Figure A10–11 Visual inspection of the denture borders may also reveal areas that need adjusting. Borders should be similar to this figure and fit snuggly into the vestibule without extending the tissues.

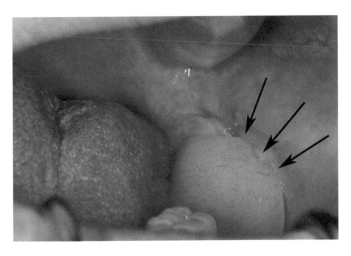

Figure A10–12 Active muscle groups should be evaluated for excessive pressure against the denture borders. In this figure, the masseter muscle can pull across the distobuccal border of the mandibular denture (arrows) and unseat the prosthesis during function. Proper adjustment of the border will eliminate that problem.

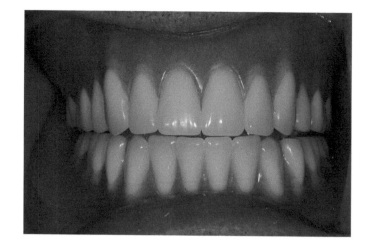

Figure A10–13 The dentures were evaluated for esthetics and proper function at the previous try-in appointment. The dentures are inserted and evaluated in a similar manner before refining the occlusion.

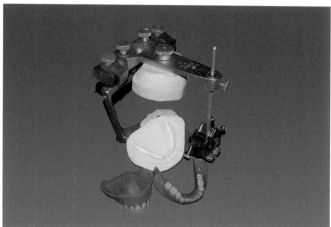

Figure A10–14 Final occlusal adjustments should be accomplished by mounting the processed dentures on a properly set articulator. The maxillary remount cast is returned to the articulator to preserve the facebow orientation. A new centric relation record is used to mount the mandibular denture in the correct horizontal position for occlusal equilibration.

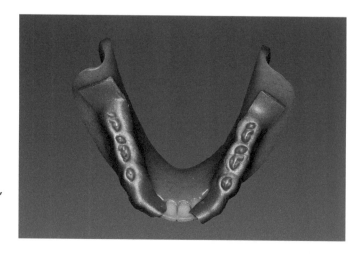

Figure A10–15 The new centric relation record can be made with AluWax™, PVS, or modeling compound. It is made at a slightly open vertical dimension (<1mm) to prevent contact of occlusal surfaces, which may introduce errors due to possible shifting of the denture bases from premature contact.

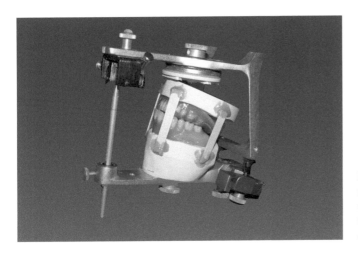

Figure A10–16 The centric relation record returns the dentures to a stable platform to make the final occlusal equilibration more accurate and easier to accomplish.

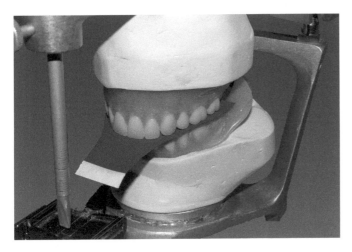

Figure A10–17 Centric relation contacts are established using marking paper, and refined using a technique established for the type of occlusal scheme present on the new dentures. See Chapter 14 (Insertion) for more detailed information.

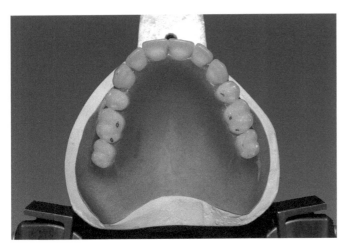

Figure A10–18 Initial centric relation contacts in a nonbalanced lingualized occlusal scheme are seen in this figure.

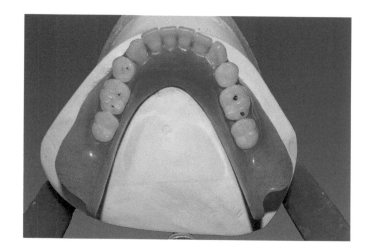

Figure A10–19 The opposing occlusal surfaces in a nonbalanced lingualized occlusal scheme are seen in this figure.

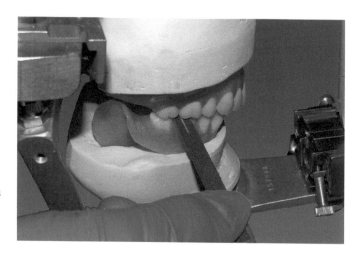

Figure A10–20 In a nonbalanced lingualized occlusal scheme, all adjustments are performed on the maxillary arch because the mandibular teeth are set on a flat plane and present a uniform flat surface to adjust against. Carborundum strips are a common instrument to use for this adjustment. The heaviest occlusal contacts are systematically reduced until all possible contacts are found and equilibrated.

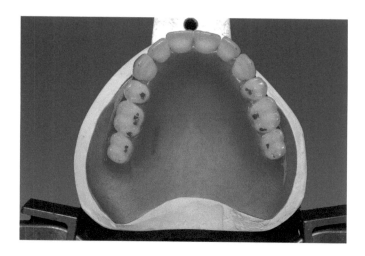

Figure A10–21 All maxillary cusp tips are now in equal contact with the opposing arch.

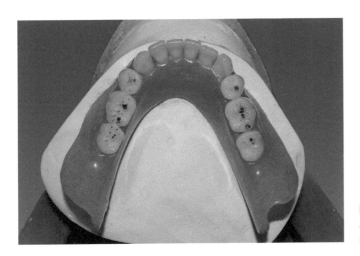

Figure A10–22   Maxillary cusp tips are now in equal contact with the mandibular arch.

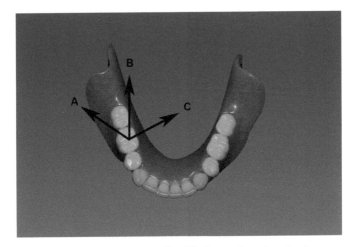

Figure A10–23   In a lingualized balanced occlusal scheme, the centric relation contacts would be refined and then the right working and nonworking, the left working and nonworking, and then protrusive eccentric movements would be refined. In balanced occlusal schemes, the adjustments are made on the mandibular arch.
A) Nonworking scribe line showing path of a maxillary lingual cusp during a left mandibular lateral movement.
B) Protrusive scribe line showing the path of a maxillary lingual cusp during a mandibular protrusive movement.
C) Working scribe line showing the path of a maxillary lingual cusp during a right mandibular lateral movement.
See Chapter 14 (Insertion) for more detailed information.

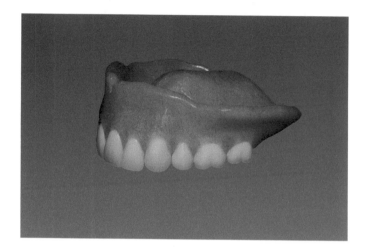

Figure A10–24 The dentures are polished, and appropriate instructions are given to the patient. (Maxillary)

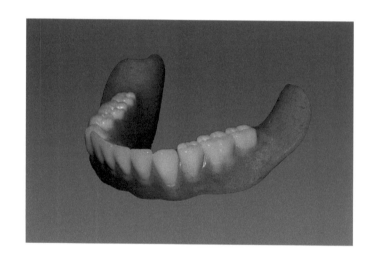

Figure A10–25 The dentures are polished and appropriate instructions are given to the patient. (Mandibular)

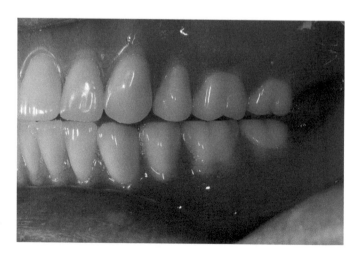

Figure A10–26 A final intraoral evaluation is performed, and the patient is scheduled for an appropriate post-insertion check.

Index

NOTE: Letter "f" denotes figures.